10 REASONS YOU FEEL OLD AND GET FAT

Also by Dr Frank Lipman

The New Health Rules: Simple Changes to Achieve Whole-Body Wellness (with Danielle Claro)

Revive: Stop Feeling Spent and Start Living Again (with Mollie Doyle)

Total Renewal (with Stephanie Gunning)

10 REASONS YOU FEEL OLD AND GET FAT

...AND HOW YOU CAN STAY YOUNG, SLIM AND HAPPY!

DR FRANK LIPMAN

HAY HOUSE

Carlsbad, California • New York City • London • Sydney
Johannesburg • Vancouver • Hong Kong • New Delhi

First published and distributed in the United Kingdom by:
Hay House UK Ltd, Astley House, 33 Notting Hill Gate, London W11 3JQ
Tel: +44 (0)20 3675 2450; Fax: +44 (0)20 3675 2451; www.hayhouse.co.uk

Published and distributed in the United States of America by:
Hay House Inc., PO Box 5100, Carlsbad, CA 92018-5100
Tel: (1) 760 431 7695 or (800) 654 5126
Fax: (1) 760 431 6948 or (800) 650 5115; www.hayhouse.com

Published and distributed in Australia by:
Hay House Australia Ltd, 18/36 Ralph St, Alexandria NSW 2015
Tel: (61) 2 9669 4299; Fax: (61) 2 9669 4144; www.hayhouse.com.au

Published and distributed in the Republic of South Africa by:
Hay House SA (Pty) Ltd, PO Box 990, Witkoppen 2068
info@hayhouse.co.za; www.hayhouse.co.za

Published and distributed in India by:
Hay House Publishers India, Muskaan Complex, Plot No.3, B-2,
Vasant Kunj, New Delhi 110 070
Tel: (91) 11 4176 1620; Fax: (91) 11 4176 1630; www.hayhouse.co.in

Distributed in Canada by:
Raincoast Books, 2440 Viking Way, Richmond, B.C. V6V 1N2
Tel: (1) 604 448 7100; Fax: (1) 604 270 7161; www.raincoast.com

Text © Frank Lipman, 2016

Indexer: Joan D. Shapiro, MLS; Interior design: Riann Bender.
Yoga sequences and illustrations © copyright 2015 by Bobby Clennell, author of
The Woman's Yoga Book, *Watch Me Do Yoga* and *Yoga for Breast Care*.
Illustrations on pages 309-326 © Alexis Seabrook.

A catalogue record for this book is available from the British Library.

ISBN: 978-1-78180-502-2

Printed and bound in Great Britain by TJ International, Padstow, Cornwall.

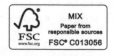

CONTENTS

INTRODUCTION:

YOU DON'T HAVE TO GET OLD AND FAT!

For most of her life, Jamie has struggled with her weight. Sometimes she's been just a few kilos over her ideal weight, and sometimes she's gone up to 5 kilos extra, but with strenuous dieting, she's always been able to get her weight back down.

Then Jamie turns 45, and suddenly, the weight she used to be able to diet off stubbornly stays on. Worse, the extra 5 kilos turns into an extra 7 . . . and then into an extra 10.

Besides her weight problems, Jamie has developed some other disturbing symptoms. She has begun to have what she calls "senior moments"—forgetting names, facts, and phone numbers; feeling spacey and unfocused; coming into a room to get something and being unable to remember what she came for. In addition, Jamie—always an upbeat person—has begun to struggle with periodic bouts of feeling listless, sad, and hopeless. Although she and her husband have always had a good physical relationship, Jamie even begins to lose interest in sex.

Frustrated, Jamie goes to see her doctor, hoping to learn some new weight-loss secret and get some help for her other problems. The doctor shrugs and advises her to eat less and exercise more, telling her that she has to exert more willpower and self-control.

"If you don't watch out, you'll just keep gaining," he warns her. "That's normal as you start to enter menopause. If you're feeling low, I can prescribe an antidepressant, but there's not much you can do about the other things. All of this is just part of the aging process."

Ever since high school, Martin has been vigorous and active. He played baseball as a teenager and college student, took up running in his 20s, and started regular gym workouts in his

30s. With his high-stress job as a corporate lawyer, Martin relies on exercise as a way to blow off steam. Except for an occasional cold or flu, he feels strong and healthy most of the time.

Then, in his early 40s, Martin is hit with a frustrating case of indigestion. He almost always suffers from gas and bloating after meals, and frequently he's constipated.

Soon after, Martin notices that the colds and flu that used to come rarely and pass quickly now seem to come far more often and last much longer. And a few years later, Martin develops arthritis in both knees, which is sometimes so painful that he can hardly walk.

To treat all these ailments, Martin's doctor has prescribed Nexium for his stomach troubles, Zyrtec for his colds, and Advil for the arthritis. "I wouldn't worry," she tells Martin each time he wonders why he's having so many health issues. "These kinds of problems just seem to crop up as you get older."

Thirty-year-old Andi has always prided herself on never having a weight problem. When the rest of her friends were angsting about diets, Andi was chowing down on chili dogs, doughnuts, nachos, and pizza. A strong swimmer, Andi got some kind of vigorous exercise every day.

Then, just before her 30th birthday, Andi gets a coveted promotion at the PR agency where she works. She's making more money than she ever dreamed of—but she's also working harder, sleeping less, and feeling way more stressed out. She starts having trouble falling asleep at night, and even when she does manage to sleep, she often wakes up at 2 or 3 A.M., her heart pounding, her mind racing.

Somehow, Andi manages to keep up her rigorous gym schedule—until she slips on an icy sidewalk and sprains an ankle. Unable to exercise and overwhelmed with stress, Andi begins to gain weight for the first time in her life. She's sure that she'll be able to get rid of the extra 10 kilos as soon as she gets back to the gym—but to her distress, the weight stays on, no matter how much she exercises or tries to restrict her food intake.

Andi feels devastated by the sudden onslaught of health problems that seem completely out of her control. Even though she's only 30, she starts describing herself miserably as "old and fat before my time!"

What *Really* Happens as You Get Older?

Jamie and Martin have both been told that their problems are the natural result of aging. You may have heard something similar from friends, family, or even your own doctor: that growing older is synonymous with getting fat, slow, forgetful, and sick. Like most people in our society, you might see the years from age 40 onward as a slow, painful decline, marked by the following inevitable outcomes:

- You gain weight.

- You slow down.

- You have to live with mysterious aches and pains.

- You get sick more often.

- It takes you longer to "bounce back" from any physical or emotional challenge.

- You develop memory issues, "senior moments," and brain fog.

- You lose interest in sex or maybe lose some of your ability to perform.

- You feel sadder, more depressed, and maybe also more anxious.

As a physician, I can agree that for many people over 40—and now, for an increasing number of folks in their 30s—these and other ailments do become more common. But I can also tell you with absolute certainty that they are not inevitable. If you know the right ways to eat, sleep, move, and de-stress, and if you commit to creating community, meaning, and passion in your life, the years of your 40s, 50s, and beyond can be some of the most rewarding and vital you have ever known.

How can I say this with such confidence? Because the real obstacle for most of us isn't age. It's *loss of function.* Our bodies are perfectly capable of remaining slim and vigorous, and our brains can absolutely stay clear and sharp—*if* we give them what they need.

The problem is that most of us don't do that. We buy into the myth that age means decline, and we buy into a lot of other myths as well. We misunderstand what our bodies need to function at their best, so we eat the wrong foods, skimp on sleep, and deprive our bodies of the movement they crave. We become overwhelmed by the pressures of our lives, burdened by an unremitting stress that saps our bodies of vitality and drains our life of joy. We take one medication after another, never realizing that they might be disrupting our bodies' own innate ability to heal, depleting our bodies of essential nutrients and draining our natural resilience. Most insidious of all, many of us lack the personal support and community we need to feel fully human.

So yes, in that case, our body's natural functions—our intricate systems of hormones, nerves, brain function, digestion, detoxification, and immune function—begin to break down. The wrong diet disrupts our gut, destroys our friendly bacteria, imbalances our hormones, and renders us vulnerable to brain fog, anxiety, and depression. A sedentary life leaves our bodies starved for movement. Lack of sleep literally shrinks our brains. Unnecessary medications cue our body to slow down and put on the pounds. And stress, isolation, and the loss of purpose create their own set of problems while making everything else worse.

That is what middle and old age look like for many of us. And for more and more of my patients, this process begins even before middle age. I have seen many people in their 30s and even in their 20s struggling with the kinds of problems Andi is facing: weight gain, stress, sleep issues, and feeling "old and fat before my time!"

But I can tell you as a physician that it's not that way for me, nor for my patients who have worked with me for a while. And it doesn't have to be that way for you.

What's the secret? It's actually quite simple:

Give your body what it needs to function at its best.

Support your body with the food, movement, and sleep it requires. Nourish your mind and spirit with the meaning, purpose, and community they crave. Whatever your age, your reward will be a healthy weight, a vast reserve of energy, and a renewed sense of resilience, vitality, and joy.

YOU DON'T HAVE TO FEEL OLD AND FAT IF YOU . . .

- Eat the foods your body needs

- Avoid the foods that stress your body

- Support your *microbiome*—the community of friendly bacteria that lives throughout your body, governing your digestion, your immune system, and your mental health

- Balance your hormones

- Give your body the movement it craves

- Find effective ways to cope with stress

- Get all the good, restorative sleep your body needs

- Minimize as far as possible the medications that can interfere with your body's natural state of health

- Supplement your diet with crucial nutrients

- Reconnect to your sense of meaning, purpose, and community

What Is Your Body Trying to Tell You?

In conventional Western medicine, we don't really have this concept of *function*—it actually comes from Chinese medicine and the relatively new Western discipline of *functional medicine*.* Both the ancient Chinese tradition and functional medicine focus less on addressing symptoms—such as weight gain, fatigue, stomach problems, or brain fog—and more on discovering the underlying problems that might be causing those symptoms. Both Chinese medicine and functional medicine have taught me not to focus on a single isolated symptom but rather to

---

* *Functional medicine* is a science-based approach to medicine that addresses the underlying causes of disease and relies on improving function rather than on medicating symptoms. Functional M.D.s sometimes prescribe conventional medications, but whenever possible, we rely on natural treatments—dietary changes, lifestyle management, herbs, and supplements—to help restore the body's own natural ability to heal.

consider the body as a whole. As a result, my go-to questions are not "What symptoms does my patient have?" and "Which pill can I prescribe for each symptom?" but rather

What is harming you and needs to be removed to permit your body to heal and function better?

What is lacking or what does your body need to promote healing and improve function?

For example, when Martin came to me after several frustrating experiences with other doctors, he was on five separate medications:

1. Nexium, a proton pump inhibitor to decrease the stomach acid that was supposedly causing his nausea

2. Zyrtec, an antihistamine for his colds

3. Sudafed, a decongestant for his colds

4. Advil, an anti-inflammatory for his arthritis

5. Celebrex, a stronger anti-inflammatory for when the Advil didn't work

Martin's other doctors had viewed each of his symptoms as a unique phenomenon to be treated with its own separate medication. I was far more interested in discovering the underlying causes that had created these symptoms. I also believed that all of these seemingly separate problems were actually related.

Let's start by considering Martin's gas, bloating, and constipation, which as you'll recall he first developed in his early 40s. These symptoms are so common that most people don't even tell their doctor about them. They might take some of the over-the-counter remedies such as Prilosec, Mylanta, and Pepto-Bismol. Or perhaps they do consult their physicians and, to reduce stomach acid, they are prescribed higher-dose Prilosec, Nexium, or Prevacid: prescription proton pump inhibitors that have become Big Pharma's latest multi-billion-dollar industry.

Despite the plethora of drugs prescribed to treat digestive symptoms, most doctors don't take these symptoms seriously, and most patients don't either. After all, doesn't "everybody" have a little indigestion? Isn't it "normal" to be a bit constipated or gassy?

I view those symptoms very differently. Partly because my background includes Chinese as well as Western medicine, I have learned that the gut is what in Chinese medicine is known as "the earth element," the central element that grounds all the others. As such, it's the center of our health, and when the gut is off, everything else is off too—or soon will be. Even if you stick to a strictly Western medical perspective, you can see that when the gut isn't functioning at its peak, you won't be properly digesting and absorbing nutrients. As a result, your entire health will suffer.

Consequently, the gut has always been a central core of my treatments, especially because most people do have some sort of gut imbalance. As we shall see throughout this Introduction and the first three chapters of this book, Jamie, Martin, and Andi's problems all began in the gut.

Problems that begin in the gut soon spread to the rest of the body, particularly to the immune system. The gut wall is a very fragile barrier that in many places is only one cell thick. Just on the other side is our immune system. As a result, the gut and the immune system are intimately involved. When the gut is out of balance, the immune system is often the next to follow. Sure enough, Martin's gut problems were followed by immune system problems: the frequent and persistent colds and flu that began to plague him.

Again, most conventional doctors don't take those types of "minor" illnesses seriously. I, however, view them as the body's cries for help—and I know that those cries are likely to get stronger and stronger if they are not attended to.

Certainly they did for Martin. In Martin's early 40s, his gut was in distress but he ignored its distress signals. A few years later, his immune system started to feel the strain, but he ignored that too. And so finally, at a relatively young age, Martin developed a seemingly age-related problem: the debilitating arthritis that made him feel old and decrepit.

Martin's doctor viewed these disorders as separate. I, by contrast, see them as related. Digestive problems can often trigger *inflammation,* an immune system response that is helpful in moderation but can cause all sorts of problems when it's either excessive or chronic. Indeed, chronic inflammation often underlies virtually every major and minor chronic disease of our time.

Martin's joint pain and frequent illnesses were two indications of that inflammation. In its early stages, inflammation can also express itself through such seemingly minor symptoms as acne, headaches, PMS, painful periods, and weight gain. As it progresses, inflammation moves on to more significant disorders, including the chronic illnesses that we associate with age: joint pain, arthritis, hypertension, stroke, heart disease, obesity, diabetes, and even cancer.

What's striking about all of these problems is that none of them actually *are* signs of age. Rather, they are signs of a body that has been allowed to go farther and farther out of balance.

Yes, the more years you are alive, the more time your body has to become imbalanced, which is why your problems *seem* to come from getting older. However, the problem is not really age but imbalance and loss of function. Once you resolve the distress and restore function—whatever your age might be—the problems disappear or at least markedly improve. Even after a lifetime of distress, your body retains a remarkable capacity to heal itself—as long as you support it in the right way.

In addition, once you improve function in one of your body's systems, your other systems are likely to benefit. For example, when we supported Martin's gut, he also began to see better function in his immune system, hormones, and nervous system. As a result, he began to find relief from all sorts of petty ailments that he had just accepted as a part of age. He had more energy. His sex life improved. He lost 5 kilos. He felt more optimistic and resilient. By changing his diet and his lifestyle, Martin began to feel the vitality and vigor he assumed were lost forever.

My focus with Martin was on helping him choose the foods, supplements, and lifestyle that supported his body in having optimal function. Sure, I could have given Martin medications for each of his symptoms, and they might even have brought him some temporary relief. But isn't it better to heal the underlying problems that cause those symptoms? And isn't it best of all to teach Martin how to keep his body feeling healthy and strong?

That's what I want to do with this book. I want you to understand what might be going wrong in your body and how that imbalance has produced the symptoms that we incorrectly associate with aging. Weight gain, memory loss, fatigue, aching joints, sore muscles—none of these are the inevitable result of middle age. Rather, they are the signs that your brain and body are in distress.

Heal the underlying dysfunctions, and your symptoms will disappear. Support your body with the right food, supplements, movement, sleep, and stress relief while you fill your life with meaning, passion, and community, and you will continue to enjoy ongoing vitality, a healthy weight, and a joyous, energized life, regardless of how old you are.

I've seen this approach work with patient after patient. Once they understand how the wrong foods drag them down and the right foods lift them up, they lose weight without even trying. Once they discover the joys of movement and the benefits of deep, refreshing sleep, they feel stronger, calmer, and happier. Once they replenish themselves with the right supplements, they feel energized, stronger, and remarkably resistant to minor ailments, aches, and pains. Once they reconnect with the purpose and meaning that each of us needs and create the communities of support that make us fully human, they discover a whole new level of fulfillment and inspiration that is enriched—not dampened—by each additional year.

This is the gift I myself have gotten from functional medicine, and from the Chinese medicine, yoga, and meditation that I have studied along the way. This is the gift that these ancient and modern traditions have enabled me to share with my patients, even as I have learned so much from them in more than 35 years of being a physician. And this is the gift I am now excited to share with you: an ongoing state of glowing health and resilience that you can enjoy for the rest of your life.

Breaking Through the Myths

Over the past 35 years of practicing medicine, I've noticed that many people—and most doctors—have bought into certain myths about what happens to our bodies as we age. In this book, we're going to break through those myths so you finally have some good, reliable information about weight loss, aging, and good health.

We've already taken apart the most deadly myth of all—the one that says aging equals decline. Once you know how to support your body through diet, supplements, and lifestyle, you don't have to dread getting older. Instead, you can welcome it, knowing that your mind and body can remain vigorous, healthy, and resilient.

We'll zero in on some other problematic myths in each chapter—specific myths that might be preventing you from making healthy decisions without even realizing it. First, though, let's look at some of the big myths about health and aging that are so prevalent in our culture.

Three Common Myths about Health and Aging

- "These problems just hit me suddenly, out of nowhere."
- "I can't do much about my health—I just have poor genes."
- "I can take meds for one issue without affecting the rest of my body."

Myth: "These problems just hit me suddenly, out of nowhere"

In conventional Western medicine, we tend to focus on end-stage disease, which does, indeed, seem to come out of nowhere. In Western medicine, the diagnoses tend to be very black and white: either you have a disease or you don't.

In functional medicine, by contrast, we view health as more of a spectrum. Instead of narrowing in on end-stage disease, we look at the long, slow decline in function that finally erupts into a serious condition . . . but that began slowly, gradually, with seemingly minor symptoms. Instead of "black" versus "white," we have a huge spectrum of gray: a whole area of suboptimal function that isn't really a disease exactly, but isn't really good health either.

Let's see how this works in practice. Suppose your doctor tests your blood sugar levels, a common way to find out whether you have diabetes. A typical Western doctor might look at your blood sugar readings and say, "Well, you're in the high-normal range, but you don't have diabetes, so you're okay." Until your blood sugar levels cross the magic line that divides "diabetes" from "non-diabetes," most conventional doctors are not concerned.

By contrast, a functional-medicine doctor might say, "I see that your blood sugar levels, although considered normal by conventional standards, are on the high side. If this continues, you might someday get diabetes. But even if you don't, that high blood sugar can lead to all sorts of other problems. It incites your body to produce excessive amounts of insulin, which leads to weight gain and also causes inflammation. That inflammation might in turn produce other symptoms, such as acne or skin eruptions, aches and pains, headaches, hormonal imbalances, fatigue, brain fog, puffiness, anxiety, and depression. Even though you don't have diabetes, your blood sugar levels are 'dark gray'—so let's look at how we can get those levels back to 'white.'"

As you can see, the functional-medicine approach is concerned with far more than simply treating disease. Instead, its focus is on helping you achieve optimal health. Even though you're not actually "sick," your relatively high blood sugar levels meant that you aren't completely well either. Getting your blood sugar to an optimal level is likely to clear up or prevent a whole slew of symptoms, restoring your energy, boosting your mood, sharpening your mental focus, and helping you lose that unwanted weight.

This approach made a lot of sense to Jamie when I began treating her for her weight problems. Jamie had thought that her inability to lose weight came suddenly, out of the blue. In fact, she had been struggling with the same dysfunction since her early twenties. As the dysfunction worsened, her symptoms progressed: from slight weight gain that was relatively easy to lose . . . to greater weight gain that was a little harder to lose . . . to even greater weight gain that was seemingly impossible to lose.

In other words, Jamie had been slowly moving downward along a spectrum, from optimal function toward disease. Her problems with weight hadn't come "out of nowhere." She had just never realized that she even *had* a problem—until it got worse.

Happily, when Jamie discovered the foods, movement, and lifestyle that supported her gut, her immune system, and the rest of her body, she was able to move back up the spectrum. With all her systems functioning at their best, Jamie could easily maintain a healthy weight, and she noticed that her other symptoms cleared up as well. Suddenly Jamie had more energy, glowing skin, and, to her surprise, a lot more patience for coping with her boss, her husband, and her kids. Her mind sharpened, her memory returned, her sex drive improved, and she no longer felt blue and hopeless. Just as dysfunction had created multiple problems, improved function created multiple benefits.

Most Western doctors are okay with you feeling "not completely well" as long as you aren't actually sick. But I want something better for you! I want you feeling terrific, all the time. And if you support your body in the right ways—the ways I will teach you in this book—that level of great health is possible for you.

Myth: "I can't do much about my health—I just have poor genes"

Most of us were raised to believe that the genes we were born with are our destiny, and that the diseases that "run in the family" are most likely coming for us too. I myself have wrestled with this demon, since my father died of a heart attack at the age of 54; my brother, who is super fit and exercises regularly, had a coronary bypass at 50; and I, now in my 60s, have many of the markers indicating that I should have heart disease as well.

Yet I have escaped the condition that seemed to be the genetic destiny of the other men in my family. Why? Because even though I have all the genetic markers for heart disease, I don't necessarily have to develop that condition. Whether I do will be determined by how I live my life: what I eat, how much I move, whether I get enough good sleep, how well I release stress, and which supplements I take. We all have a lot more control over our health than we think.

Where does our control lie? True, we can't change our genes. But in the vast majority of cases, we can change how our genes express themselves. The science of genetic expression is known as *epigenetics,* and it is one of the most exciting frontiers of medical science.

Of course, some of our genes will always express themselves in the same way. For example, the genes that determine eye color are fixed by the time we emerge from the womb. No matter what we eat, we can't turn our brown eyes blue! Likewise, certain genetic conditions, such as sickle-cell anemia or Tay-Sachs disease, are not affected by diet or lifestyle. If you have the genes for those conditions, you'll suffer from those disorders no matter what you do.

The good news is that these "fixed" genes make up only about 2 percent of the total. The other 98 percent can be turned on or off. This is true for most of the disorders we associate with aging—Alzheimer's, cancer, arthritis, diabetes, heart disease, and hypertension. What you eat, how you exercise, whether you get enough sleep, how well you release stress, and which supplements you take to address your particular nutrient needs can all have an enormous impact on whether you develop these conditions—regardless of your genetic destiny. Your exposure to environmental toxins and your ability to detoxify your body also affect your genetic expression. Whether you know it or not, you are affecting your own genetics daily and perhaps even hourly through the foods you eat, the air you breathe, and even the thoughts you think.

For example, you might have been born with a "fat" gene causing a tendency to obesity. Guess what—you can overcome your "fat" gene by avoiding sugar, refined starches, and the many other foods that disrupt your metabolism and imbalance your gut. (You'll learn more about this in Chapters 1, 2, and 3.)

Or perhaps you were born with a gene giving you a predisposition to diabetes, or autoimmune disorders, or, like me, heart disease. Yes, you are more likely than other people to develop those disorders. However, you can turn off those genes by making the healthy choices that will maintain a healthy gut, support your friendly bacteria, and heal your inflammation.

Several studies have shown that lifestyle changes, both good and bad, trigger changes in gene expression. We have already seen how my own lifestyle changes have so far prevailed over my genetic tendency to heart disease. Likewise, many people have family histories of obesity and/or diabetes, yet with the right diet and lifestyle, they can avoid these chronic conditions.[1]

It works the other way too. Your genetic inheritance includes at least some genes that improve your resilience, increase your longevity, and help you fight cancer. But if you smoke cigarettes or eat junk food rather than *real* food, you shut those genes down and inhibit their expression. Both good and bad choices continually "speak" to our genes and thereby modify the way our genes express themselves.

This is another reason why I am confident that you don't have to get fat and you don't have to feel old. Even if your parents suffered from an age-related disease—hypertension, heart disease, arthritis, diabetes, stroke, or even cancer—you don't have to go down that road. When you learn how to support your body, you are also learning how to shape your own genetic expression. Every day—maybe even every hour—your genes are responding to the food you eat, the air you breathe, the stress you encounter, the choices you make. This is epigenetics, and it allows functional medicine to make an extraordinary promise:

Feed your genes the right "information" and you will modify the expression of your genes, improving the way your whole body functions.

So that is another reason why you don't have to get fat and feel old, no matter what your family history might be. By following the precepts in this book, you can reshape your genetic destiny, avoid age-related diseases, and live a life of glowing health.

Myth: "I can take meds for one issue without affecting the rest of my body"

Western medicine—and Western thinking in general—promotes a kind of linear approach to the human body. We are taught in medical school and in our subsequent training to zero in on symptoms and to medicate them. If the medication affects the symptom as we would like, we consider it successful. If it has any other effects, we call them "side effects," and, in most cases, downplay their importance.

But in fact, there are no "side effects"; there are only effects! Each of us is an intricate ecosystem, and we can't alter any one aspect of our body without other aspects being affected. This is why, whenever possible, I prefer to use natural treatments, adding in the nutrients that will improve function while removing the foods and habits that impede function.

The key word in this regard is *balance*. So much of the time, what a patient needs is not necessarily a "higher" or "lower" level of a hormone or biochemical, but rather more balance.

For women going through menopause, for example, the conventional medical approach is to prescribe synthetic estrogen, the female hormone whose levels decline at that time. But balancing estrogen and progesterone (another key female hormone), and making sure that all the other hormones—especially insulin and the thyroid hormones—are in balance as well are far more effective and much safer. Just increasing estrogen levels can lead to all sorts of problems, including a greater risk of cancer. Balancing estrogen and progesterone is a much wiser course, while balancing thyroid and insulin guarantees improved function and ongoing vitality with few or none of the symptoms typically associated with menopause.

I learned about this notion of balance very early when I was growing up in South Africa. It was a key concept in the management of the large game reserves that exist in my home country, which are home to many endangered species, including rhinos and elephants.

Someone who is aware that these types of animals are in short supply would naturally want to increase their population. They might think that targeting predators—the leopards and lions that feed on the endangered animals—is the most effective course of action.

But in fact, looking at only one portion of the whole system is not the best way to proceed. If you get rid of too many predators, other animal populations, including elephants, become too numerous. They devastate the vegetation on which they feed—with ruinous consequences. If the vegetation can't grow back quickly enough, the increased population of elephants face the risk of starvation. Now the predators are gone, the vegetation is devastated, and the elephants are at even greater risk than they were before. Following this unbalanced approach means that the whole ecosystem might be destroyed.

A wise caretaker understands that a healthy ecosystem needs balance: predators as well as prey, lions as well as elephants. Preserving the ecology of the game reserves requires that sort of wisdom—and so does preserving the ecology of our bodies.

However, this model of the ecosystem does not fit so well with the way conventional medicine is usually practiced. Instead of seeing the body as a coherent whole, conventional medicine chops up the body into separate systems, each with its own different specialist, completely ignoring the ways all our body parts are interconnected.

Specialization may have some advantages when it comes to promoting certain types of knowledge, but it all too frequently creates fragmented and ineffective medical care. For example, if you have acne or psoriasis, the standard medical response would be to send you to a dermatologist. But as you'll see in Chapters 1 and 2, I would view both conditions as a type of inflammation presenting in the skin, reflecting an underlying problem with digestion and immune function. Moreover, that underlying problem is probably also causing a whole other set of symptoms and disorders, such as gas, bloating, constipation, diarrhea, hormonal imbalances, anxiety, depression, brain fog, and memory problems. If these symptoms persist, a conventional physician might send you to a gastroenterologist for the digestive issues and a psychiatrist for the emotional/cognitive issues. But again, all of the symptoms would be coming from the same underlying dysfunction—which none of the specialists would address!

As you will see, this book takes quite a different approach. Throughout each chapter, you will see how each of your body's systems "talk" to each other and interact with the others to create either wellness or dysfunction. You'll see how some actions, such as eating too many sweets and starches, create dysfunction in multiple systems of your body, while other actions—such as taking probiotics—improve function in multiple areas. Instead of seeing your body as carved up into separate specialized domains, you'll come to view your body as an ecosystem in which—as in the game reserves I grew up with—every organ and system affects the functioning of the whole.

Getting the Most from This Book

Often, people ask me for a simple and direct way to improve their health. It has taken me many years, but I have finally found a way to boil down the complex, individual treatments that I give to each patient into one accessible book.

So I invite you on a journey throughout this book's ten main chapters—each of which corresponds to one of the ten reasons you feel old and fat. The book then culminates in a 2-Week Revitalize Program and a lifelong Maintenance Program. Each chapter addresses a key reason why we feel old and fat, breaking through the myths that lead us to make poor choices. And at the end of these chapters, I offer some quick fixes—immediate action that you can take to address the problem.

The first chapter explains how the food you eat can make you fat while creating a host of symptoms that make you feel old. Sugar, artificial sweeteners, and the wrong types of fat all weigh your body down, tax your immune system, and disrupt the healthy function of your brain. An insufficient amount of healthy fat in your diet has the same problematic effects. As a result, you might struggle with memory problems, loss of focus and concentration, brain fog, anxiety, and depression, as well as putting yourself at risk for such age-related diseases as cancer, heart disease, and diabetes.

In Chapter 2 you will learn still more about how eating the wrong foods makes you feel old and fat before your time. Specifically, you will find out about the problems of insulin resistance and carbohydrate intolerance, an underacknowledged disorder that plagues many of my patients and from which I also suffer. It turns out that even "healthy" grains and dried pulses are hard for some people to handle, as are too many fruits. If you are one of those people, your weight gain and your "age-related" symptoms might be fixed simply by switching out the rice for cauliflower and exchanging apples for kale.

At the root of our problems with diet, however, are the gut and the *microbiome,* the community of bacteria that is crucial to our weight, our metabolism, and our overall health. So in Chapter 3, you'll learn how to balance your microbiome and heal your gut. You'll also find out about some common foods—including gluten, dairy, corn, and soy—that might be stressing your microbiome, your gut, and your immune system. And you'll learn why preservatives, processed foods, and, again, sugar, starch, and artificial sweeteners are all making you feel old and fat.

Adjusting your diet, supporting your microbiome, and healing your gut are typically the three most effective ways to achieve a healthy weight and avoid the symptoms of age. Once you've mastered those tools, you're ready to look at Chapter 4, which explains how to balance your hormones. Hormonal issues are at the heart of many seemingly age-related problems, especially for women, and this chapter offers a lot of insight into how you can restore your energy, boost your mood, and improve your sexual function.

With a healthy diet and balanced hormones, you're ready to move! So Chapter 5 explains the kinds of movement your body craves and shows you why giving yourself chances to use your body—from strength training to yoga—is one of your best ways to stay slim and feel young. You'll also discover the importance of *fascia,* the connective tissue that binds your muscles, blood vessels, and nerves and that can make a tremendous difference in your flexibility, openness, and relaxation.

On to Chapter 6, where you consider all the ways stress weighs you down, burdening your body, mind, and emotions. No matter how busy or burdened you feel, I'll help you figure out practical ways to de-stress so you can bring some restorative balance back into your life.

The most healing medicine of all is deep, restful sleep, which you'll learn about in Chapter 7. If you have begun eating the right foods, balancing your hormones, getting the movement your body craves, and coping more effectively with stress, many of your sleep problems will already be solved. You'll learn how to remove any remaining obstacles in this restful chapter.

Sadly, our medical system too often creates as many problems as it cures, and that is the topic of Chapter 8. You'll find out how some of the medications you're taking might be affecting your health, potentially causing the weight gain and "senior moments" that you attribute to simple aging. You'll learn how to work with your doctor to safely get off the medications you no longer need, and how to compensate for the side effects of the meds you're still taking.

If you are taking medications, you almost certainly need to take nutritional supplements, which is the topic of Chapter 9. Even those of us who aren't taking meds need to supplement, and in this chapter I'll explain why. You'll also learn about the key anti-aging supplements I recommend for feeling vital and energetic at any age.

Finally, in Chapter 10, we come to a term I first learned in South Africa: *ubuntu*. Ubuntu is a Xhosa word that basically means "What makes us human is the humanity we show each other." In other words, "I can't be fully human without being part of a community." So in this chapter, you'll learn why a supportive community is so important to good health, as well as learning some ways to find or build that community if you don't already have it. You'll also find out why passion and meaning are crucial aspects of your health.

To put these ten chapters into practice, you can follow my 2-Week Revitalize Program, your step-by-step guide for supporting your body with the food, supplements, movement, sleep, and community that it needs. Speaking of community, I've drawn on mine to create this book, including one of my health coaches, Kerry Bajaj, who wrote the introduction to the program. A wonderful trainer, Jim Clarry, created the exercise plan, while Dr. Keren Day, a skilled Active Release Technique practitioner who works with me at my wellness center, supplied the fascia release exercises. Senior Iyengar Yoga teacher Bobby Clennell supplied the yoga exercises, and the terrific chef Tricia Williams is responsible for the delicious menus and meal plans.

Although I'm a big advocate of balance, I humbly request that you follow my 2-Week Revitalize Program to the letter. Why? Because I think that's the best way for you to get the full impact of what I've learned in the past 35 years. I want you to fully experience how terrific you *could* feel once you've improved your body's function and put yourself on the road to health.

In my office, we have health coaches who work with patients on this program, answering questions and offering support. My coaches have come up with a wonderful phrase—*the barrier of belief.* They tell me that often, people are reluctant to try this program simply because they can't bring themselves to believe that it can really make a difference. Indeed, many of us are so used to feeling old and fat that we've basically given up the hope of ever feeling terrific.

If that's your response to my program, let me make a deal with you. Just give me two weeks—only 14 days—in which you try what I'm suggesting. You don't have to believe that it will work. Just suspend your disbelief and take the experiment. I'm willing to bet that at the end of two weeks, you're going to feel so much better that you don't even need to listen to me anymore! Your own body will be telling you what feels good and what feels bad, and you'll be able to listen to your own instincts and responses to choose your healthiest path. You'll find some suggestions to help you on your way in the Maintenance section at the end.

Throughout this book, I focus on a key concept that I personally have always found to be a source of inspiration: *resilience.* Resilience is your capacity to respond effectively to a stressor or hardship—to bounce back, with energy and determination, after even the most crushing blow. Resilience is what enables you to endure the inevitable losses and tragedies that do tend to come with age, along with whatever health challenges you might face. Resilience is what allows you to emerge stronger, wiser, and more open to life than before, ready to appreciate the good things in your life as you move forward toward a new future.

None of us can be immortal. None of us can avoid at least some loss or hardship, especially as we get older. And all of us—if we're lucky!—*will* get older; we can't stop the aging process.

What we *can* do is change *how* we age. If we know how to support our bodies, minds, and spirits, we can greet our challenges with resilience, and go on to years of vitality, meaning, and joy.

Sound good? Then let's get started. I can't wait for you to feel terrific!

REASON #1:

YOU'RE NOT EATING THE RIGHT FOODS

When Madeleine first came to see me, she was in despair.

"I'm only fifty-six, but I feel like I'm a hundred and six," she told me. "I'm carrying at least 12 kilos of extra weight, and sometimes it seems like I can barely move. I know I should eat less, but I just can't seem to control myself. I guess I just don't have any willpower."

I could see how ashamed Madeleine was of what she viewed as her own personal failing, and how hopeless she felt about it.

"I do the best I can," she said. "I never put dressing on my salads, and I only ever eat low-fat. But no diet has ever really worked for me—and believe me, I've tried them all! Even when I starve myself, I don't really lose any weight, and after a few weeks, I get so hungry I end up eating everything in sight."

She sighed. "My mom and my sisters and even my grandmother all have the same problem," she said. "We just pack on the pounds and nothing ever seems to work. Our family must just have fat genes."

She looked at me miserably, sure that I was about to give her the same scolding she had heard all her life, including from her doctors: *Control yourself. Eat smaller portions. Cut out the fat. Try harder.*

But I wanted to give Madeleine a very different message.

"Madeleine," I told her, "this is not your fault. Your problem is not willpower, or self-control, and it's not your genes either. Your problem is that you've been given the wrong information about food."

My patient Amber was also in despair. At 35, she was used to being slim and trim—"a gym rat from way back." But for months, Amber had been feeling dragged out, exhausted, and "just not myself." Her skin was starting to break out. She wasn't sleeping well. Recently she, too, had begun gaining weight—and she, too, found herself constantly craving sugar.

"I only ever eat sugar-free," she assured me. "Diet sodas, sugar-free yogurt, Splenda in my coffee, sugar-free desserts. So why am I gaining weight? Plus, I find myself thinking about sweet things all day long. No matter how much I get, it's never enough."

She laughed uncomfortably.

"Even though I never eat sugar, I feel like I've turned into a sugar addict," she told me.

"That's not surprising," I replied. "There's a good chance that's exactly what has happened."

Myths to Break Through

- "I don't have any willpower."
- "Sugar-free products and artificial sweeteners are a healthy way to lose weight."
- "I have fat genes."
- "Weight loss is mainly about cutting calories."
- "Fat is bad for my health and weight."

Myth: "I don't have any willpower"

Believe it or not, scientists have actually discovered not only that sugar is addictive, but that sugar substitutes are too.[1] Both Madeleine and Amber were suffering not from lack of willpower or some kind of psychological compulsion, but from a very real biological syndrome.

If you feel out of control around food, and particularly if you feel compelled to eat sweet things, a sugar addiction might be your problem.

There are three possible causes for the hold sweet and starchy foods have on you—and you might suffer from one, two, or all three:

Cause #1: You're on the "blood sugar roller coaster."

I see this all the time; in fact, I must be careful not to fall prey to it myself! If you eat a sugary food—or in some cases, a starchy one—you can flood your blood with *glucose,* a type of sugar.

Glucose is a vital substance, and your whole body depends on it. Your muscles, organs, and even your brain all need a nice, steady supply of glucose, which ideally you get from having a small, healthy meal or snack every few hours.

When your glucose cycle functions optimally, everything is fine. Your weight stays at a healthy level, and you only ever experience the right degree of hunger to keep you at your healthy weight.

⬥——— What's a Healthy Glucose Cycle? ———⬥

Your optimal cycle begins when you eat some healthy food—say, a fresh green salad. Your digestive tract breaks the salad down into its component parts, including *glucose,* a type of sugar. (Yes, lettuce and fresh vegetables contain sugar too!)

As the digestion process continues, the glucose is released into your bloodstream. This triggers a moderate release of *insulin,* a hormone that helps move the glucose out of your bloodstream and into your cells.

Eventually, insulin has moved most of the glucose out of your blood, causing another set of hormones to trigger the feeling of hunger. That hunger leads you to eat another healthy meal . . . your glucose rises again . . . and once again, a moderate amount of insulin is released. When this system is working optimally, you get only moderate, pleasant ups and downs—and no roller coaster.

Your Optimal Sugar Cycle

You feel hungry.

You eat some food.

In your digestive tract, the food breaks down
into glucose (and other ingredients).

The glucose leaves your digestive tract
and enters your bloodstream.

Glucose in your bloodstream (blood sugar)
triggers a moderate release of insulin.

Insulin moves the glucose out of your
bloodstream and into your cells

When your blood glucose levels fall
("low blood sugar"), you feel hungry . . .
. . . and the whole cycle starts again.

So far, so good. But what happens when you eat something sweet or starchy—a cookie, some white rice, or a white potato? Those types of food tend to break down into glucose very quickly. As a result, foods that are too sweet and starchy slam your blood with a whole load of glucose at once, abruptly jolting your blood sugar levels too high—what you might know as a "sugar rush."

That excess sugar triggers not a healthy, balanced, moderate release of insulin but instead a massive flood. All that extra insulin moves the glucose out of your bloodstream way too quickly—and now you've got a "sugar crash."

A sugar high can feel so good! You might feel happy, excited, keyed up, and powerful. Or you might feel satisfied, relieved, or comforted. You might also feel dizzy, anxious, wired, or out of control.

These might seem like psychological states, but they are actually *physical* responses to an overload of glucose, just as a cocaine high is a physical response to a hit of cocaine. (As we'll see in a moment, cocaine and sugar have a lot in common!)

A sugar high might feel terrific, but a sugar crash is pretty awful—and again, it has a lot in common with a cocaine crash. As that sudden wave of excess insulin abruptly jerks the sugar out of your bloodstream, you are likely to feel depressed, dizzy, foggy, and tired. You might have trouble keeping your eyes open, causing you to reach for some coffee or soda—creating a caffeine cycle in addition to your sugar cycle! You might have trouble concentrating on your work, keeping your temper, or thinking clearly at all. Like Madeleine, you might feel obsessed with food, overwhelmed by your cravings for bread, cake, doughnuts, or potatoes.

Once again, these are *physical responses,* programmed into your body over the millennia of human evolution. When your blood glucose levels are low, your body thinks it's starving. As a result, you desperately want food. Your whole body is frantic to get hold of anything that will push those blood sugar levels back up to normal.

The Blood Sugar Roller Coaster

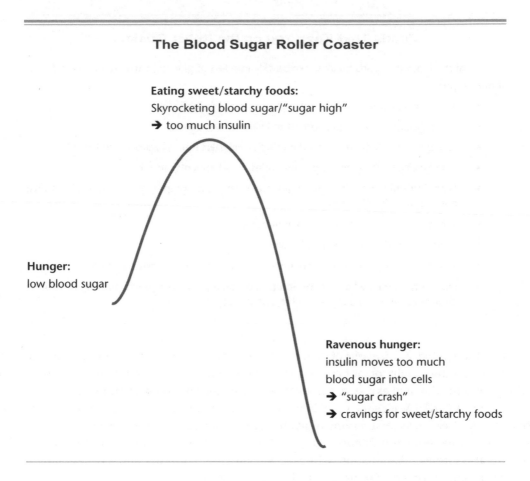

Eating sweet/starchy foods:
Skyrocketing blood sugar/"sugar high"
➔ too much insulin

Hunger:
low blood sugar

Ravenous hunger:
insulin moves too much
blood sugar into cells
➔ "sugar crash"
➔ cravings for sweet/starchy foods

Of course, the foods that will most quickly boost your glucose are the sweet and starchy foods that gave you the sugar high in the first place. That's why Madeleine—and perhaps you too—craved sweets and starches, rather than, say, a nice kale salad: that cookie, bagel, or doughnut that quickly breaks down into lots of glucose and will boost your blood sugar a lot faster than the salad will. So once you get onto the roller coaster, you might find it very hard to get off.

This has nothing to do with willpower, however. It's a simple matter of biology.

Foods That Keep You on the Roller Coaster

All of the following foods break down quickly into lots of glucose, causing your blood sugar to spike:

- Table sugar, confectioner's sugar, or any kind of refined sugar
- Honey, agave, cane sugar, and other "natural" sweeteners
- Rice syrup, maltodextrin, and the other sweeteners found in processed foods
- Dried fruits, such as raisins, prunes, dates, dried apricots, and the like
- Fresh fruits that are very high in glucose, such as figs, grapes, and most tropical fruits: banana, mango, pineapple
- White flour: pasta, baked goods, white bread
- White rice and other processed grains
- White potatoes, which are high in starch and so convert quickly to glucose
- For many people, whole grains and pseudo-grains, including such supposedly healthy choices as brown rice and oats (see Chapter 2)

Besides making you feel out of control, this roller coaster practically guarantees that you will keep gaining weight, or, at best, you won't be able to lose any. Why? Because it will keep stimulating insulin, and excessive amounts of insulin cue your body to store fat.

That was part of Madeleine's problem. Even when she stuck to a low-calorie diet, just a few bites of a fat-free cookie or a serving of white rice sent her glucose levels rising too far too fast. In response, her body was flooded with insulin . . . which cued her body to store fat. Excess insulin also creates inflammation, which, as we saw in the Introduction, creates many of the symptoms and disorders that make us feel old (see page xiv).

Even with a low-calorie diet, too many sweet and starchy foods cause your body to be flooded with insulin . . . which cues your body to retain fat.

Excess insulin also creates inflammation . . . which creates the symptoms and disorders that make you feel old.

Cause #2: Sweet and starchy foods are addictive.

It's not just that glucose and insulin keep us hooked. Sweet foods are also *literally* addictive, setting off the same biological mechanisms that are triggered by cocaine.

When I said the word "addictive" to Madeline and Amber, both of them thought I was using a metaphor. They thought I was saying something like, "These foods taste so good, you can't help wanting them."

But no: I'm using the word exactly as I would if I were talking about cocaine. In fact, experiments with animals have shown that sugar might even be *more* addictive than cocaine. Even more remarkably, artificial sweeteners share that same addictive power.

For example, in 2009, a group of French scientists gave lab rats the choice between pressing a lever that gave them an intravenous dose of cocaine and one that gave them the chance to drink sugar water.[2]

You would think that most if not all of the rats would choose cocaine. After all, cocaine is a highly addictive substance that floods the brain with intense pleasure signals. Once you've had a taste of that cocaine high, it's very difficult to resist.

But it turns out that resisting sweetness is even harder. An overwhelming 94 percent of the French rats chose water sweetened with saccharin over cocaine. They did so even though they were given the chance to try the cocaine lever two separate times before making their final decision. Still, all but a few of the rats still chose sweetened water. Apparently just the *taste* of sweetness can be addictive, even when the blood sugar roller coaster is not involved.

This is why both Madeline and Amber felt out of control around sweet things. Whether you're drinking a caramel mocha latte or a Coke Zero, the sweetness gets you hooked.

Why? The French scientists hypothesized that we evolved in a world where sweetness was usually associated with a type of food that cues the body to store fat. To avoid starvation, we evolved special "sweetness receptors" that flood our brains with unusually intense pleasure signals whenever we taste something sweet. For most of our time on this planet, sweet things were rare—basically, you could only get sweetness from fruit—so this part of our brains didn't get the chance to create an addiction.

Now, however, you can get a sugar fix on every corner—and for many of us, obesity is a far greater health risk than starvation. Instead of helping us survive, our "sweet receptors" are actually threatening our health.

A study at The Scripps Research Institute in Florida makes it even clearer that sugar addiction is a real biological phenomenon.[3] The defining characteristic of addiction is that you need more and more of the addictive substance to achieve the same response. Today, you're satisfied with one square of chocolate. Tomorrow, you need a whole bar. Next week, you need two bars.

If you've noticed this response—as I have!—you might have thought you were just "weak" or "undisciplined." But when the team at Scripps put a bunch of rats on a sweet diet, they noticed that eating sugar actually changed the rats' brains: their pleasure centers were literally getting smaller. As a result, the rats needed more and more sweetness to produce the same response—so they kept eating more and more and more. Eventually, according to Scripps Research Associate Professor Paul Kenny, "the animals completely lost control over their eating behavior, the primary hallmark of addiction."

These rats weren't turning to sweets out of any deep-seated psychological problem. They hadn't just broken up with their boyfriends or lost a big promotion. They were responding to sugar the same way they responded to cocaine: with a physical addiction. And, as with cocaine, they were even willing to brave electric shocks to get to the sweet stuff. In the words of yet another team of scientists who have studied this issue, both drugs and sweet foods seem to "'hijack' the brain."

Do you feel as though *your* brain has been hijacked? My 2-Week Revitalize Program will help you free yourself. Just as eating the wrong foods has turned you into a sugar addict, eating the right foods can reshape your brain. You will get to a place where you won't need willpower—because you simply won't crave sugar. Instead, you'll enjoy a pleasant hunger, a balanced appetite, and a healthy weight.

Cause #3: Your gut is overgrown with certain types of unfriendly bacteria. When they crave sweets and starches, so do you.

One of the ways sugar hijacks your brain is through your gut bacteria. Certain types of gut bacteria actually produce biochemicals that cue your brain to crave sugar. If your gut is overgrown with those types of bacteria, you'll turn into a sugar addict.

And guess what—artificial sweeteners also disrupt your gut bacteria. As we'll see in Chapter 3, that was part of why Amber was gaining weight, feeling run down, and having trouble sleeping: her gut bacteria were out of balance.

Luckily, my Revitalize Program will kill the bad bacteria and help you focus on the right kinds of foods—the ones that rebalance your gut bacteria and eliminate your cravings. In just two weeks, you'll start to feel the difference, and within a few months, you'll feel calm, centered, and healthy once more. (You'll learn more about your gut bacteria in Chapter 3.)

Myth: "Sugar-free products and artificial sweeteners are a healthy way to lose weight"

Once you know that sweet and starchy foods disrupt your insulin response and cue your body to store fat, you might think that sugar-free foods are a safe haven. After all, if they're low in glucose, they can't trigger insulin. And if they're low in calories, they can't pack on the pounds.

That all sounds logical—but it's actually not true. As we just saw, our brains respond to sweetness with an overpowering desire for . . . more sweetness. So even if your only source of sweetness is a diet Pepsi or a sugar-free yogurt, you—like Amber—will probably find yourself craving sweet and starchy foods. You might indulge or you might not, but either way, you're going to *feel* like an addict. And if you do indulge, as Amber had begun to do, those doughnuts, chips, and pasta are going to make you fat.

To make matters worse, artificial sweeteners keep you from knowing when you're full. At least when you consume actual sugar, your blood sugar rises, so your body understands that it has eaten a high-sugar food. Until your blood sugar crashes again, you feel sated.

When you eat a no- or low-cal sweet, however, you crave more sweetness—*and* you're still hungry. Your body gets very confused when it eats something—especially something sweet—but does not feel full. (In scientific terms, the hormones signaling "hunger" and "fullness" become *dysregulated.*) Eventually, you lose your capacity for knowing when you are really hungry and when you just want more sugar.

When I asked Amber about this, she agreed that her meal portions were getting larger and larger. Even if she resisted the sweets, she was still eating more food—and gaining more weight.

More insidiously still, the popular sweetener known as *aspartame*—which you find in Equal or NutraSweet—is made primarily of two amino acids (phenylalanine and aspartic acid) that stimulate our old friend insulin. Even though you haven't consumed any actual sugar, aspartame cues your body to react as though you have—and you get fat anyway.

These amino acids also stimulate *leptin,* which normally would be a good thing because leptin is the hormone that makes you feel full. You depend upon leptin to feel satisfied enough to stop eating, and a healthy, balanced leptin response is the key to a calm and healthy appetite.

However, when you consume a lot of Equal or NutraSweet, your body is flooded with too much leptin, and you might develop the syndrome known as *leptin resistance.* When you become leptin resistant, your cells stop "hearing" the leptin message. As a result, you lose your ability to feel full, even when you've just eaten an enormous meal. (We'll be talking more about leptin in Chapter 2.)

Finally, artificial sweeteners disrupt your body's friendly bacteria, which, as we've just seen, causes weight gain and creates a host of other problems. (We'll learn more about that in Chapter 3.)

Artificial Sweeteners Make You Fat!

- In its mammoth study of 80,000 women, the American Cancer Society found that those who drank diet soda gained more weight than the women who drank full-sugar soda. Numerous other studies have supported this finding. (Now, please don't start drinking full-sugar soda—that's just as bad! See www.bewell.com/blog/give-up-soda for a list of healthy beverages you can enjoy.)

- The popular sweetener aspartame spurs weight gain, especially *visceral fat,* the deadly fat that accumulates around your organs and makes your abdomen stick out. Aspartame also has negative effects on your glucose-insulin cycle and increases a problem known as *insulin resistance,* which you'll learn about in Chapter 2.

- Animals that consumed yogurt sweetened with aspartame or saccharin actually gained *more* weight than those who ate yogurt sweetened with sugar—even when the two groups of animals ate the same number of calories. (Again, please don't take this as a cue to eat sugar-sweetened yogurt!)

- Sucralose—used in making Splenda and prevalent in diet sodas—also seems to cue people to feel hungrier and crave more sweet foods, disrupting metabolism and leading to weight gain.

- If you drink diet soda while you're pregnant, you're putting not only yourself but your baby at risk: recent animal studies have shown that exposure to aspartame in the womb is bad for a child's future ability to learn and remember. And if that's what it does to your child's brain, imagine what it's doing to yours![4]

⬥—— HIGH-FRUCTOSE CORN SYRUP: ——⬥
THE "HIDDEN ASSASSIN"

There is one other sweet culprit that disrupts your metabolism, inflates your appetite, fuels your addiction, and packs on the pounds: *high-fructose corn syrup,* or HFCS. This industrial sweetener, which began to be widely used in the 1980s, is used to sweeten sodas, baked goods, and many other products that you might not even consider sweet, such as ketchup, barbecue sauce, and even soup.

As the name suggests, HFCS is primarily composed not of *glucose* but of another type of natural sugar, *fructose.* Fructose bypasses your normal insulin response and goes straight to your liver. (The sugars in wine and other alcoholic beverages behave in the same way.) There are three problems with this ubiquitous sweetener:

1. Because it's extremely high-calorie—and the wrong type of calorie—it contributes significantly to weight gain.

2. Because it bypasses your normal insulin response, you can consume a lot of it and still feel hungry. So you're eating way more of these "bad" calories than your body was ever designed to consume.

3. Because it's sweet, it helps create the same type of sugar addiction that both glucose and artificial sweeteners produce.

If you want to stay slim and feel young, avoid HFCS like the plague. For many reasons, I want you eating primarily whole, fresh foods—but if you must eat packaged foods, read the labels carefully for HFCS and its sneaky cousin rice syrup, another type of "natural" sweetener that creates sugar addiction, inflated hunger, and weight gain.

By the way, fructose can also be found in fruits, usually in combination with glucose. We'll see in Chapter 2 that if you have a condition known as *carbohydrate intolerance,* even too much fresh fruit can also sometimes make you feel old and fat.

Myth: "I have fat genes"

We've already broken through this myth in the Introduction, on pages xvii to xix. So I'll just reaffirm what I tell my patients: You might well have a genetic tendency to put on weight. However, you can transform that tendency, and you can do so in just a few months. Food, supplements, movement, sleep, and stress relief can make the difference between your genes frantically shouting "GAIN WEIGHT" and those same genes remaining calm and silent.

Throughout this book, you'll learn the strategies that will help you silence your "fat genes." Then, when you get on your 2-Week Revitalize Program and your lifelong Maintenance Program, you'll start practicing the habits that enable you to reshape your genetic destiny.

You are not the prisoner of your genetic inheritance.

Diet, supplements, and lifestyle can reshape the behavior of your genes.

Myth: "Weight loss is mainly about cutting calories"

Yes, calories are important. But they are very far from the whole story. If you eat mainly sweet and starchy foods, you're going to throw your metabolism out of balance—even if you cut back on the number of calories. Ultimately, the *number* of calories you consume is far less important than the *type* of calories.

You might have heard that 3,500 calories equals half a kilo of body fat. In theory, that's true, but your body isn't an account book—it's more like an ecosystem. Everything you eat affects numerous interactive systems—metabolism, digestion, immune system, hormones, brain—with multiple complex effects. You can't just count calories; you have to look at the metabolic impact of the calories, since different foods have vastly different biological effects in your body.

Sugar, for example, stimulates the insulin response. So 220 calories of sugar—or even fewer—will trigger a process that often leads to weight gain and other symptoms. (For more on how insulin affects your weight, see Chapter 2.)

By contrast, 220 calories of kale will *not* stimulate your insulin response in the same way. Kale is also full of fiber that feeds your healthy bacteria, and it contains loads of antioxidants that reduce stress on your body and improve function.

So, eating 220 calories of sugar will make you feel old and fat. Eating 220 calories of kale will make you feel vital and help you maintain a healthy weight. You can't just swap them out by the numbers. You have to look at how they affect your whole ecology.

Amber found this out the hard way. She used artificial sweeteners to restrict calories—but those same sweeteners cued her body to store fat, slowed down her metabolism, and sabotaged her feelings of hunger and fullness. She gained weight, she felt lousy, and she began to see herself as powerless and addicted.

Madeleine, too, stumbled over her calorie counting. Before she came to me, she would sometimes swap out a big portion of vegetables for a single cookie or a few bites of cake, reasoning that the calories were ultimately the same. However, those sweet and starchy calories set off an insulin response, put her on the blood sugar roller coaster, inflamed her addiction, and cued her body for fat storage.

By contrast, when Madeline and Amber began to follow the Revitalize and Maintenance programs, they discovered that clean proteins, healthy fats, raw or lightly cooked vegetables, and an occasional serving of fresh berries turned the whole equation around. Both women lost weight and regained their sense of control.

All calories are *not* created equal!

Myth: "Fat is bad for my health and weight"

That's the overall myth—but actually, it's made up of a number of different myths. Let's break them down and look at them one by one.

Myths to Break Through about Fat and Weight

- "High-fat foods are fattening and generally bad for my health."
- "Saturated fats are bad for me because they raise my cholesterol and cause heart disease."
- "All vegetable oils are healthy choices."

Myth: "High-fat foods are fattening and generally bad for my health"

Okay, there is a grain of truth in this myth: *some* dietary fats are bad for you. But many others are not only good for you—they are absolutely crucial for your brain and body to function at their best. In fact, increasing the amount of healthy fat in your diet is actually one of your best weight-loss weapons.

How can you tell the difference between healthy and unhealthy fat? A good rule of thumb is that fats you can find in nature are good for you, whereas fats that have been created in laboratories and factories are likely to be bad for you. I want you to start making friends with friendly fats:

- Avocados and avocado oil
- Coconuts and coconut oil (virgin or expeller pressed)
- Olives and olive oil (extra virgin)
- Palm oil
- Fish oil
- Flaxseeds and flax oil
- Raw nuts
- Nut butters
- Unheated nut oils like walnut oil and macadamia oil
- Seeds, such as chia seeds
- Cold-water fish like wild salmon, mackerel, herring, anchovies, and sardines
- Organic grass-fed or pastured meats
- Organic pastured egg yolk
- Pasture-raised duck fat
- Grass-fed butter or ghee (clarified butter)
- Goat's and sheep's milk cheese*

What's So Healthy about Healthy Fats?

All of your cell walls are made of fat, which means that your cells require fat to maintain their integrity. Without enough healthy fat, your cells—particularly your brain cells—don't function properly. As a result, you feel old, tired, cranky, and forgetful, and perhaps also anxious, foggy, unfocused, or depressed. You might also have trouble falling or staying asleep.

Healthy fat is also crucial to your gut, and therefore to your immune system. When your body is deprived of healthy fat, the cells that line your stomach and intestines don't function properly, compromising your ability to digest and absorb nutrients. The single cell wall that separates your gut and immune system doesn't work properly either.

For these reasons, a lack of healthy fat in your diet might be contributing to all sorts of seemingly unrelated symptoms, including digestive difficulties, acne and skin eruptions, hormonal issues, frequent colds and flu, and perhaps even more serious problems such as heart disease, diabetes, autoimmune disease, and cancer.

---

* Although these are generally healthy fats, you won't be eating them during your 2-Week Revitalize Program because they can be reactive and stress your gut, as you will see in Chapter 3. Once your gut is in better shape, you can add these healthy fats into your lifelong Maintenance Program.

Healthy fat is also necessary for getting the most out of your food. Many key vitamins are *fat soluble,* meaning they dissolve not in water but in fat.

This scientific fact leads to a conclusion that many of my patients find surprising:

If you are eating salad without dressing or steamed vegetables without a light coating of olive oil or grass-fed butter, you are basically missing a good part of the nutritive value of those otherwise healthy vegetables.

For example, vitamins A, D, E, and K are all fat soluble, so if you don't put a little healthy fat on your veggies, you are not going to absorb any of those vitamins. Even if you are taking vitamin D supplements, if you take them on an empty stomach or with a fat-free meal, you are missing almost the entire value of the vitamin.

So please, add a light coating of olive oil, flaxseed oil, or walnut oil to your salads, and either lightly sauté your cooked vegetables or throw on a little grass-fed butter or olive oil when you steam them. Healthy fat is your best friend when it comes to nutrient absorption.

To sum it all up, healthy fat is crucial to staying slim and feeling young.

If you're not getting enough healthy fat, you will find it nearly impossible to maintain a healthy weight.

When You Skip the Fat, You Get Old and Fat!

Healthy fat:

- Keeps your brain sharp

- Helps balance your mood

- Supports your gut—which is key to overall health (see Chapter 3)

- Helps you to absorb nutrients, so you can eat less food for the same benefit

- Allows your cells to achieve optimal function

- Soothes your hunger, so you are less likely to crave sweets and starches, which *do* make you fat (see above, and also Chapter 2)

- Fights inflammation, which is the primary underlying reason people feel old and get fat.

That's why one of the first things I told Madeleine to do was to increase her intake of healthy fat. After years of eating plain steamed veggies and salads without dressing, she found it almost impossible to believe that adding fat to her diet would help her subtract fat from her hips. But I assured her it was true. The myths about fat—unfortunately shared by many doctors—are part of the reason why so many of us are getting old and fat.

Myth: "Saturated fats are bad for me because they raise my cholesterol and cause heart disease"

Saturated fats are "saturated" with hydrogen molecules, which affects the molecular structure of the fat. One of the ways you can tell whether a fat is saturated is that it's usually solid at room temperature.

Typically, saturated fats come from animals in such forms as red meat, chicken skin, milk, butter, cheese, yogurt, eggs, or lard. Other saturated fats include coconut oil and palm oil.

The American Heart Association (AHA) has long promoted the idea that saturated fats are bad for us on the grounds that they increase *cholesterol*—a type of fat found in the blood. Following conventional medical wisdom, the AHA argues that cholesterol is a major contributor to cardiovascular disease—high blood pressure, heart attacks, atherosclerosis (hardening of the arteries), and stroke.[5] The solution, according to this view, is to limit your consumption of saturated fat and focus instead on unsaturated fat, typically found in fish, poultry (without the skin), nuts, and seeds.

Unfortunately, this view simply isn't accurate, and in Chapter 8 I'll give you the full, true story on cholesterol, weight, and health. Here let me just say two things:

1. **Cholesterol is actually a healthy substance that your body makes to perform many vital functions.** It is not the cause of heart disease or any other disorder. Even if, like me, you are at risk for cardiovascular disease, your cholesterol levels are not what you should be focusing on. Instead, you should work to lower your levels of inflammation, which you can do by following the recommendations in this book.

2. **You don't get high cholesterol levels from eating fat, whether saturated or any other type.** You get excessively high cholesterol from eating too many sweets and starches. If you take in more glucose in one meal than your body can use, your body either stores that glucose as *glycogen* in the liver, converts it to blood fat (cholesterol), or converts it to the body fat that shows up on your abdomen, hips, and thighs. Eating healthy high-fat foods—whether saturated fat or any other type of fat—does not play a significant role in raising your "bad" cholesterol.

⟨— So red meat, dairy products, and eggs —⟩ are good for me, and I can eat as much as I want?

Well, yes . . . and no. The AHA is actually correct here—but not for the reasons it says. Ideally, you would avoid most conventionally farmed red meat, dairy products, and eggs. But that's not because the fat is saturated. It's because the animals on factory farms are raised in such an unhealthy fashion, fed the wrong foods, and injected with all sorts of drugs.

Those poor animals are stuffed full of corn, soy, and other grains rather than being given the grass and plant food that would be healthier for them—and us. Because they're raised in such close, unsanitary quarters, they're shot full of antibiotics, which are bad for both their health and ours.

Besides protecting the animals from disease, antibiotics are actually used to fatten them. As we'll see in Chapter 3, antibiotics make us fat by destroying our healthy bacteria and thereby disrupting gut function. If you want to lose weight, skip the "antibiotic" meat, dairy, and eggs and go organic and pasture raised instead.

To make matters worse, factory-farmed animals are also given lots of hormones to make them fatter or to speed up their production of milk and eggs. Those hormones don't do your health any favors, and they're terrible for your weight as well, especially if you're a woman.

Finally, conventionally raised cows, pigs, and chickens are exposed to a huge toxic burden in the form of pesticides, fertilizer, and a slew of other industrial chemicals—and all of those toxins are stored in their fat. They live and are slaughtered under conditions of extreme stress, so that the stress-induced chemicals affect their meat and their fat as well. Is it any wonder that these cruel and unnatural ways of treating animals give us obesity, heart disease, and cancer? It is a true example of how the macrocosm affects the microcosm!

But none of these problems are caused by saturated fat per se. If you eat only the products of humanely raised animals—grass-fed cows, pigs, goats, and lambs and free-range chickens raised without chemicals, toxins, hormones, or antibiotics—you will be consuming healthy types of fat.

With regard to the saturated fats in coconut and palm oil, the AHA warnings are simply wrong. Both are fantastic friendly fats that will support your brain, gut, immune system, and hormones as they help heal your inflammation. As a result, they'll protect your heart and your health while helping you lose weight.

So, to sum it all up:

Healthy fat is one of your best weapons against feeling old and getting fat. You just need to know which types of fat are healthy.

Myth: "All vegetable oils are healthy choices"

Many healthy fats come from plants, including olive oil, walnut oil, coconut oil, palm oil, and avocado. However, some of the unhealthiest fats around are also plant based, including many types of vegetable oil, which are actually not made from vegetables, but rather grains, seeds, and beans.

Unhealthy Fats: Trans Fats

Trans fats, aka *partially hydrogenated fats* or *partially hydrogenated vegetable oils,* are one of the unhealthiest foods on the planet. These fats—and the processed foods in which they are found—are so destructive to our health that fortunately the FDA took steps to ban them and gave manufacturers three years to remove such fats from their products.

Trans fats are produced by injecting extra hydrogen into vegetable oils to extend their shelf life. This makes them very handy for the companies that want to sell you packaged foods—but the modification is absolutely terrible for just about every aspect of your health. Unlike healthy fats, which can actually improve your blood lipid profile, trans fats increase both triglycerides and "bad" LDL cholesterol while also lowering "good" HDL cholesterol. (As you'll see in Chapter 8, not all LDL is unhealthy, but small, dense LDL particles are bad for you.)

Trans fats also promote systemwide inflammation. As a result, they vastly increase your chances of suffering from a whole host of symptoms, including aches, pains, forgetfulness, brain fog, and obesity. Eventually, that inflammation can lead to heart disease, diabetes, auto-immune conditions, and cancer. If you don't want to get old and fat, stay away from trans fats!

Unhealthy Fats: Industrial Oils

Almost as bad as trans fats are such vegetable oils as canola, corn, cottonseed, safflower, sunflower, rice bran, and soy. I call them "industrial oils" because they were never part of the human diet until we developed food factories to produce them. Because this type of oil is so prevalent—especially in restaurant, processed, and packaged foods—it might even be *worse* for your health than trans fats, simply because you may be consuming it in such high quantities.

These deceptive fats threaten your health in several ways:

Problem #1: They are often made from genetically modified crops.

Genetically modified organisms (GMOs) can have harsh consequences for your health, destroying your healthy bacteria and altering your microbiome. As we'll see in Chapter 3, an imbalanced microbiome leads almost immediately to weight gain and inflammation, with all the symptoms and disorders that inflammation brings.

Problem #2: They imbalance your ratio of omega-3s and omega-6s.

Omega-3s are a type of fat found in coldwater wild fish, pasture-raised meats, pasture-raised or omega-3–enriched eggs, flax, nuts, and chia seeds. Omega-6s are a type of fat found most frequently in factory-farmed meat and eggs from grain-fed chicken—but predominantly in industrial oils and all the products made with them.

Ideally, your ratio of omega-6s to omega-3s is 1:1. But our modern consumption is more like 10:1 or even 25:1.

What is causing this lack of balance? Two things:

1. Most of us eat too much industrially raised meat and poultry and not enough grass-fed meats, wild fish, nuts, and seeds. Industrially raised animals are fed corn, soy, and other grains, which turns their fats into omega-6s. So most commercially available meat, eggs, butter, milk, and cheese are full of omega-6s. Grass-fed and pasture-raised animals, by contrast, are high in omega-3s. That is one of the many reasons why free-range, pasture-raised animals produce much healthier meat, eggs, and dairy products. Wild fish are also high in omega-3s, while farm-raised fish are far less so.

2. Restaurant food—especially fast food—contains high quantities of industrial oils, as do packaged and prepared foods. These oils are high in omega-6s, so our frequent consumption of them is throwing off our healthy balance of omega-3s and omega-6s.

Of course, we need some omega-6s in our diet, to properly balance the omega-3s. But the use of industrial oils in processed and prepared foods means that many of us consume far too many omega-6s. When the balance is off, those omega-6s have an inflammatory effect—and, as we have seen, inflammation is at the root of most of the reasons why we feel old and fat.

Problem #3: They are unstable, which makes them inflammatory.

Saturated fats are more stable fats because of their molecular structure. Unsaturated fats are less stable—and polyunsaturated fats are the least stable of all.

When a fat is unstable, that means it is vulnerable to *oxidation*—that is, to penetration by molecules of oxygen. Oxidation causes a fat to go rancid and to create *free radicals:* atoms with an odd number of electrons that can cause extensive damage to your cells.

Any fat can be oxidized and create this damaging effect, but because polyunsaturated fats are so unstable, they are the most prone to it. Polyunsaturated fats like the industrial oils can become rancid simply from exposure to light through a clear glass bottle, which means that they've often gone bad even before you take them home from the store.

Heat also oxidizes these types of fats, so if you eat anything cooked in an industrial oil, you're exposing yourself to free radicals that can cause quite a lot of cellular damage.

Problem #4: *They are highly refined, which makes them even more inflammatory.*

It's not an accident that we didn't consume industrial oils before we had factories; in their natural state, they don't taste or smell very good, and many of them are not even digestible. In order to make an industrial oil fit for human consumption, it has to be *refined*—that is, processed in such a way that the taste and smell are removed.

This refining process must be done at a high heat, and as we just saw, this oxidizes an unstable oil and turns it into a nest of free radicals just waiting to do damage to your cells. To remove oil's natural flavor and aroma, chemical solvents must be used, and these solvents aren't especially good for you either.

For example, canola oil—which has been sold to us as a healthy choice—is quite a dangerous substance. First, it's a made-up food. Despite the pictures of pretty fields on the label, there is no canola plant found in nature. "Canola" stands for "Canadian oil low acid," because it was originally developed in Canada and the word "canola" sounded good for marketing at the time.

Although canola oil does come initially from nature—from a plant called rapeseed—we can't actually digest it in its natural form. For years, we used rapeseed only for industrial purposes, until someone got the bright idea of processing it at high heat with *hexane,* a harsh chemical solvent. As a result, the fats in the rapeseed are oxidized, become rancid, and create inflammation. Inflammation, as we have seen, is at the bottom of just about every chronic disease, as well as every symptom that we associate with aging: weight gain, suppressed immune function, and all the aches, pains, fatigue, and brain fog that make you feel so old.

Bottom line: this oil is not recognized in the body as food, and it's questionable whether it's even remotely fit for human consumption. And what is true for canola oil goes for all the other industrial oils too, especially soy oil, which has also deceptively been sold to us as a health food. (See Chapter 3.)

By contrast, extra-virgin olive oil is cold pressed, so it isn't exposed to high heats and chemical solvents. It is often sold in dark bottles, so it has less exposure to light. Even though it, too, contains a lot of polyunsaturated fat, it is a very healthy choice, as are the more stable saturated fats, as long as you don't cook with it at high temperatures. Save the olive oil for salad dressings, sauces, and light sautéeing, and use coconut oil or avocado oil for high-temperature cooking.

Making Friends with Fat: The Bottom Line

I've thrown a lot of information at you, but here's the main thing I want you to remember:

Every cell in your body depends upon healthy fat.

Cell membranes are made from fat, which means that if you don't eat enough healthy fat, your cells don't have strong, healthy membranes. They become vulnerable to any invader—any virus, bacteria, or toxin that you happen to encounter. They also become vulnerable to cancer, which threatens the integrity of healthy cells.

If you consume a lot of unhealthy fat—particularly trans fats and industrial oils—you weaken the integrity of your cell membranes. It's like building a house on a foundation of substandard concrete. The house might be tall and beautiful—but the foundation is shaky, and at the first storm, flood, or other challenge, the whole house might totter and, eventually, collapse.

Give your cells the support they need, and build your house on a strong foundation! Eat a lot of healthy fat, avoid the unhealthy fats, and enjoy a healthy life at a healthy weight.

The Skinny on Fats

- Try to keep your ratio of omega-3 and omega-6 fats as close to 1:1 as possible.

- Keep your home free of industrial oils and canola, and stay away from restaurant foods that have been fried. Focused on grilled, baked, or broiled instead.

- For cooking, choose coconut oil or avocado oil, because they can withstand higher heat.

- For cooking at low temperatures (sautés, stir-fries), use extra-virgin olive oil; for dressings and sauces, use extra-virgin olive oil, walnut oil, or flaxseed oil.

- Coat your vegetables with a healthy fat—olive oil, grass-fed butter, or ghee—to get the benefit of the vitamins they contain.

Transforming Your Diet, Your Appetite, and Your Weight

When Madeleine started her 2-Week Revitalize Program, she was somewhat anxious about what it would be like to go for 14 days without sugar, baked goods, pasta, and some other foods she was used to. "I'm afraid I'll just be hungry all the time," she told me. "And I've already told you I don't have any willpower."

"Madeleine," I said, "I know that getting started isn't necessarily going to be easy, and you might have a few rough days at the beginning because you'll be going through sugar withdrawal, which can sometimes be a painful experience. But it *will* get better—and you *can* do it."

When Madeleine came into my office two weeks later, she was exhilarated.

"I won't lie to you, Dr. Lipman—the first three days were pretty awful," she said. "I had a headache one day and felt kind of shaky and out of it the other two. But then I started to feel better—and *then* I started to feel *great!* I wasn't hungry all the time—I was hungry around mealtimes, just like a normal person instead of a ravening maniac. I didn't care if I had sugar or not. I actually felt good about mealtimes instead of like they were this big trap or this awful test. And look!—I lost 5 kilos!"

Madeleine's experience on the Revitalize Program is typical of what my patients experience. Although some sail through the first few days with no problem and others struggle a bit, by the end of the two weeks, just about everyone describes feeling liberated, energized, and lighter. This lightness isn't just a matter of the scale. Feeling free—perhaps for the first time in years—of cravings and an outsized appetite is a huge relief to many patients. Feeling energized yet also calm is an exciting experience for many others.

Amber was also delighted with her experience on the Revitalize Program. Like Madeleine, she had a few bad days at first, but was quickly rewarded with weight loss, blazing energy, improved sleep, and clear, glowing skin. "Yeah, I hated giving up chips and salsa," she told me. "And I still miss Diet Coke. But this is *so* worth it—it's not even close."

I'd like to take you through the next nine chapters so you can really understand what the Revitalize Program is all about and why it works so well. But if you're looking for three quick fixes to get you started right away, you'll find them at the end of the chapter. And in Chapter 2, you'll learn more about how even carbs that *seem* healthy might be making you feel old and fat.

You're Not Eating the Right Foods: Three Quick Fixes

1. Cut out addictive foods: all those that contain processed sugar.

2. Cut back on starchy foods: potatoes of all types, including sweet potatoes; rice, including brown and wild rice; corn; pasta, including whole-wheat pasta; bread, including whole-grain bread; baked goods of all types; and any soups, sauces, or gravies that are thickened with wheat flour or corn starch.

3. Eat lots of healthy fat.

REASON #2:

YOU'RE EATING TOO MANY CARBS AND STARCHES

My patient Ricardo was frustrated.

A successful software executive with a high-pressure job, Ricardo was used to being in control of his environment, his work life, and himself. He stuck to what he considered a healthy diet, and he expected his weight to remain healthy too.

Yet when he came to me in his mid-40s, Ricardo had noticed a disturbing tendency to put on weight. He was also concerned about the bouts of fatigue that typically hit him at about three or four o'clock each afternoon and about the light-headed feeling he got when he was hungry.

"If I don't have a couple of lattes, I'm falling asleep at my desk," he told me. "But if I do have them, I can't fall asleep till two or three A.M. and I'm wiped out the whole next day."

Ricardo told me that he was ravenous with hunger several times during the day. Although he was eating substantial, healthy meals, he found that he was often starving soon after each one.

I have found all of these symptoms—the weight gain, fatigue, and ravenous appetite—to be typical of patients who consume too many sweets or "white" foods. But when I questioned Ricardo about his diet, he proudly informed me that he ate the healthiest possible diet, cooking for himself and even bringing food to work from home. In fact, he told me, he was a "pescatarian" who basically ate only fish, whole grains, beans, fresh fruits, and vegetables.

I asked Ricardo to tell me what he normally ate. He said he started the day with steel-cut oatmeal or homemade unsweetened granola loaded with bananas and perhaps with a side of fruit "because I know I need the fuel to get me through the day!" For lunch, he had a salad with lentils or rice and beans. His afternoon snack was an apple, occasionally with some peanut butter. Dinner was a stir-fry of brown rice, tofu, and veggies or maybe some fish, a sweet potato, and greens, followed by a fruit salad or some melon.

"I never eat dessert," Ricardo told me proudly. "I don't even want it. Only fruit."

Another piece of the puzzle showed up in Ricardo's hemoglobin A1c test, which is a blood test showing the average level of blood sugars over the previous three months. According to this test, Ricardo's blood sugars were high—just on the verge of indicating diabetes. This reading, along with his weight gain, the light-headed feeling he got when was hungry, and fatigue, all added up to tell the same story.

"Ricardo," I said to him, "I believe you are suffering from a very common problem that so many of us have yet almost nobody knows about. I call it *carbohydrate intolerance.*"

Myths to Break Through

- "Whole grains and high-fiber carbs are healthy for everyone."
- "Eating a few servings of fruit a day is healthy for everyone."

⊸—— WHAT IS A CARBOHYDRATE? ——⊸

When you hear the word "carbohydrate," you might think "bread" or "grains," but in fact, carbohydrates are also the main ingredient in vegetables, fruits, and dried pulses (beans and peas), as well as grains and sweeteners.

Basically, if it's not animal protein (meat, poultry, fish, eggs) or fat (nuts, seeds, olives), it's a carb.

Carbohydrates that still contain their natural fiber—whole grains, beans, and raw or lightly cooked fruits and vegetables—are known as *complex* carbohydrates. The "complex" refers to the fiber.

If a food has been refined—such as white flour or any type of sugar or syrup—it's known as a *simple* carbohydrate. When you consume these foods, they break down very quickly into glucose because there's no fiber to slow the process. White potatoes are also simple carbs, although when eaten with their skins, they contain somewhat more fiber.

Drying, cooking, or juicing fruit destroys or removes a lot of the fiber and concentrates the glucose and fructose. So while fresh fruits are complex carbs, "processed" fruits are much closer to simple carbs.

Do You Know What a Carb Is?

- Grains, and everything made with grains: baked goods, pancakes, cereals, pastas.

- Beans of all types. Beans contain both protein and carbs.

- Dairy products. Dairy products contain a combination of protein, fat, and sugars. Low-fat and no-fat dairy contains less fat but consequently more carbs.

- Vegetables of all types, including lettuce and leafy green vegetables.

- Fruits.

- Virtually all types of sugar and sweetener, including the ones listed on page 6 and high-fructose corn syrup. However, a non-calorie sweetener is *not* a carb.

Myth: "Whole grains and high-fiber carbs are healthy for everyone"

Sometimes I think that every time we break through a myth about diet, another myth springs up to take its place.

Many people are aware, for example, of the dangers of sugar and "white" foods. They know that sugars and starches are "simple carbohydrates," and that these are harder on your body than "complex carbohydrates"—the whole grains, dried pulses, vegetables, and fresh fruits that are generally considered part of a healthy diet.

But what very few people realize is that even complex carbs can be extremely challenging for many people, who need to avoid or limit them almost as much as they limit their sugar or starch intake.

Moreover, even if you *can* tolerate carbs, you might not be able to tolerate as many as you think. Each of us has our own metabolic set point for the amount of carbs—including grains, fruit, and starchy vegetables—we can healthily consume. Hit that set point and your body will function just fine. Exceed that set point and your function will be compromised. Over time, you're likely to develop *insulin resistance* and *leptin resistance* (see below), your body will become inflamed, you'll put on weight, you'll feel fatigued, and—just as if you were eating doughnuts and bagels instead of quinoa and yams—you'll be riding that blood sugar roller coaster.

To make matters even more complicated, your carbohydrate set point isn't fixed either. Exercise more and you might be able to tolerate more carbs. Experience more stress and your tolerance might go down. And as we get older, most of us become more carbohydrate intolerant.

As we have seen, your body is a dynamic, ever-changing ecosystem that is always striving to find its balance. Depending on stress, mind-set, sleep, exercise, toxic exposure, and the rest of your diet, your ability to tolerate carbs might vary from day to day, or even from hour to hour.[1]

Myth: "Eating a few servings of fruit a day is healthy for everyone"

Just as not everyone can easily consume a lot of grains or sweet potatoes, many of us can have trouble with too much fruit. Fruit contains both fructose and glucose—two types of natural sugars—which puts some people on the blood sugar roller coaster.

As with other types of carbs, this is more of a spectrum than a hard-and-fast rule. Some people never have trouble with fruit. Some people always do. Some of us had no trouble in our youth but begin to notice problems as we get older. Or our ability to tolerate fruit might depend on a host of other factors: sleep, stress levels, amount of exercise, and the rest of our diet.

One of my goals with this book is to help you become more aware of your own individual body—how you respond to different foods, what you need, what works for you and what doesn't. Becoming aware of how fruit affects you is one part of your journey away from "old and fat" and toward "feeling young and slim."

⬥—— My Own Carbohydrate Journey ——⬥

I know this problem very well because I recently discovered that I myself am carbohydrate intolerant. Although I wasn't a pescatarian—I often enjoyed grass-fed beef or organic free-range chicken—I did eat a lot of whole grains and beans, and a good amount of fruit. Like Ricardo, I was surprised to find out that there was anything wrong with what I considered a very healthy diet and a decent level of exercise.

Yet in my late 50s, I began mysteriously putting on weight, struggling with late-afternoon fatigue, and generally feeling out of sorts. When I reviewed my own labs, I found that my blood sugar levels were creeping up toward the prediabetic range even though I didn't eat much sugar, sweets, or "white" foods. It just didn't make any sense.

Eventually I realized that the so-called healthy carbs I was consuming were at the root of the problem. I simply couldn't tolerate the brown rice, quinoa, beans, sweet potatoes, gluten-free oatmeal, and all the fruit that had been my mainstays. An occasional dish of fresh berries was okay, but my mid-morning apple and my watermelon or fruit salad dessert were not. My system just couldn't handle all the sugar.

My wife, Janice, is much better able to handle complex carbs than I am. So she continued to consume whole grains, black beans, garbanzos, and fresh fruit while I cut back. Sure enough, within two months, I had lost all the excess weight, regained my usual blazing energy, and achieved healthy blood sugar levels. Meanwhile, Janice was eating foods that I could not tolerate—and enjoying her own glowing health, healthy weight, and stable blood sugar.

The moral of the story is that we are each individuals, each with our own unique—and ever-changing—tolerance for carbs. Since my own experience, I've frequently seen that my young or active patients who exercise regularly are more likely to be able to tolerate carbs.

With age, however, your challenges begin. And even in your 30s and 40s, too much stress, too little exercise, and not enough sleep can set off a bout of carb intolerance that produces weight gain, fatigue, and excessive appetite, along with a host of other inflammatory symptoms: aches and pains, skin eruptions, hormonal issues, and digestive problems.

I told you at the beginning of this book that age doesn't have to doom you to poor health, and I meant every word. Age might mean that you have to make some adjustments, however, in order to remain healthy. For me—and, as it happened, for Ricardo—cutting back the carbs was one of those adjustments.

From Too Many Carbs to Just Enough

Ricardo's Old Breakfast	Ricardo's New Breakfast
Oatmeal or granola Bananas and other fruit	Eggs or a protein smoothie with at most a few berries Except for the berries, no fruit in the morning—too much sweetness to start the day!
Ricardo's Old Lunch	**Ricardo's New Lunch**
Rice and beans	Wild Salmon
Salad and lentils	Vegetables or salad
Ricardo's Old Snack	**Ricardo's New Snack**
Apple and peanut butter	Celery sticks and almond butter
Ricardo's Old Dinner	**Ricardo's New Dinner**
Stir-fry with brown rice & tofu	Steamed veggies and fish
Ricardo's Old Dessert	**Ricardo's New Dessert**
Melon, mangoes, or pineapple	Fresh berries of any type

When Your Insulin Goes Out of Balance

So what exactly happens when you consume more carbs than your system can handle, whether your carbs take the form of cookies, bagels, beans, sweet potatoes, fruit, or quinoa?

Well, as we saw in Chapter 1, carbohydrates of all types are broken down by your body into glucose. This glucose enters your bloodstream, where it triggers your pancreas to release insulin.

In ideal conditions, the glucose enters your bloodstream slowly and gradually, and your pancreas releases exactly the right amount of insulin needed to move your glucose efficiently into your cells.

When you eat sweets and starches, the glucose is likely to enter your bloodstream too quickly, setting off a blood sugar spike. This spike triggers an excess of insulin, which in turn produces a blood sugar crash.

When you eat high-fiber carbs, the extra fiber slows the process down, and you're less likely to get the spike and crash. But if you're eating more carbs than your system can handle, you are still likely to provoke more insulin than is healthy. If your system is flooded with too much insulin—either because you are eating carbs too often or because you are eating too many of them—you could develop a condition known as *insulin resistance.*

Insulin resistance occurs because your cells are already full of all the glucose they can handle—and yet, thanks to all those carbs you ate, there is still quite a lot of glucose in your bloodstream. Where can it go?

At this point, your body becomes a bit frantic. It doesn't understand why the glucose isn't moving properly into the cells. So your continued high level of blood glucose triggers your pancreas to release more insulin.

If your cells are *still* full of glucose, however, the second wave of insulin won't help—so perhaps your pancreas releases a third wave of insulin, or even a fourth or fifth. Because you've loaded up your system with more glucose than your body can handle, your insulin response goes way out of balance.

If this just happened once in a while—say, after the occasional large holiday meal—it would probably be no big deal. Eventually, your blood glucose and insulin would balance out and everything would go back to normal. But if it's a chronic problem—if, like me or Ricardo, you are consistently consuming more carbs than your body can handle—you end up with chronically high levels of insulin.

This is the point where insulin resistance kicks in. It's as though the insulin in your bloodstream were knocking at your cells' door. The cells don't want to open up because they're already full of glucose and they can't take in any more. But the insulin doesn't get it, so it keeps knocking, louder and louder. Eventually, the cells stop listening. (What literally happens is that your cell shuts down some of its insulin receptors to resist all that excess insulin in your bloodstream.)

Now you've got a bloodstream full of both glucose and insulin, which drives your pancreas absolutely wild. It keeps producing more and more insulin—making your cells more and more resistant. If the situation continues long enough, your pancreas could go from producing *too much* insulin to producing *not enough* insulin—and now you've got adult-onset diabetes.

Meanwhile, all that excess insulin is causing havoc in your body. First, the insulin itself cues your body to store fat. Second, excess insulin is probably the single most important factor that leads to premature aging. Third, it's causing inflammation, which leads to obesity and a host of other symptoms, including acne, digestive issues, immune problems, hormonal imbalance, brain fog, memory problems, and sleep difficulties.[2] Finally, it's stimulating a stress hormone called *cortisol,* which also produces inflammation and cues your body to store fat.

As you can see, insulin resistance is one of the surest recipes for getting old and fat. Transforming unhealthy insulin resistance into healthy *insulin sensitivity* is your recipe for staying vital and slim. One of the key goals of my 2-Week Revitalize Program is to help you start regaining your insulin sensitivity, which is one of the main reasons why I have you cut out all grains and many dried pulses and fruits during that 14 days. Once you've given your insulin response a chance to reset, you can figure out what level of carb intake is right for you.

Another approach to insulin resistance is a practice known as *intermittent fasting,* in which you eat all three meals within a limited time frame, say, between 11 A.M. and 7 P.M., for 8 hours of eating and 16 hours of fasting. It is best to do this three or four times a week rather than every day. For more on intermittent fasting, visit www.bewell.com/blog/intermittent-fasting/.

When Your Leptin Goes Out of Balance

Insulin isn't the only hormone to go out of balance when you consume more carbs than your system can handle. A hormone called *leptin,* which regulates your feelings of fullness, is also disrupted.

You've already seen in Chapter 1 how artificial sweeteners can throw your leptin out of balance. Too many carbs can also imbalance your leptin, with problematic effects on your hunger, your metabolism, and your weight.

Leptin is a great example of how your body is always seeking balance. When your levels of body fat are low, your leptin levels are also low, meaning that it takes longer for you to feel full; that is, you end up eating more. When your levels of body fat are high, so are your leptin levels—so, in theory, you feel full sooner and eat less.

However, when your leptin levels are too high for too long, you develop *leptin resistance.* Like insulin resistance, leptin resistance represents a major disruption in your metabolism. Because of the high amounts of leptin circulating in your bloodstream, some of the leptin receptors in your cells shut down.

Now you've entered a vicious cycle: the more leptin in your bloodstream, the less receptive your cells become . . . but the less receptive your cells become, the more leptin your body produces. Again, that leptin is knocking frantically on the door—and when your cells won't open the door, the leptin just keeps knocking, louder and louder and louder.

This is why knowing your ideal level of carbohydrates is so important. Eating too many carbs for your personal metabolism—even if you haven't consumed many calories—disrupts both insulin and leptin sensitivity, cuing your body to gain weight (from the excess insulin) and to remain perpetually hungry (from the leptin resistance).

Another cause of leptin resistance is high *triglycerides,* a type of blood fat. Too many sweets and starches—and perhaps too many complex carbs and fruits as well—raise your triglyceride levels. So do trans fats.

This is why processed foods, sweets, and starches are so disastrous for your weight, even if you're restricting your calories. The biochemistry of these foods triggers a series of responses that end in weight gain, inflammation, and a ravenous appetite, making it nearly impossible for you to lose weight.

Your first step in overcoming leptin resistance is to cut out sugar, sweeteners, and refined carbs. Your second step, however, might well be to avoid or at least to cut back on grains, dried pulses, starchy vegetables, and fruit.

By the way, another factor contributing to leptin resistance is insufficient sleep. We'll talk more about sleep when we get to Chapter 7, but this is a good reminder to take off the weight by spending more time in bed!

Working the Spectrum

Remember: we each have our own set point. When it comes to carb consumption, we must avoid thinking in terms of black and white and instead think of a spectrum. Some of us, like me, can barely tolerate any grains or fruit at all. I have some patients (mostly young and very active) who tolerate them well. Many of us fall somewhere in between. And depending on our genetics and life circumstances—how much sleep and exercise we get, how stressed we are, and what else we've been eating—our tolerance might vary from week to week, from day to day, or even from hour to hour.

To some extent, this is a matter of genetics, and it's a great example of how epigenetics can work. Ricardo and I were probably both born with a genetic predisposition to carbohydrate intolerance. My wife, Janice, almost certainly was not. So she has a greater tolerance for grains, dried pulses, and fruit, whereas Ricardo and I have to be more careful. Neither of us is doomed, however. We simply have to be aware of what our bodies are telling us, and modify our diets accordingly.

I have seen this issue with fruit as well. I personally have a lot of trouble metabolizing the sugars in fruit, so I have to watch my fruit intake. A daily dish of berries is fine, but more than that and I get into trouble. Janice, by contrast, has no trouble whatsoever; she often eats two or more fruits a day and still maintains a healthy weight and healthy levels of blood sugar.

Moreover, my relationship with carbs and fruit varies from week to week, depending on how hard I'm working, how stressed I feel, and how often I've made time to go to the gym or otherwise exercise. When I'm in a more vulnerable place, I make sure to avoid fruit, grains, and dried pulses. When I'm stronger and functioning more optimally, I can indulge a bit more. Through awareness coupled with trial and error, I've learned how to manage my own personal spectrum.

When Ricardo learned to work *his* spectrum, his health problems disappeared, along with his excess weight. During the 2-Week Revitalize Program, Ricardo cut out grains, dried pulses, and most fruits. He felt so much better that he decided to stay low-carb for the next few months. His energy came flooding back, his weight melted away, and his appetite returned to normal.

About six months after he began the program, Ricardo went on vacation with his family. He found himself adding some quinoa or lentils to his noon meal, though he still started the day with a breakfast that focused on proteins and healthy fats rather than oatmeal, granola, or other grains.

"If I start the day with a grain, I crave sugar all day," he told me on his last visit. "But when I'm relaxed and getting plenty of sleep, I can tolerate some more carbs during the day. If I have them at dinner, though, they seem to rev me up. I get really hungry just before bed, and then I can't sleep. And if I'm stressed out at work, I can't handle grains or lentils at any time, even at noon."

Ricardo had really learned how to listen to his body, fine-tuning his carb intake based on what his body was telling him. I was proud of him for taking charge of his health in this pro-active way—and he felt empowered, confident, and strong. Working the spectrum had worked for Ricardo.

Are You Eating More Carbs than Your Body Can Handle?

Learning what your body needs can be challenging at first, but with practice, you'll soon become your own best expert on how best to nourish yourself. These questions can help you get started:

- Do you gain weight easily when your diet includes a lot of "healthy" carbs: whole grains, dried pulses, and fresh fruit?

- Do you feel tired shortly after consuming carbohydrates?

- Do you feel foggy-headed after meals?

- Do you frequently crave sweets?

- Do you frequently crave starchy foods?

- Do you have a difficult time controlling how much sugar or carbs you eat?

- Does your weight fluctuate easily?

- Do you have dramatic energy ups and downs throughout the day?

- Do you feel light-headed or irritable when you're hungry?

- Do you tend to gain weight in your face and around your abdomen more than on your hips and thighs?

• Do you turn to sweets or carbs when you're feeling anxious, tired, or depressed?

If you answered yes to three or more of these questions, you might be eating more carbs than your system can handle. Your first line of defense is to cut out the sweet and starchy "white" and refined foods. If you've already done that, try cutting back or avoiding altogether all grains, including whole grains, dried pulses, and fresh fruit, although a small amount of berries each day might be okay.

You might need to experiment a bit to find the right amount of carbs for you, and to find out how your life circumstances affect your ability to tolerate carbs. Stress, sleep, exercise, and other factors can all affect your tolerance.[3] Maybe you can enjoy oatmeal and bananas for a relaxed Sunday brunch but have to cut them out on a high-stress workday. Maybe you can manage sweet potatoes for dinner on a day when you've had good sleep but have to stick to or sub in broccoli or cauliflower after a night of dealing with a colicky baby.

Some people find it simpler—or perhaps necessary—to cut out high-carb foods altogether. Others learn how to read their own bodies and adjust their carb intake accordingly. After two weeks on my Revitalize Program, you'll be able to make your own healthy choices around high-carb foods.

You're Eating Too Many Carbs and Starches: Three Quick Fixes

1. **Start fresh.** Cut out all sugars and grains for two weeks, including brown rice, corn, oats, and even quinoa. Let your grain-free experience help guide you toward finding the right carb level for you.

2. **Eat more green leafy vegetables and healthy fats.** These foods will fill you up while providing you with vital nutrients. You'll have a better chance of finding your healthiest level of grains if you're also getting enough other types of food.

3. **Exercise.** You might be able to tolerate more carbs if you give your body the vigorous movement that it craves. A sedentary life and a high-grain diet burden your body with the worst of both worlds.

REASON #3:

YOUR MICROBIOME
IS OUT OF WHACK

When I first met Laila, a bubbly social worker in her mid-30s, I was immediately struck by her enthusiastic attitude and her warm, open smile. Yet as we talked about her medical history, I could see that she was struggling not to give in to a growing sense of confusion and discouragement.

"I've always been healthy," she told me earnestly. "But this past year, so many things have gone wrong. I've had terrible gas and bloating—so bad that it keeps me up at night! I've started to get these weird breakouts on my face and chest. My monthly cycle has gone way out of sync—and I've always been so regular! I get cramps too, which I never got before. Worst of all, I've picked up an extra 7 kilos, which is just unreal. I can't figure out what's happening to me."

Laila was one of many young people I've seen with increasing frequency over the past ten years, coming in with complaints that I used to hear only from folks in their 40s, 50s, and beyond. Like my patient Andi, whom you met in the Introduction, Laila was feeling old and fat before her time.

I looked again at Laila's medical history and noticed that in the past year she had had three courses of antibiotics to get rid of a chronic sinus infection (sinusitis). Then, after the antibiotics, she developed acid reflux, so her doctor prescribed a proton pump inhibitor.

"Oh, yeah, all of that was such a hassle—but I'm all right now," she told me when I asked her about it. But now I knew I had found the answer to the mystery.

"Antibiotics are one of the great discoveries of modern medicine," I replied, "and I'm grateful that we have access to them. But they can also be one of the biggest disrupters of our health—and perhaps even one of the major factors behind the obesity epidemic."

"Antibiotics? Why?" Laila asked.

"We use antibiotics to kill dangerous bacteria," I explained, "and they often do that job very well. The problem is, they also kill *friendly* bacteria—they basically devastate your *microbiome*. And since you depend on your microbiome for good health, good gut function, and a healthy weight, throwing it out of balance has terrible consequences for your entire ecosystem."

"So the medicine that was supposed to make me better made me sicker?" Laila asked.

"Not only the antibiotics," I told her. "When they disrupted your digestion, you developed acid reflux, so you were prescribed Nexium, a proton pump inhibitor—called PPI for short. PPIs are also bad for your microbiome. Between that and the antibiotics, your microbiome got a double whammy!"

I was eager for Laila to understand just what had happened because the microbiome is such a crucial aspect of our health, vitality, and well-being, as well as being a major factor in our ability to maintain a healthy weight. Most of my patients have never even heard of the microbiome and have barely any idea of the importance of gut bacteria. Yet the state of your microbiome is probably the single most important factor in whether you are feeling old, fat, unfocused, and sad or young, slim, sharp, and optimistic.

If you don't like the idea of getting old and fat, balance your microbiome!

Myths to Break Through

- "Bacteria are my enemies."

- "If I don't have celiac disease, I can safely eat foods with gluten—foods made from wheat, rye, barley, and some other grains."

- "If I don't have any food allergies, all foods are safe for me to eat, including dairy products and corn."

- "Soy is a health food."

Myth: "Bacteria are my enemies"

Sometimes it seems that every advance in medical science is balanced by a downside. When 19th-century scientists discovered that many diseases were caused by bacteria, or germs, this represented a huge step forward in Western medicine. Rather than believing that illness was caused by a "miasma"—a hovering cloud of unhealthy air—doctors began to understand that many disorders were triggered by unfriendly bacteria. Identifying the true causes of such diseases as tuberculosis, cholera, and typhoid eventually enabled scientists to find cures for illnesses that had once devastated whole communities.

The downside, though, was that we began to view all bacteria as our enemies. When antibiotics were discovered, their ability to destroy dangerous bacteria seemed like a miracle.

Unfortunately, along with the dangerous bacteria, antibiotics also kill off the friendly bacteria upon which we depend. Killing off these helpful bacteria has terrible consequences for our health and our weight, as well as for our memory, mental focus, mood, and energy.

How is this possible? The key lies in understanding the importance of your microbiome.

Antibiotics: A Double-Edged Sword

If your doctor prescribes antibiotics for you, confirm that they are absolutely necessary for your health. Sometimes there are other alternatives that your doctor may be willing to consider. In Laila's case, antibiotics probably weren't needed, as most cases of sinusitis can be treated without them. If antibiotics *are* the correct medical treatment for you, be sure to follow my protocol for protecting your microbiome on pages 41–42.

◆—— WHAT IS THE MICROBIOME? ——◆

The microbiome is the community of bacteria that lives within every one of us. Each of us contains a whole inner ecosystem composed of trillions of microbes. These bacteria outnumber our human cells by a factor of 10 to 1. Their genes outnumber our human genes by a factor of 150 to 1. It's no exaggeration to say that each of us is actually more bacteria than human!

We begin developing our microbiome in the womb, as our mothers pass on bacteria to us during pregnancy. As we pass through the birth canal, we acquire still more bacteria. Breastfeeding provides us with still more. (That's one reason why bottle-fed babies are at somewhat of a disadvantage.)

As we grow, we continue to acquire more bacteria—from our food and water, but also from our environment and from the people with whom we come in contact. These bacteria can be friendly, unfriendly, or a mix of the two. In a healthy body, you have mainly friendly bacteria.

The microbial community within our bodies is absolutely crucial in maintaining optimal function—or indeed, in maintaining function at all. Every human and animal on this planet has a microbiome, with the odd exception of experimental lab animals deliberately raised in artificially sterile environments. Without their microbiomes, these animals do not develop or function normally. And without a healthy microbiome, *you* can't achieve optimal function either.

The bacteria in your microbiome are your crucial partners in digesting your food, supporting your immune system, protecting your gut, and maintaining a healthy weight. Certain components of these micro-organisms even trigger anti-inflammatory responses, whereas others promote inflammation.

As a result, having a balanced microbiome is your best weapon against inflammation—and your best means of preventing all the symptoms that inflammation can produce. As you'll recall from previous chapters, inflammation is the chief reason you feel old and fat, since it produces weight gain, aching joints, loss of energy, brain fog, memory loss, and a host of other problems that we tend to associate with age but are really caused by inflammation. Inflammation is also the main culprit behind such chronic diseases as diabetes, heart disease, Alzheimer's, autoimmune disorders, and even cancer.

Healing inflammation is the secret to staying young and slim.
And balancing your microbiome is the key to healing inflammation.

When your microbiome is balanced, most other things in your body go right. But when you eat the wrong kinds of food, are exposed to a lot of toxins, skimp on sleep, undergo a lot of stress, or take too many medications—particularly antibiotics and PPIs—you throw your microbiome out of balance. As a result, many other things go wrong as well, including problems with digestion, immune function, hormones, and your ability to process thought and emotion.

What throws your microbiome out of balance? You probably won't be surprised to learn that it's the usual suspects.

Factors That Throw Your Microbiome Out of Balance

- Sweets

- Starches

- Unhealthy fats: trans fats, industrial oils

- Artificial sweeteners

- Toxins

- Stress

- Lack of sleep

- Antibiotics

- Many common medications, including antidepressants, antianxiety medications, antacids, proton pump inhibitors, and pain medications

- Genetically modified organisms found in such GM crops as corn, soy, papaya, sugar beetroot, as well as some of the plants used to make industrial oils, including canola (rapeseed) and cotton

---

✧── WHY IS MY MICROBIOME ──✧ IMPORTANT TO MY HEALTH?

When I explained the importance of the microbiome to Laila, she was shocked to learn that this microscopic community could play such a vital role in her health and well-being, including her weight, her mental state, and her mood. Many of my patients have the same reaction.

If you, too, are wondering how these invisible creatures can affect you so deeply, consider that our bodies did not evolve independently. Rather, we *co*-evolved with the bacteria that were on this planet long before we got here. As a result of this joint evolution, there are many functions that we cannot perform on our own. Even our ape ancestors depended on the microbiome, and we humans certainly do. From our very first moments as *Homo sapiens,* our bodies have relied upon its community of bacteria not just to remain healthy, but to survive.

Consider one of the microbiome's primary tasks: enabling us to digest our food and metabolize nutrients. Isn't it remarkable to think that without the trillions of bacteria that live within us, we couldn't absorb the nutrients we consume? And that when that bacterial community is out of balance, we don't absorb *enough* nutrients?

Another key job of our microbiome is to maintain a healthy gut by nourishing the cells of the gut wall. This wall is only one cell thick and most of your immune system is just on the other side of it. So it, too, relies upon the microbiome to function at its peak. When your microbiome is out of balance, your immune system struggles and you're likely to suffer from frequent colds, allergies, joint pains, acne, and, potentially, more serious disorders.

We need the microbiome to keep our gut healthy because the gut is so vital to our overall health. Besides its role in digestion, it also helps us process thought and emotion—so much so that it is often referred to as "the second brain." To take just one example, 70 percent of your *serotonin*—a feel-good chemical that promotes emotional well-being, self-confidence, and good sleep—is made in the gut.

When your microbiome is in good shape, chances are your gut is too—and your serotonin and other neurochemical levels are more likely to be optimal. As a result, you feel calm, balanced, optimistic, and confident and you are likely to sleep well.

But when your microbiome is out of balance, your gut suffers. Your production of serotonin and other neurochemicals drops, leaving you vulnerable to depression, anxiety, self-doubt, and sleep problems. We think of these issues as "brain problems," but in fact, the biochemicals that govern them are more densely populated in the gut. So really, they could be "gut problems."

Every day, we are learning more about how the microbiome and the gut affect our emotions and our brain. In fact, while I was preparing this book, a new study revealed that the microbes within us literally evolved to affect our food choices! By releasing signaling molecules into our gut, the bacteria in our bodies can actually engineer our cravings.

One of the researchers, Athena Aktipis of Arizona State University Department of Psychology, explains: "Microbes have the capacity to manipulate behavior and mood through altering the neural signals in the vagus nerve, changing taste receptors, producing toxins to make us feel bad, and releasing chemical rewards to make us feel good."[1]

Gut bacteria have such a huge influence on our thoughts, feelings, and mood that some people even call them "mind-altering micro-organisms." Fortunately, through our own diet and lifestyle choices, we can choose which microbes will be manipulating us! Following my 2-Week Revitalize Program and my Maintenance Program thereafter will ensure that you populate your microbiome with friendly bacteria that keep you craving vegetables and other healthy choices, rather than unfriendly bacteria that will crave sugar and unhealthy fats.

Your Microbiome and Your Brain

Healthy Microbiome	Unhealthy Microbiome
Calmness	Anxiety
Optimism	Discouragement
Self-esteem	Self-doubt
Balance	Depression
Clear thinking	Brain fog
Sharp memory	Memory issues
Healthy sleep	Trouble falling or staying asleep
Craving vegetables and other healthy choices	Craving sweets, starches, and unhealthy fats

HOW DO ANTIBIOTICS AFFECT MY MICROBIOME?

Laila was fascinated to learn about this entire ecosystem that had been living inside her, but she still didn't understand why the antibiotics she had been given a year ago were still having such a destructive effect on her health.

"Antibiotics kill all bacteria—not just the unfriendly ones," I explained. "To treat your sinusitis, you were given antibiotics, but that devastated your microbial community. It's as though you sprayed a whole lake with poison trying to get rid of the mosquitos breeding in that lake. You probably would kill a lot of mosquitos—but you would also kill a lot of other creatures as well. The ecology of the whole lake might suffer, just as your inner ecology is suffering now."

In the developed world, antibiotics are prescribed with disturbing frequency. By the time your child has turned eighteen, he or she will likely have gotten 10 to 20 courses of antibiotics, setting the stage for the kinds of problems Laila was facing and perhaps cuing your child's body to develop an early pattern of obesity.

In fact, one of the most dramatic effects of antibiotics is weight gain. Even before we understood the science of *why* this was so, farmers knew that giving antibiotics to their livestock helped fatten them up. When we humans are given antibiotics, we tend to gain weight as well. In fact, a study published in November 2014 showed that even when a mother takes antibiotics during her pregnancy, her child is at greater risk of obesity.

As we saw in Chapter 1, conventionally farmed meat, chicken, and dairy products are all laden with antibiotics as well as hormones—which also disrupt your microbiome. And because antibiotics are such an integral part of factory farming, you might end up consuming quite a few of them even if you are never given them by your doctor. So, while we are fattening up our farm animals, we are fattening ourselves up as well, not to mention creating many other symptoms of aging and dysfunction.

Microbial damage from the antibiotics had probably also caused Laila to develop acid reflux—leading her doctor to prescribe her a PPI. That PPI then damaged her microbiome still further. Laila's situation was a classic example of the way that Western medicine tries to solve problems with medications . . . which cause further problems . . . which require still more medication. It's a truly vicious cycle that is a big part of why so many of us—even young people like Laila—are feeling old and getting fat.

So here's your takeaway:

Your microbiome helps protect your brain, your gut, and your metabolism.

When antibiotics or some other factor throws your microbiome out of balance, your brain and gut health suffer, your metabolism slows down, and your whole body becomes inflamed. This inflammation produces weight gain as well as many other symptoms, including the gas, bloating, reflux, acne, and hormonal issues that had brought Laila to my door.

How an Imbalanced Microbiome Makes You Feel Old and Fat

Brain: anxiety, depression, brain fog, sleep issues, memory problems
Digestive system: gas, bloating, indigestion, constipation, loose stools, heartburn
Hormones: menstrual and premenstrual issues, symptoms of perimenopause and menopause (hot flashes, skin problems, sleep difficulties, mood swings)

Immune system: frequent colds and flu; difficulty recovering from illness; allergies; acne; rosacea (a reddening of the skin); eczema (dry, flaky skin); psoriasis (scaly patches of skin); joint pain

Overall function: fatigue, muscle pain, weight gain

⟡ —— How Do GMOs Affect My Microbiome? —— ⟡

Another threat to your microbiome is genetically modified organisms (GMOs). I consider the genetic modification of our food one of the most disturbing developments of the past few decades, so let's take a closer look.

Genetic modification began with the giant corporation known as Monsanto, which had developed a weed-killing herbicide known as Roundup. The only problem was that Roundup tended to kill the crops as well as the weeds.

So Monsanto invented a genetically modified soy that was able to resist the herbicidal poison—the so-called "Roundup-ready" soybean. Farmers began to shower their crops with vast quantities of the Monsanto herbicides, with potentially disastrous consequences for the neighboring soil and water, as well as for any livestock or humans who might consume the soy.

Genetic modification developed quickly. As of this writing, a number of crops are grown almost exclusively in genetically modified form, including soy, corn, sugar beetroot, rapeseed (used in canola oil), and cotton (used in cottonseed oil).

I'd love to be able to tell you exactly what effect this has on our health, or on the health of the livestock we consume, but unfortunately, I don't know—nobody does. We've been genetically modifying food for such a relatively short time that we don't have a comprehensive picture of how it affects us.

However, a number of disturbing pieces of information have come to light. If they don't add up to a conclusive picture, they at least suggest the need for concern:

- Danish pigs, German cows, and other European livestock have suffered from various gut problems and digestive issues since the introduction of Roundup-ready soy. In some cases, the problems might be caused by the ways in which the soy itself damages the beneficial gut bacteria of the animals. In other cases, problems seem to result from the ways that Roundup, the herbicide used in conjunction with GMO crops, destroys beneficial bacteria while leaving intact the deadly bacteria that cause *E. coli* and botulism—which are reaching epidemic levels among European livestock.

- Some evidence suggests that Roundup and similar herbicides destroy beneficial microbes that live in the soil, affecting the soil's fertility and perhaps also affecting the nutrient content of plants grown in that soil.[2]

- In 2010, Monsanto registered glyphosate as an antibiotic, so when we eat these foods, we are consuming antibiotics.[3]

The study of GMOs—and of the microbiome itself—is in its infancy. Given that each of us contains trillions of bacteria and hundreds of trillions of microbial genes, trying to protect the health of the microbiome feels like a bit of a crapshoot. We simply don't know enough.

However, I made a few recommendations to Laila—concerning GMOs and much more— that I can make to you too.

Protect Your Microbiome

- Avoid GMOs whenever possible—we simply don't know enough. For a full listing of genetically modified foods, see www.nongmoproject.org/learn-more/what-is-gmo/.

- Avoid sweet and starchy foods.

- Avoid junk food and processed food, almost all of which contains trans fats, GMO corn, GMO soy, or industrial seed oils.

- Avoid gluten, a protein found in wheat, rye, barley, and some other grains, as well as in soy sauce, seitan, beer, and many packaged and processed foods. (For more about gluten, see page 44.)

- Avoid preservatives and artificial ingredients, which also disrupt your microbiome.

- Avoid conventionally farmed meat, poultry, dairy products, and eggs, which likely contain antibiotics and hormones, and which likely have been fed on genetically modified corn or soy.

- Whenever possible, avoid antibiotics or use herbal antibiotics, which seem to kill the unfriendly bacteria while leaving the friendly microbes alone.

- Avoid artificial sweeteners: they disrupt your microbiome.

- Add water filters to your home taps and drink filtered water whenever possible. We know that the chlorine in tap water kills microbes in soil, so it's only logical to think that the chlorine in unfiltered water will alter *your* bacterial balance.

- Take a daily *probiotic,* a capsule or powder containing friendly bacteria that can replenish your own microbiome. Taking a probiotic is especially important if you are taking antibiotics.

- Eat fermented foods—sauerkraut, kefir (fermented milk), kimchi (Korean fermented vegetables), or other fermented vegetables. Fermented foods contain natural bacteria that also protect your microbiome.

- Incorporate *prebiotics* into your diet: foods that contain the fiber on which friendly bacteria feed. Key prebiotics include tomatoes, garlic, onions, radishes, leeks, asparagus, and Jerusalem artichokes. Make sure to eat the stalks, not just the tips—the stalks are full of healthy prebiotics that your microbiome will love.

- Find effective ways to cope with stress (see Chapter 6).

- Get enough sleep (see Chapter 7).

◆——— How Does My Microbiome——◆ Affect My Gut Health?

A healthy, balanced microbiome is crucial for optimal function and vital health—but unfortunately, very few of us reach adulthood with our microbiome in good shape. Between antibiotics and other medications, junk food, GMOs, conventionally or factory farmed meats, and all the other assaults on our inner ecology, it's quite a challenge to keep our microbiome healthy!

All of the factors that impair our microbiome disrupt gut health as well, acting either directly on the gut or indirectly through the microbiome. We've come to think of digestive symptoms as normal—doesn't "everyone" have a bit of gas or bloating?—but in fact, these symptoms are the first signs of trouble in one of our most crucial systems.

When the microbiome goes out of balance, it releases toxins and other substances that trigger inflammation. This inflammation almost inevitably leads to a condition known as *leaky gut* or *increased intestinal permeability,* in which the cells of the gut lining—which is only one cell thick—begin to come apart. Instead of holding in all the partially digested food in our intestines, they allow some to leak through.

Along with this undigested food come any toxins we have ingested. When these toxins find their way into our bloodstream, they further disrupt function. Meanwhile, the imbalanced microbiome continues to release toxins of its own, as well as other substances that promote inflammation. That is how an imbalanced microbiome creates the symptoms that Laila experienced, and many others besides (see box on pages 39–40).

Leaky gut also means that we're not digesting our food properly, since a damaged gut wall cannot absorb all the nutrients from our food. This has further negative consequences for our health—and for our weight. As I told Laila, an imbalanced microbiome—which virtually all of us have—sets off a whole slew of processes that triggers inflammation, leading to all sorts of diseases and imbalances. That's why one of the most important things you can do for your health is to protect your microbiome (see pages 41–42).

◆—— Your Microbiome and Artificial Sweeteners ——◆

As I was completing this book, a startling new study emerged from Israel, where researchers found evidence that artificial sweeteners disrupt the microbiome—with disastrous results for blood sugar levels and the risk of diabetes.

The study, published in the prestigious *Nature* magazine, was conducted by Eran Elinav, Eran Segal, and their team at the Weizmann Institute of Science.[4]

The scientists began by feeding mice some common zero-calorie sweeteners, including saccharin, aspartame, and sucralose. In response, the mice developed glucose intolerance, a typical precursor to diabetes.

The researchers then used antibiotics to destroy the mice's intestinal bacteria—and saw the blood sugar readings return to normal. They even transferred fecal samples from the high–blood sugar mice into other mice—and within six days, the other mice developed glucose intolerance.

It seemed highly likely that the altered microbiome—in response to the artificial sweeteners—had pushed up the mice's blood sugar readings. Indeed, the glucose-intolerant mice showed high counts of a species of microbe known as *Bacteroides fragilis.*

The scientists followed up by analyzing the blood sugar readings of some 400 subjects who frequently consumed artificial sweeteners and discovered that indeed, they had elevated levels when compared to a control group.

Finally, they found seven volunteers who agreed to consume the equivalent of about ten sugar packets during a single week. Even this short-term exposure seemed to produce prediabetic blood sugar readings in four of the seven subjects.

The Israeli study is only a first step in the efforts to discover the effects of artificial sweeteners on the microbiome and on blood sugar. But as we saw in Chapter 2, artificial sweeteners are correlated with weight issues. Their effect on the microbiome might well be one of the primary reasons why.

◆—— Your Microbiome and Leaky Gut ——◆

An imbalanced microbiome gives you leaky gut, but if you get leaky gut in some other way, it will also give you an imbalanced microbiome. To see all the factors that might give you leaky gut, check out the list on pages 36–37. Yes, those are the factors that threaten your microbiome—and they are also the factors that threaten your gut. Basically, what is bad for your microbiome is bad for your gut, and vice versa.

So, you should assume that if you have a leaky gut, you also have an imbalanced microbiome; likewise, if you have an imbalanced microbiome, you almost certainly have developed a leaky gut. We need to heal them both at the same time, and my 2-Week Revitalize Program gets that process started, while my Maintenance Program keeps you on a healthy, gut-healing course.

◇——— HEAL YOUR GUT WITH BONE BROTH ———◇

One of the most effective ways to heal your gut is with a wonderful concoction known as "bone broth"—a nourishing broth made from the bones of poultry, fish, shellfish, beef, or lamb (of course, only pastured, organic, and grass-fed animals and wild-caught fish). A staple of the human diet for thousands of years, bone broth is full of gelatin and collagen, which soothe the intestinal tract and help heal leaky gut. Its rich array of nutrients (especially gelatin) supports your immune system. Bone broth is also full of *bioavailable* minerals—minerals that may be easier for us to absorb than those that come in other forms. Calcium, magnesium, potassium, silicon, sulfur, and phosphorous are all abundant in bone broth.

Bone broth is also a powerful anti-aging food. It's full of glucosamine, chondroitin, collagen, and gelatin, all of which support your joints and bones, as well as reducing inflammation throughout your body. And the amino acids it contains—glycine and proline—as well as the collagen (the ultimate skin food) can make your skin more elastic, which helps keep the wrinkles away.

You'll see that you can incorporate bone broth into your Revitalize and Maintenance meal plans, with some delicious recipes on pages 226–227.

Myth: "If I don't have celiac disease, I can safely eat foods with gluten—foods made from wheat, rye, barley, and some other grains."

One of the most common causes of both a leaky gut and an imbalanced microbiome is *gluten,* a protein found in wheat, rye, barley, and many other grains. Gluten is probably one of the most misunderstood health issues of our day, so let's break through the myths around that too.

You might have heard about gluten in connection with celiac disease, a painful, dangerous condition that damages the lining of the small intestine and prevents it from absorbing nutrients. Consuming gluten triggers a celiac reaction, which can provoke cramps, internal bleeding, and a host of digestive issues, not to mention fatigue, anemia, malnutrition, and wasting.

You only get this particular response to gluten if you are genetically prone to celiac, an autoimmune condition that currently affects only about 1 percent of the population. One of the key symptoms of celiac is weight loss—caused by the inability to absorb nutrients—so if you are normal weight and particularly if you are overweight, you are unlikely to have celiac.

However, just because you don't have celiac doesn't mean you can safely consume gluten. Far from it! According to the groundbreaking research of Dr. Alessio Fasano, gluten triggers the release of a substance called *zonulin,* which then causes the tight junctions holding your gut cell walls together to open slightly. If you consume enough gluten, or if you are sensitive enough to gluten, that space between your cell walls remains open—and now you have leaky gut.[5]

Part of the challenge with gluten is that at this point in our industrial food culture, it is *everywhere.* A surprising number of packaged and processed foods use gluten as a preservative—often hidden under some clever name, such as "natural flavoring"—so that it is often impossible to detect. Gluten is frequently added to such nonstarchy foods as ice creams, sorbets, and puddings, as well as to thicken soups, sauces, and gravies. We are so bombarded with gluten that many of us who might have been able to consume it under other circumstances have become overly sensitive to it and need to avoid it.

Now at this point you might be wondering how bread, the staff of life, can be the evil bane of your existence. After all, we have been eating bread for thousands of years!

The answer is that bread today is a far cry from the bread of our ancestors or even the bread from just 50 years ago.

According to Dr. William Davis, author of *Wheat Belly*, modern wheat has been hybridized and altered to increase yields. It is not really wheat anymore but the transformed product of industrial research. Although it looks and tastes the same as the bread we once knew, it is biochemically very different, and it is causing havoc with our health.

The new strains of wheat have been bred to have more gluten in them than previous types, because gluten is what makes foods light and fluffy. Industrial scientists have also figured out how to remove one of the key amino acids from wheat, to give the gluten it contains a longer shelf life. As a result, gluten is now widely used as a preservative, which means we're being exposed to it at a level that wasn't even imaginable 50 years ago. Moreover, today's gluten-bearing flour, pasta, bread, and baked goods are all highly addictive and designed to stimulate your appetite. And the gluten they contain is highly inflammatory.

Perhaps even more importantly, wheat and many other gluten-bearing grains now contain glyphosate, the toxic ingredient used in common herbicides. We are beginning to discover that glyphosate exposure is highly correlated with the rise in celiac disease. Moreover, glyphosate is a huge killer of healthy gut flora, creating the kind of microbial imbalance that produces inflammation and all of its attendant problems, including leaky gut. Maybe that's why glyphosate has also been seen to cause many chronic diseases of the gut.

In other words, we can't be sure if it's the actual gluten or the herbicide that's been added to it that is causing the problem. Either way, what you are being offered these days is not your grandmother's pasta or your mother's bread. It is a *Frankengrain!*

❖⸺ "I DON'T HAVE CELIAC —SO CAN I EAT GLUTEN?" ⸺❖

I'm often asked by my patients whether it's safe for them to consume any gluten at all, and you may be wondering the same thing. Is it possible to safely consume gluten if you don't have celiac?

If you have an autoimmune condition, my answer is an unequivocal *no.* Due to a phenomenon known as *molecular mimicry*, your immune system frequently mistakes gluten for your own cells. It develops antibodies to attack the gluten . . . and those antibodies trigger an attack on your own body tissue instead. Avoiding gluten minimizes the danger of autoimmune destruction.

If you are carbohydrate intolerant, I would also steer you away from gluten. In addition to the problems of zonulin and leaky gut, gluten-bearing grains are going to trigger all the problems we discussed in Chapter 2.

If you have any type of health issue, including excess weight, I'd advise against gluten as well. On my Revitalize Program, I want you to spend at least two weeks completely gluten free so you can really get all the health threats out of your system and feel what it's like to enjoy complete vitality and glowing health.

Having said all of that, although I don't recommend it, if you are in perfect health, at a healthy weight, and don't have an autoimmune condition, you *might* be able to occasionally tolerate small amounts of gluten—say, once or twice a week. However, it's possible that even in small amounts, gluten will leak through your gut—or cause other foods and toxins to do so—producing the same types of symptoms that result from a disrupted microbiome (see pages 39–40).

If you are otherwise healthy, and if it's important to you to eat gluten, you might give it a try while monitoring your body for signs of fatigue, indigestion, acne, hormonal upsets, or any other symptom. Be aware that your tolerance for gluten is, as with most health issues, on a spectrum, and that it might change depending on how balanced your microbiome is; your levels of stress, sleep, and exercise; the rest of your diet; and any other health challenges you might encounter. What you could tolerate today might not work for you tomorrow.

As you can see, I'd love to steer you away from this problematic food—but more importantly, I want you to have the tools to decide for yourself how it affects you and whether you can tolerate it in small doses. A good rule of thumb, however, whenever you are stressed or recovering from a physical or emotional challenge, is to protect your gut, support your immune system—and pass the gluten by.

Where Gluten Is Found

- Wheat, rye, barley, and many variations of wheat, including durum, graham, kamut, triticale, semolina, spelt, and oats, unless they are specifically labeled gluten free (see www.bewell.com/blog/gluten-FAQ-2 for more detail)

- Any product containing those grains: baked goods, fried foods, pastas, cereals

- Soy sauce (unless it's marked "gluten free")

- Many condiments, including ketchup—so check the labels

- Packaged, processed, and canned foods, including soups. "Natural flavoring" often indicates gluten.

- Seitan

- Beer (unless it's marked "gluten free")

Myth: "If I don't have any food allergies, all foods are safe for me to eat, including dairy products and corn"

When I explained the 2-Week Revitalize Program to Laila, I told her that for two weeks, she would be avoiding all grains (both gluten and gluten free, including corn), all dried pulses (including soy), and all dairy products.

Laila now understood why she would do well to avoid gluten, but she was surprised to hear she would have to avoid all grains, corn, soy, and dairy.

"I don't have any food allergies," she assured me. "When I started getting these weird breakouts, I got tested for allergies, and I was told I'm allergy free."

I explained to Laila that allergies are one type of immune system response, the result of aggressive antibodies known as *immunoglobulin E,* or IgE. If you are allergic to foods or other substances, these antibodies leap into action within a matter of minutes and you immediately see the inflammation—the pain, redness, heat, or swelling that your immune system has produced. Swelling of the airways is what produces the anaphylactic reaction—being unable to breathe—that makes a peanut allergy so deadly.

However, your immune system has a bigger tool kit than just the IgE antibodies. You're also equipped with immunoglobulin G (IgG) antibodies, which work much more slowly and less intensely. If you consume a food that provokes an IgG reaction—commonly referred to as *food sensitivity* or *food intolerance*—your symptoms might not show up for several days. Laila's acne breakouts, hormonal issues, and weight gain are typical food sensitivities caused by IgG reactions.

Because of the time lag, you can easily have difficulty relating the symptom to the offending food that triggered it. But once you are aware that food sensitivities exist, you come to see that the symptoms are often provoked by your immune system's response to a reactive food.

What's going on? Well, once you have leaky gut, partially digested food can leak between the cells of your gut wall and into your bloodstream, where it doesn't belong. This strange "invader" provokes your immune system to make antibodies designed to zap the intruder. As a result, you become reactive to that food in any form.

Your immune system responds with inflammation, a "killer" response that includes some collateral damage. Minor inflammation produces symptoms: digestive issues, acne, hormonal imbalances, frequent colds and flu, achy joints, brain fog, memory problems, sleep issues, anxiety, and depression. Chronic, sustained inflammation can lead to more serious disorders, including autoimmune conditions, heart disease, diabetes, and cancer. Inflammation also generally provokes weight gain.

So if you've developed leaky gut and you have, say, a dish of yogurt, some of the undigested yogurt might leak through your intestinal walls into your bloodstream. Your immune system goes on alert and creates an antibody so that it will recognize the intruder again and "zap" it with killer chemicals. Now every time you eat a food containing the milk protein found in yogurt, your immune system goes on alert. You develop symptoms, gain weight, and generally feel under par.

If you don't do anything to heal your leaky gut and rebalance your microbiome, you are setting yourself up for even more serious disorders down the line—and that's another reason why people confuse age with decreased function. The problem isn't that you've gotten older. It's that for years, your leaky gut has been allowing partially digested foods to escape into bloodstream, provoking your immune system and creating low-grade chronic inflammation. Sooner or later, your symptoms will get worse—but you can reverse the situation at any time by rebalancing your microbiome and healing your gut.

Certain foods seem to provoke the immune system more than others. Apart from gluten, the three most reactive foods tend to be dairy, corn, and soy.

Dairy products are highly inflammatory—cow's milk, cheese, and yogurt even more so than products from goats, sheep, or buffalo—so if you have leaky gut, dairy is possibly one of the foods that gives you trouble.

Both dairy and gluten also frequently provoke the phenomenon I touched on earlier known as *molecular mimicry,* in which your immune system confuses molecules of dairy products with your own body's tissue. As a result, the antibodies that your immune system makes to attack dairy or gluten molecules sometimes go after your own body as well, provoking a wide range of disorders, including autoimmune conditions.

Corn is another challenging food, very likely because the vast majority of corn available in the United States has been genetically modified.[6]

In my clinical experience, even nongluten grains can sometimes be challenging to digest, particularly for people who suffer from autoimmune conditions. To a lesser extent, dried pulses (beans of all types, including garbanzos/chick peas and string beans) can also pose digestive challenges. While beans in particular can be an extremely healthy food, gut and immune issues can turn grains and beans into reactive foods.

In response, I have my patients avoid these digestive challenges for the two weeks of the Revitalize Program and then see whether it works for them to resume eating grains, dried pulses, or both. Eggs can also sometimes be reactive foods until your gut and microbiome are functioning optimally, and in some cases, so can nightshades (white potatoes, tomatoes, aubergines, peppers). Joint pains are often a clue that nightshades are causing you problems.

So, as I explained to Laila, your first step for gut healing and microbiome support is to cut out dairy, corn, soy, grains, dried pulses, eggs, nightshades, and all the other foods that might provoke a reaction from your immune system. The foods themselves are not necessarily the problem—the problem is the poor function in your gut and immune system. As your gut heals and your immune system recovers, foods that once created problems for you might become easier to tolerate.

Meanwhile, you will be taking supplements to kill the "bad" bacteria, and later, *probiotics* to replenish your friendly bacteria, so that your gut can heal. Depending on the severity of the problem, your gut might be fully healed within four to six weeks, or you might need somewhat longer.

Laila wondered if this meant she could never eat grains, corn, soy, or dairy again. She also wondered whether she might be reacting to other foods as well.

I'll tell you what I told her: you might need to cut out reactive foods for a few weeks, or even for a few months. In some cases, you might need to cut some foods out permanently—that's something else you will discover as you listen to your own body and find out what it needs. If you're like most people, once you have healed and balanced the gut, your food sensitivities resolve. That's because the problem is not necessarily the food, but rather the microbiome, which has been thrown out of balance by all the factors I identified on pages 36–37. Often, once your microbiome is balanced and your gut is healed, you can go back to eating foods that might have given you problems before.

However, as I told Laila, one step at a time. Your first step is to cut out reactive foods during your 2-Week Revitalize Program so you can find out what your body feels like when it is not being continually assaulted with inflammation and challenges to your gut. Once your gut has begun to heal, you'll feel much better—and you'll have a lot more information about what your body needs.

Myth: "Soy is a health food"

Laila was open to the idea that gluten, corn, and dairy products might be provoking her symptoms and her weight gain—but she was surprised to hear my objections to soy.

"I thought soy was a health food!" she told me. "In fact, I've been making a point to switch out the beef and chicken for some tofu whenever I can."

Unfortunately, "soy is a health food" is an extremely common myth, which, not surprisingly, has been promoted primarily by the soy industry. This again is one of the unfortunate by-products of living in an economy of factory farms. Until very recently, soy was used primarily for animal feed because we humans don't digest it well. Then the soy industry figured out that by isolating soy protein and selling it to the food-processing industry, it could increase its share of the market. Now soy is in just about every packaged or processed food you can think of.

The only cultures that ate soy before our current manufactured health craze were Asian cultures. There, soy is used as a condiment, not as the mainstay of a meal. It's also frequently used in fermented form, and the fermentation increases its health benefits. However, the vast majority of U.S. soy has been genetically modified, so even if it is prepared in a healthy way, the soy itself might be challenging our microbiome and our gut.

On top of everything else, there are a number of other problems with soy:

- It disrupts your endocrine system, which regulates your hormones, particularly your thyroid and estrogen, possibly creating such issues as fatigue, constipation, and issues with menstruation, perimenopause, and menopause.

- It interferes with leptin sensitivity, predisposing you to leptin resistance as well as carbohydrate intolerance.

- It blocks your body's ability to absorb certain minerals.

- It is a common allergen and frequently triggers inflammation.

As I told Laila, we're trying to correct certain key functions in your microbiome, your gut, your immune system, and your hormones. Soy disrupts almost all of the things that we're trying to get back on track! Best to simply avoid it.

If you do feel strongly about eating soy, I recommend organic tempeh. Tempeh is fermented, which makes it easier to digest and adds to its health benefits. And if you buy organic, you know the soy has not been genetically modified.

However, if you have any thyroid challenges, or any family history of female cancers, you really should avoid soy altogether. We know it disrupts your thyroid, and while the evidence on female hormones is controversial, you are better off being safe than sorry.

Where Soy Is Found

Edamame

Tofu

Tempeh

Natto

Soy sauce and tamari

Meat substitutes, such as soy hot dogs, "vegan chicken," or soy bacon

Many protein bars, protein powders, and protein shakes—so read the label

Virtually every packaged or processed food, so again, read the label

Healing the Gut, Regaining Your Health

Once she understood how her symptoms were all part of the same underlying problem—an imbalanced microbiome and a leaky gut—Laila was eager to do whatever she could to rebalance her microbiome and heal her gut. She jumped enthusiastically into her two weeks on the Revitalize Program, and was rewarded with almost instant results. This, I think, had something to do with her relative youth—sometimes, when you're older, it can take a bit longer to reverse the problems that you have spent more time creating. Laila, however, felt energized and revitalized almost immediately, and she quickly began to lose her excess weight.

On her last visit, Laila told me that she had decided to stay permanently gluten free.

"To be honest, I can probably handle it some of the time," she told me. "The problem is, I never know when that time will be. I might be having a quiet week, and then suddenly a big crisis comes and I'm regretting that pasta I had last night because I can feel that it's slowing me down a bit. Or I think I'm in good shape, and then I'll feel a little gassy, and I'll realize that I overestimated what I can handle. Easier just to cut the gluten out completely—then I don't have to think about it."

As with Ricardo, I was proud of Laila for listening to her body and learning so much about what she needed. My happiest days as a physician are when I hand the reins back over to my patients and watch them take complete charge of their own health!

Your Microbiome Is Out of Whack: Three Quick Fixes

1. Take a daily probiotic.

2. Eat a serving of a fermented food three to four times a week.

3. For at least two weeks, cut out reactive foods: sugar, processed foods, gluten, dairy products, corn, all grains, dried pulses, eggs, nightshades (potatoes, tomatoes, aubergine, and peppers), and soy.

REASON #4:

YOUR HORMONES ARE OUT OF BALANCE

As Quinn dragged herself into my office, I could see how thoroughly exhausted she was. She looked at me miserably, running a hand through her limp hair, and shook her head.

"I watched my mother run down as she got older," she said as soon as we had exchanged introductions, "and I swore it was never going to happen to me. I eat healthy, I go to the gym—I really thought I was taking good care of myself.

"But look at me! My hair is all stringy no matter what I do. I actually think it's getting thinner. My skin's a mess. My nails keep breaking. I'm constipated. I've put on 7 kilos in the last two years. I'm so worn out, I can barely make it through the day—but at night, when it's time to go to bed, my mind starts racing and I'm wide awake. I look terrible, and I feel worse—and I'm only forty-five!"

She took a deep breath. "Plus, my cycle is completely off. I've always had some issues with PMS, but now it's off the charts! My periods are heavier than they've ever been, and I get terrible cramps that I never used to get. I don't even feel like myself anymore. My last doctor told me that this is all part of approaching menopause and I just have to accept it. Well, I don't accept it! But I don't know what to do about it either."

"You're quite right not to accept it," I told Quinn. "Once we figure out where the underlying problems are, we'll know how to make you feel the way you used to—and possibly even better."

Listening to Quinn's symptoms, I suspected four different types of hormonal imbalance:

1. Her fatigue and difficulty sleeping suggested possible problems with her *adrenals,* the glands that produce *stress hormones,* such as *cortisol.*

2. Her fatigue—along with her constipation, thinning hair, brittle nails, and weight gain—also suggested possible problems with her *thyroid,* the gland that produces *thyroid hormone.*

3. Her perimenopausal and menstrual issues suggested possible problems with *estrogen, progesterone,* and *testosterone,* the *sex hormones.*

4. Her weight gain could be the result of all three hormonal imbalances, but it also led me to suspect that she was eating too many sweets and starches and/or was carbohydrate intolerant, indicating problems with the hormone *insulin.*

When I shared my thoughts with Quinn, she told me that her doctor had tested her adrenals, thyroid, and blood sugars and found nothing wrong. This did not surprise me. It was yet another instance of conventional medicine viewing health in black-and-white terms rather than on a spectrum. I knew from long experience that Quinn might test "normal" by conventional measures and yet still not have *optimal* levels of balanced hormones. Despite her suffering, most conventional physicians would insist that there was "nothing wrong."

More subtle tests would confirm that, like many women in their 40s and 50s, Quinn was in the midst of a hormonal firestorm—but not necessarily because she was getting older. True, our hormones change as we age, with men experiencing a drop in testosterone and women seeing declines in their estrogen, progesterone, and testosterone levels. However, when your whole body is enjoying optimal function, these changes are relatively easy to ride out.

When your body is stressed, however—by too many sweets and starches, unhealthy fats, gluten and other reactive foods, an imbalanced microbiome, lack of sleep, ongoing exposure to chemicals, and psychological or emotional stress—your stress hormones are frequently out of balance. When you eat too many sweets, starches, and perhaps also too many grains, dried pulses—and for some folks, even fruit—your insulin could be out of balance as well. And when your stress hormones and insulin are out of whack, they often send your thyroid and sex hormones spiraling out of control.

All of these might *look* like age-related problems—but really, they are a problem of function.

Fix the underlying dysfunctions, and your hormones find that nice, healthy balance, no matter how old you are.

What Throws Your Hormones Out of Balance?

- Too many sweets and starches
- If you are carbohydrate intolerant, too many grains, dried pulses, and fruits

- Not enough healthy fat
- An imbalanced microbiome
- Leaky gut
- Gluten and other reactive foods that challenge your immune system and your gut
- Not enough sleep
- Too much caffeine in the form of coffee, energy drinks, sodas, and sometimes even tea or chocolate
- Ongoing low-level exposure to common chemicals in your food, air, water, household cleaners, personal-care products, and cosmetics
- Ongoing exposure to medications, including both over-the-counter remedies and prescription drugs
- Unremitting life challenges that pile up and don't seem to ever go away

Luckily, my 2-Week Revitalize Program could help Quinn begin the process of bringing her hormones back into balance: healing her adrenals, rebalancing her insulin, and restoring order to her thyroid and sex hormones. The first step, though, was to help Quinn see for herself what was going on with her body so she could learn how to restore its function.

Myths to Break Through

- "Feeling tired is a natural part of getting older."
- "As I approach and go through menopause, I have to expect some unpleasant symptoms."
- "The environment has no effect on my hormones."

Myth: "Feeling tired is a natural part of getting older"

When my patients tell me that they are feeling fatigued—and particularly if they also say that they feel wired, especially in the evening, or unable to fall asleep at night—I usually suspect an adrenal problem. When they seem to have the classic symptoms of a thyroid issue (see the questionnaire on pages 62–63), I usually suspect an adrenal problem as well, since many thyroid problems start with adrenal dysfunction. So let's begin where I do with my patients: by focusing on the adrenals.

How Your Adrenals Help You Manage Stress

The adrenal glands sit on top of the kidneys, just about in the small of your back. They produce a number of different *stress hormones,* including dopamine, adrenaline (aka epinephrine), noradrenaline (aka norepinephrine), and cortisol.

The word "adrenaline" might get you to thinking about the "adrenaline rush" that many of us feel when we are stimulated, excited, or challenged. Adrenaline is indeed part of the stress response, but so are several other hormones.

One of the most powerful stress hormones is *cortisol,* which gets involved pretty much whenever your body faces any type of challenge, from a hard-to-digest food to a pressing deadline at work. Whenever you have to put in some extra effort—physical, emotional, or both—cortisol is the hormone that keeps you motivated and focused.

In fact, cortisol literally gets you up in the morning. Ideally, your cortisol levels are highest right around the time you wake up—they are actually what help you wake up, full of energy to face the day. Then, ideally, they follow a gently downward-sloping curve, until finally, by evening, they are low enough to send you drifting peacefully off to sleep.

Throughout the day, you might be called upon to face particular short-term challenges—an urgent call from your boss, a tough problem to solve, a challenging conversation with your mother. For each of these challenges, your cortisol levels might spike as you mobilize your resources. In primitive times, you might have faced more physical challenges—a predator to flee, a boulder to push out of the way, a fishing boat to pull from the surf. For any and all challenges, cortisol is there to spike up when you need some extra energy, and settle back down again when the challenge is done . . . all while following this overall pattern of high in the morning and sloping down to low at night.

That's what a healthy, balanced cortisol response looks like. Unfortunately, for many of us, life is not like that at all!

How Chronic Stress Makes You Old and Fat

Our bodies were designed to face *acute* stress—short-term challenges that arise, are settled, and disappear. You encounter a predator, run away, and then relax. Your fishing boat comes in to shore, you pull it from the surf, and then you relax. The healthiest way to live, if you can manage it, is to have a life full of short, engaging challenges that are over by the end of the day so you are pleasantly challenged all day and pleasantly relaxed all night.

Unfortunately, for many of us, acute stress is only the punctuation for a low-level underlying *chronic* stress—a stress that never goes away. Your child has been diagnosed as learning disabled and you never really stop worrying about it. Your boss is hard to please, and you never know when you'll be asked to stay late at work or meet an impossible deadline. Your schedule is jam-packed from morning till night, and weekends are even worse. Chronic, unremitting stress becomes a way of life for many of us.

To make matters worse, we put our bodies under chronic stress as well by eating too many sweets, starches, and unhealthy fats; exposing them to the low-level toxins found in our food, air, water, and household products; skimping on sleep; and in some cases, taking medications that, whatever their other benefits might be, stress our microbiome and our gut and cause numerous other problems in our bodies.

This is not the one-time acute stress of fleeing a predator or pushing a boulder out of the way. This is chronic, unremitting stress, and our bodies weren't really designed for it.

Well, actually, our bodies do know one thing about chronic, unremitting stress. They know that it probably means we are facing both a shortage of food and an ongoing physical challenge, such as trekking across the tundra or fleeing from an invading horde. These were the kinds of challenges that our ancestors evolved to deal with, so our bodies figured out a very effective response to chronic stress. They shut down every function they possibly could— including reproduction—and they focused on retaining body fat so that when the lean times inevitably came around, we would have some extra weight to see us through.

So this is a big reason why so many of us feel old and fat. If we put our bodies under chronic, unremitting stress, they shut down the sex drive and focus on food. Reproduction is a luxury; survival is not. When you stress your body day in, day out—not just with emotional challenges, but with the wrong food, insufficient sleep, and environmental toxins— your body responds by holding on to fat.

In fact, I have been struck by how well my patients can handle ongoing, unremitting emotional challenges—*if* they are supporting their bodies with the right food, supplements, movement, and sleep. We're used to thinking of stress as an emotional issue. But I have found that many of my patients—including Quinn—are actually suffering more from the *physical* stressors of a poor diet, lack of sleep, and exposure to too many chemicals. Once these physical problems are resolved—once my patients follow the 2-Week Revitalize Program and continue on with the Maintenance Program—they are actually able to find a whole new depth of emotional and mental resources to face even the toughest challenges.

By this point it probably won't surprise you that excess cortisol cues your body to retain fat. Cortisol in balanced amounts won't have this effect. But excess cortisol—the steady drip, drip, drip of it as you keep stressing your body with the wrong foods, too many toxins, and not enough sleep—cues your body to gain and retain weight while also disrupting your digestion, immune system, nervous system, and the rest of your hormones, including your insulin response.

That's right. Excess cortisol disrupts your insulin response, while insulin resistance and blood sugar fluctuations provoke excess cortisol. And both insulin and cortisol cue your body to retain fat. Talk about a vicious cycle!

How Chronic Stress Makes You Old and Fat

Poor diet, lack of sleep, toxic exposure, many medications, emotional stressors, isolation, lack of purpose and meaning

▼

Chronic ongoing release of stress hormones, including cortisol

▼   ▼   ▼

| Disruption of other hormones: thyroid, sex hormones, insulin response, skin problems, achy joints, immune issues, digestive issues | Weight gain | Symptoms: anxiety, depression, brain fog, memory issues, mood swings, fatigue |

This, I believe, is what happened to Quinn. And if you want to know what was triggering the chronic stress response, just compare the "hormonal stressors" on pages 54–55 with the "gut and microbiome stressors" on pages 36–37. The problems always go back to these same usual suspects because very often, whatever disrupts your microbiome and your gut also provokes a cortisol response.

Likewise, when your blood sugar spikes and crashes, that provokes a cortisol response. And when your body is flooded with excess insulin—typically from eating too many sweets and starches or from consuming more carbs than your body can tolerate—that provokes a cortisol response as well.

If you chronically disrupt your microbiome and stress your gut, you will flood your body with a constant drip of cortisol. And if you chronically overdo the sweets, starches, and carbs, you will provoke both excess insulin and excess cortisol (which both cue fat storage). Eventually, the excess cortisol will disrupt all your other hormones—while also making you fat.

Are You Suffering from Adrenal Dysfunction?

- Have you been gaining weight or unable to lose excess weight?
- Do you routinely get less than your ideal amount of sleep?
- Are you frequently tired?
- Do you wake up tired?
- Do you have trouble staying awake—during a movie, while watching television, after a meal?
- Do you rely on caffeine—coffee, energy drinks, sodas, tea, chocolate—to get you through the day?
- Do you rely on sweet and/or starchy foods for energy to get you through the day?
- Do you have trouble falling or staying asleep?
- Do you often feel wired—mind racing, heart pounding—especially at night?
- Do you feel cold all the time?
- Do you periodically or frequently feel dragged-out, listless, unmotivated?
- Do you feel frayed, frazzled, at the end of your rope?
- Would your friends, family, or coworkers describe you as short tempered or someone who easily flies off the handle?
- Do you often feel overwhelmed?
- Do little things get to you far beyond what you think they should?
- Does exercise make you feel more exhausted?

A yes to three or four of these questions could indicate some adrenal dysfunction. A yes to at least six or most suggests that you almost certainly have some adrenal imbalance. Following my 2-Week Revitalize Program along with the suggestions in Chapters 5, 6, and 7 should make a big difference. See Appendix B for some suggested supplements as well.

MANAGING CORTISOL: THE IMPORTANCE OF BALANCE

Conventional medicine typically recognizes only two types of problems with cortisol: Addison's disease, in which your adrenals produce significantly low amounts of cortisol, and Cushing syndrome, in which they produce significantly high amounts.

Both of these conditions are relatively rare—and neither is really on a continuum with the type of adrenal dysfunction suffered by Quinn and so many of my patients. You don't get

Addison's disease from routine levels of stress; it results from structural damage to the adrenal cortex, possibly as the result of a tumor, an autoimmune condition, or an infection, such as tuberculosis, HIV, or fungal infections.

Likewise, Cushing syndrome is usually the result of a tumor somewhere in the endocrine system. You don't get it from diet, lifestyle, or any of the other factors we have been considering.

If you ask your conventional doctor to test you for adrenal issues, he or she will likely look only for Addison's or Cushing. If you test normal for those two conditions, your doctor will tell you you're fine—even if you are plagued by exhaustion, anxiety, and sleep problems. Possibly your doctor will suggest an antidepressant or a sleep aid.

What you probably need instead is to rebalance your cortisol levels. They might be too high, too low, or too high or low at the wrong times. Frequently, adrenal dysfunction follows a pattern whereby your adrenals produce too much cortisol . . . and eventually become so exhausted that they can't produce enough. In that case, they might compensate for low cortisol by producing excess adrenaline or dopamine, so that even though you are exhausted, you still feel wired.

Another possibility is that your adrenals are producing cortisol at the right levels but at the wrong times, so you're exhausted when you wake up but wired when it's time to go to sleep.

There are still more possibilities because there are so many stress hormones, and their interaction with the rest of the body is so complex. Luckily, we don't always need an exact diagnosis to address the problem. If you've answered the questions on page 59 and think you're struggling with adrenal dysfunction, following my 2-Week Revitalize Program should start to make a significant difference, along with taking the suggestions in Chapters 5, 6, and 7 with regard to exercise, stress, toxic exposure, and sleep. If your adrenal dysfunction is more pronounced, you probably need some additional support. Check out Appendix B, where I recommend some supplements that my patients have found to be very helpful.

Caffeine: A Double-Edged Sword

Many of my patients ask me whether they can continue to enjoy their favorite lattes or caffeinated tea. As in the case of other "problem" foods, my answer usually sends them back to their own sense of self-awareness rather than to any rule I might come up with.

In my view, caffeine is a drug—but I believe that in moderate amounts, it's not dangerous for most people. By "moderate," I mean, at most two daily 250ml cups of coffee, or four daily 250ml cups of caffeinated black or green tea.

However, if you don't metabolize caffeine well—as a good number of people, me included, don't—even less caffeine than that is enough to disrupt your sleep, stress your adrenals, and cue a flood of excess cortisol, leaving you wired, anxious, and prone to put on weight.

Moreover, if your adrenals are struggling, you aren't doing them any favors by jolting them into life with caffeine. What they really need is calm, rest, and support—not a high-voltage charge to stress them further.

In addition, most of my patients have become so used to ingesting caffeine that they've lost their sense of how it might be affecting their sleep, mood, or emotional balance.

So my suggestion is that you follow the 2-Week Revitalize Program by going caffeine free, and ideally, stay in the no-caffeine zone for at least a month. That way, you can find out how much more deeply you might sleep or how much calmer and yet more energized you feel without the artificial stimulant on which you've come to rely.

When you have gone a month without caffeine—or when your adrenal issues have completely cleared up—feel free to experiment with adding back in a cup of tea or coffee if it still appeals to you. By that point, you'll be able to see for yourself how that additional caffeine affects your body and you can decide whether caffeine is a healthy choice that works for you.

WHAT ABOUT TESTING?

If your doctor tests you for adrenal issues, he or she will probably give you a blood test to measure your overall levels of cortisol. This will help determine whether you have Addison's or Cushing, but it won't actually reveal much else. Cortisol levels fluctuate so much during the day that a one-time test doesn't tell you everything you need to know.

There is a saliva test, taken four times in a day, that can measure the level of cortisol and other stress hormones, but I don't like to focus on it. Although it can be helpful in some cases, there's no guarantee that you'll actually get the information that helps you devise the right treatment. The issue isn't what the numbers say—it's how you feel.

So many problems clear up or start improving after the 2-Week Revitalize Program that I almost always begin there, perhaps with some of the supplements in Appendix B for extra support for the more severe cases of adrenal dysfunction. If that approach doesn't get results for you, I suggest you seek out an experienced functional-medicine physician or naturopath who can work with you to fine-tune the supplements.

WHERE YOUR THYROID FITS IN

The thyroid, located at the base of your throat, controls the way your body uses energy, helping regulate your metabolism and governing your responsiveness to other hormones. Thyroid dysfunction is extremely common among people, especially women, in their 40s, 50s, and beyond. Again, thyroid problems are not the inevitable result of aging; rather, they are usually the outcome of many years of dysfunction.

Conventional doctors miss subtle thyroid problems to a truly shocking extent. As a result, these men and women drag themselves through their days fatigued, cold, depressed, and struggling with weight—feeling old and fat before their time, when the real problem is an underperforming thyroid.

There are a number of reasons conventional doctors might tell you that your thyroid is normal when you could really use some more support. First, as we have already seen, Western medicine tends to view illness in black-and-white terms rather than recognizing a spectrum. You might have thyroid levels that read as normal on conventional tests—but that are not normal *for you,* or more accurately, that are not *optimal* for you. As a result, your conventional doctor might tell you that your thyroid symptoms are the natural result of getting older or perhaps are caused by some underlying depression, rather than recognizing that you need thyroid support.

Another common problem is *thyroid resistance,* in which your blood levels of thyroid hormone are normal, but your cells are not correctly metabolizing the hormone or not responding effectively to the hormone. As a result, your tests look fine, but your actual condition is very far from optimal.

Yet another reason for misleading test results is that conventional tests measure the presence of T4, but not of free T3. T4 is the inactive form of thyroid hormone while free T3 is the active form. Your body needs to convert T4 to T3 for the thyroid hormones to be active in the body. So, if you are having problems converting T4 to T3—as many people do—your T4 levels can be normal even while you suffer some or all the symptoms of an underperforming thyroid. Measuring free T3 is the most accurate way to see if you are effectively converting T4 to T3.

So many of my patients come to me with symptoms of low thyroid function, even though they are already on thyroid medication. When I raise the subject, they tell me that their conventional physicians insisted that their blood tests for thyroid came back normal and everything was fine. But when I tweaked their thyroid hormone prescription to include T3, or added adrenal support, their symptoms disappeared and they had a new lease on life—old and fat no more!

Treating thyroid fully is complicated—beyond the scope of this book—but I will say that when you take gluten and soy out of your diet and resolve your adrenal dysfunction, your thyroid problems can often improve. If my 2-Week Revitalize Program and the adrenal supplements recommended in Appendix B don't have the effect you'd like, I urge you to find a good functional-medicine practitioner to help you make some more changes. While thyroid problems can be complicated to treat, you *can* solve them in almost every case—with the right kind of help. (For suggestions on how to find a functional-medicine practitioner, see Resources.)

Are You Suffering from Thyroid Dysfunction?

- Are you frequently tired?
- Do you get cold easily?
- Is your hair thinning or falling out?

- Are your nails brittle?
- Are you constipated?
- Have you been gaining weight in spite of eating well?
- Are you struggling with depression?
- Do you frequently experience menstrual irregularities?
- Do you suffer from aches and pains?

If you answered yes to three or more of these questions, follow the 2-Week Revitalize Program and take the supplements recommended in Appendix B. If you don't get the results you'd like, find a good functional-medicine practitioner to help you further (see Resources).

Myth: "As I approach and go through menopause, I have to expect some unpleasant symptoms"

Of all the destructive myths about aging, perhaps the one that does the most damage is the myth insisting that women going through menopause or perimenopause are doomed to have a miserable time.

As we have seen, age does bring some hormonal changes. But as we have also seen, these changes don't have to create a raft of unpleasant symptoms, make you feel old, or cause you to put on the pounds. If you are maintaining optimal function—through diet, supplements, sleep, and exercise—you can easily ride out these hormonal changes.

One of the most common hormonal issues I see in women is an imbalance between the two primary female hormones: estrogen and progesterone. As progesterone levels fall—often made worse by adrenal dysfunction—the estrogen-progesterone ratio goes out of balance. One of my major concerns is to restore that balance.

Another common problem is estrogen levels that fall too far, again often because of adrenal dysfunction. From your teens through your 40s, you rely on your ovaries to make estrogen. As your ovaries begin shutting down in preparation for menopause, your adrenal glands take over. If your adrenals are functioning optimally, perimenopause and menopause can be smooth, symptom-free transitions. If your adrenals are stressed and overwhelmed, they can't make the estrogen you need—and symptoms like Quinn's can be the result.

Estrogen issues can also provoke problems with your thyroid. This is another example of how epigenetics comes into play. If you have the genetic predisposition for an autoimmune condition known as Hashimoto's thyroiditis, fluctuating estrogen might trigger you to develop that condition. However, if your gut is in good shape, your levels of inflammation are low, and your hormones remain balanced, you have a good chance of defeating your genetic tendencies and maintaining a healthy thyroid.

Unfortunately, many conventional doctors don't look at hormonal *balance*. They focus instead on hormonal *levels*. When women struggle with hormonal symptoms, their physicians often prescribe estrogen alone. In many cases, though, estrogen levels have fallen a little—but progesterone levels have fallen even more, throwing the balance off and producing hormonal symptoms.

As I tell my patients, your hormones are like a symphony orchestra. When one instrument is out of tune, it throws off the whole orchestra. If the horn section is too loud, the violins might go off course as well; if the oboe misses a cue, the entire piece sounds wrong, no matter how well the rest of the ensemble is playing. To achieve hormonal balance, we always have to look at the entire hormonal symphony and make sure that every hormone is coming in at the right level and in the right relationship to all the others. Insulin, the stress hormones (including cortisol), thyroid hormones, estrogen, and progesterone must all be in balance for any one of those hormones to play its part correctly.

⟡ —— How Can You Treat Hormonal Issues? —— ⟡

You actually have lots of options. Some women opt for hormone replacement therapy. If that is your choice, I highly recommend that you avoid commercially prepared hormones, some of which are made from horse's urine and many of which are too strong for humans. Nor can these commercial hormones be tailored to each individual.

Instead, try bioidentical hormones, which are designed to match your own hormones more completely. A functional-medicine practitioner and a compounding pharmacy can work with you to come up with exactly the right hormonal doses and composition to fit your particular needs.

Often a good starting option is progesterone cream, which is sometimes helpful for rebalancing the estrogen-progesterone ratio because a relative drop in progesterone often happens first. Herbal treatments can also be helpful (see Appendix C), as can *acupuncture,* an ancient technique of Chinese medicine that relies on tiny needles to stimulate the body's energy pathways. The needles are about the width of a hair and they don't hurt much. The experience of acupuncture is very relaxing and has multiple health benefits over and above treating any specific ailment.

I treat most of my patients with acupuncture, and I love getting the treatments myself when I need them. A single acupuncture treatment can feel so relaxing and restorative that I sometimes think of it as an entire day at the spa, condensed into less than an hour.

Before you try any of these other remedies, though, I suggest you begin with the 2-Week Revitalize Program. This approach to diet and lifestyle will help you reboot and boost overall function, which will go a long way toward bringing balance and vitality to your hormones.

Myth: "The environment has no effect on my hormones"

Quinn listened intently as I explained the various ways her hormones were interacting. "I understand everything except the part about the toxins," she told me. "I work in an office. I live in a suburb. I don't think I really come into contact with any toxins, do I?"

Unfortunately, even those of us with white-collar jobs and nice homes live in a toxic world, encountering thousands of industrial chemicals, heavy metals, and pollutants in our air, food, water, home cleaning products, and personal-care items.

These chemicals are all the more distressing because, in addition to their general toxic burden, they work specifically to disrupt our hormones. In fact, many common chemicals are known specifically as "endocrine (hormone) disrupters."

Where Endocrine Disrupters Hide

- Personal-care products: Cosmetics, moisturizers, shampoos, and conditioners often contain ingredients that disrupt your hormonal balance.

- Drinking water: atrazine, arsenic, and perchlorate are three endocrine disruptors that pervade many communities' supply of drinking water.

- Canned foods: many food cans are lined with BPA, a common endocrine disruptor.

- Conventionally farmed fruits and vegetables: pesticides, herbicides, and industrial runoff turn even healthy produce into endocrine disruptors.

- Conventionally farmed meat, poultry, and dairy products: these commercial foods contain disruptive antibiotics, hormones, and industrial chemicals.

- High-mercury fish: shark, swordfish, king mackerel, marlin, and tilefish are high in mercury and other heavy metals, which disrupt hormonal balance and function.

- Kitchen products: common hazards include nonstick cookware, plastic wrap, and plastic containers, especially when heated.

- Home and office cleaning products: these are frequently loaded with industrial chemicals that disrupt your hormones.

- Office products: toner, solvents, and ink cartridges likewise can throw hormones out of balance.

- The plastic coating on many cash-register receipts: these contain bisphenol-A (BPA).

- Furniture: many types of woods and finishes release toxins into the air of your home or office.

- Carpeting: this is frequently loaded with disruptive industrial chemicals.

- Buildings: toxic molds, fumes from building materials, and airborne pollutants from factories can toxify your office or home.

To find out specifically where toxins might lurk in your personal-care products, see www.
bewell.com/blog/personal-care-products-chemicals. For more on where endocrine disruptors
lurk in your kitchen, see www.bewell.com/blog/endocrine-disruptors-kitchen. For more
on endocrine disruptors elsewhere in your home, see www. bewell.com/blog/endocrine-
disruptors-house.

As you can see, endocrine disrupters are everywhere. If you only encountered them once
or twice, they probably wouldn't cause you much concern, but because they are so prevalent, you run the risk of constant low-grade exposure. Many of these toxins either block or
promote your estrogen and other hormones, so either way they throw off your hormonal
balance. In some cases, they affect the *levels* of your hormones. In other cases, they affect the
function of your hormones. Either way, they can cause numerous problems that you might
have been attributing to age.

It's hard to find good information about how these chemicals or toxins affect us because
whatever research has been done focuses only on individual toxins. The problem is that there
isn't just one toxin—there are thousands, and no one really knows how they interact with one
another or how years of exposure are disrupting our hormones.

No one really knows—but we can guess. As a physician, I can tell you that I am seeing
more and more young women with breast cancer, a disease that used to be almost completely
confined to women over 50. And my guess is that because these young women have gotten
such a massive exposure to endocrine disrupters starting with their time in the womb, they are
now struggling with hormonal issues that used to take decades to develop.

I don't want to stress you out or frighten you unduly, so let's focus on what you can do to
protect yourself. Here are the guidelines I gave Quinn and that I give all my patients.

How to Protect Your Hormones from Environmental Toxins

Here are some first, basic steps toward protecting your hormones. For more complete
information, visit www.bewell.com/blog/personal-care-products-chemicals, www.bewell.com/
blog/endocrine-disruptors-kitchen, and www.bewell.com/blog/endocrine-disruptors-house.

- Avoid plastics wherever possible, especially plastics made with BPA. Storing food in
  plastics is probably okay, but at all costs, don't heat your food in plastics. Molecules
  from the plastic make their way into your food—and disrupt your hormonal balance.

- Avoid plastic water bottles. As the water sits in the bottle, especially in the sun or in a
  warm environment, plastic molecules seep into the water.

- Use only "clean" personal care products. Avoid products that contain parabens,
  phthalates, DEA (diethanolamine), MEA (monoethanolamine), TEA (triethanolamine),
  sodium lauryl sulfate, and sodium laureth sulfate. For more information on which
  products to avoid, see www.bewell.com/blog/personal-care-products-chemicals.

- Avoid hand sanitizers and antibacterial soap—they destroy the bacteria on your skin, which disrupts your microbiome. A strong microbiome is one of your best protections against any type of disorder or dysfunction. Washing your hands with a good, pure soap is just as good as using an antibacterial.

- Get a water filter for each one of your home faucets, including the bath and shower; you absorb disruptive chemicals through your skin as well as by drinking them.

Nurturing Your Hormones

Quinn was enormously relieved to learn that she was not doomed to decades of feeling exhausted, miserable, and out of control. She was eager to start the 2-Week Revitalize Program and see what difference it could make. Although she wasn't thrilled about giving up some of her favorite pastas and desserts, she told me bluntly, "Anything is worth not feeling this way anymore. If you told me to live on kale and water, I would do it!"

I laughed. "Actually, I think you'll find the Revitalize meals very satisfying," I told her. "As a former pasta and dessert lover, I feel your pain. But within a few weeks, I don't think you'll even miss those foods."

Beyond the physical causes of stress, Quinn and I talked about the emotional issues that were stressing her out. I reminded her that exercise (which we'll discuss in the next chapter) is an amazing anti-inflammatory stress reliever with multiple benefits for your adrenals and just about every other system in your body. When you're struggling with adrenal fatigue, you sometimes have to take it easy on the exercise for a while—you want to feel pleasantly tired after your workout, not miserably exhausted—but the gentle exercise in your 2-Week Revitalize Program can help you find the kind of movement that is right for you.

Quinn and I also talked about one of the most stressful experiences we humans face: isolation. It's no accident that the worst punishment they can mete out in high-security prisons is to put someone in solitary confinement. We humans are social animals, and we need the company and support of others. As you'll see in Chapter 10, finding community and a sense of purpose is a huge stress reliever, as is seeking out ways to make life better for others.

The ultimate drug for stress, however, is meditation, which you'll learn more about in Chapter 6. Like exercise, meditation has multiple health benefits and can make an enormous difference in gut function, hormonal balance, and overall well-being.

When I saw Quinn six weeks later, she looked like a different person. Her hair was thicker and shiny, her skin glowed, and the harried, desperate look was gone from her eyes. She had started, very slowly, to lose some of her unwanted weight. Most importantly, as she told me, "I'm finally starting to feel like myself again."

It had taken several years for Quinn's adrenals to go out of balance, and it might take several months for her to put the balance right again. With the strong start she'd gotten, however, I knew there was no stopping her now.

Your Hormones Are Out of Balance:
Three Quick Fixes

1. Avoid or minimize disruptive, stressful foods: sweets and starches, gluten, reactive foods, and, as necessary, caffeine.

2. Go through your kitchen and bathroom and get rid of as many endocrine disrupters as you can, using the information on my website to guide you: www.bewell.com/blog/endocrine-disruptors-kitchen, www.bewell.com/blog/endocrine-disruptors-house. If you can't do it all at once, give yourself three months to allow the problematic products to run out and then replace them with safer ones.

3. Relieve your stress: find a funny movie and laugh uproariously, put on some music and "dance it out," or treat yourself to a night out and have fun!

REASON #5:

YOU DON'T MOVE ENOUGH

Aisha was a tall, striking woman, but when she inched into my office, I could see how awkwardly and tentatively she moved. "I know, I know, I move like an old person," she said before I had even introduced myself. "Isn't it awful? Aren't I too young to hobble around like this?"

Aisha explained that she'd had painful arthritis in both knees for the past three years. "I used to be a runner, and I used to love to walk," she said in her exuberant voice. "But no more. It's disgusting!" At age 46, Aisha's skin was smooth and unwrinkled, and she told me that she still worked long hours for the consulting business she had founded, a profession that took her around the world on frequent globe-hopping trips. She was discouraged, though, because the arthritis kept her from moving freely, and she frequently struggled with the many physical demands of travel—lifting a suitcase to the overhead compartment on the plane, walking down the long airport corridors, even making her way from her hotel to a nearby restaurant where a client had asked to meet.

"I don't want to slow down," she said wistfully. "But, I don't know, maybe my body is trying to tell me something. . . ."

I told Aisha that I was almost 15 years older than she was and have arthritis in both knees from soccer injuries in my youth—in fact, I've been told I need a knee replacement. Yet I regularly do yoga, go hiking, bike about 10 to 15 miles a few times a week during the warmer months, and go to the gym a few times a week during the colder months. "Movement is what keeps you feeling young and strong," I said. "As soon as we settle down that arthritis, we can get you moving again."

Aisha made a face. "I have to say it—I *hate* the gym," she announced dramatically. "I hate working out, I hate lifting weights, I hate exercise of all types. I'll eat whatever you tell me to eat, Dr. Lipman, and I'll follow anything else you tell me to do—I promise. But the way I see it, life's too short to waste it on a treadmill."

"Maybe so," I agreed, "but if you want to feel strong and empowered when you travel—if you want to be lifting your own suitcase or enjoying the chance to walk around a new city—staying active is the way to get there. Let's clear up the inflammation that is causing your arthritis, and then let's work on finding a type of movement that you really love. Your body was born to be active, and right now, it's starved for movement."

Aisha looked at me skeptically.

"I'll make a deal with you," I said. "As soon as your arthritis is cleared up, you find some kind of movement you really like—or at least, something you can stand. It doesn't have to be a treadmill—you could bike, or swim, or learn aikido, just so you're using your body. Stick with it for one month, just 30 days. If at the end of those 30 days, you still hate moving, then we'll figure out what to do next. But I'm betting that after just one active month, your body is going to be giving a very different message from the one you're hearing now."

Myths to Break Through

- "Exercise is for the young and healthy."
- "Your main focus in exercise should be to develop strength and stamina."
- "To exercise optimally, you have to go to the gym."
- "The main reason to exercise is to keep your body in shape."

Myth: "Exercise is for the young and healthy"

This is an attitude I've noticed among a lot of my middle-aged patients, and it's one of the myths that contribute most toward making us old and fat. Many people think that exercise is for the young—a matter of bench-pressing a record amount of weight, or running a marathon in a respectable time.

In fact, our bodies crave movement, and when we don't give it to them, *that's* when the aging process really takes off. Have you noticed that when you were younger, you used to spring up out of your chair, but now you get up slowly, awkwardly, defending against the stiffness and maybe some lurking aches and pains? When you were younger, did you stride through the world without thinking about it, but now you cut your errands short because you can't face walking another step? When you were younger, did you feel energized and vigorous, but now, increasingly, you feel stiff, achy, and fatigued?

I told Aisha, and I'll tell you: *You don't have to feel that way—IF you keep moving.* If you move, you feel like moving more. If you spend all day sitting at your desk and all night sitting in front of the television, all you'll feel like doing is continuing to sit—and that's when you start feeling old.

That's also when a host of physical problems begin. Our bodies were never meant to keep sitting; in fact, some people believe that our bodies were never meant to sit in chairs at all. Chairs are a relatively recent invention in human history, never mind desks and jobs that must be done at them. A growing body of research suggests that if you sit for longer than an hour at a time, you run the risk of heart disease, poor circulation, and joint pain. Sitting can cause your blood to pool in your legs, so that it doesn't properly reach your heart. Even as little as one hour of sitting can impair blood flow by as much as 50 percent.

However, as a new study out of Indiana University shows, you can reverse the potential damage by taking a five-minute walking break every hour or so. The men studied by the Indiana researchers spent five minutes each hour walking on a treadmill, which probably isn't so practical for most people in our current office culture.[1] However, even just a brisk walk around the block or in the halls of your office building—even a quick trip to the restroom and back—can get your blood flowing again.

When I suggest this to patients, they often look at me in disbelief.

"You have no idea how hard it is to leave my desk," my patient Marcia told me. "I get dirty looks even when I *have* to go to the bathroom. In my office you're supposed to keep your nose to the grindstone."

I suggested that if she got her blood flowing for only five minutes once an hour, her mind would be sharper and her productivity would increase. Reluctantly, she agreed to give it a try—and called me two weeks later to report.

"You were right!" she said. "I had way more energy, I didn't get so tired, and I could see my mind was clearer. A couple of people have even stopped giving me dirty looks and started taking 'walk breaks' of their own!"

Even that little bit of movement had made a significant difference to Marcia and her coworkers. I know from my own experience you can get even better results from a vigorous workout in the morning to get you going or a less vigorous one at the end of the day to relieve stress. The workout doesn't have to be on the treadmill, either—it can be a bike ride, a swim, a brisk walk, or even putting on some music in the privacy of your bedroom and dancing as hard as you can. Your body craves movement, so why not fulfill that craving?

I actually feel more passionate about getting my middle-aged and older patients to exercise than I do with patients who are younger. That's because physical exercise is one of the best ways to keep your brain healthy, to prevent Alzheimer's and other types of dementia, and to keep your mind sharp. If you're concerned about "senior moments," forgetfulness, or brain fog, your first line of defense is to get moving. Your brain needs more oxygen and blood flow than it can get when you are sedentary. And, along with your whole body, your brain will benefit greatly from exercise's ability to lower inflammation.

Inflammation is the culprit behind so many of the problems of aging. We've seen that it's at the root of chronic illnesses such as autoimmune disorders, heart disease, diabetes, and cancer, and that it leads to such apparently age-related symptoms as aches, pains, menopausal symptoms, and sleep issues. Inflammation also affects our mental health, promoting anxiety and depression. And it affects our cognitive health, promoting memory issues, brain fog, and, ultimately, dementia.

Exercise serves not only to heal inflammation and keep it at bay, but it also literally helps your brain cells to regenerate. That process is called *neurogenesis*—the creation of new brain cells. This is a terrific anti-aging discovery because when I was in medical school, we were taught that once you've lost brain function, it's gone forever. Now we know that you can literally regrow the cells in your brain—and one of the best ways to help that process is along is through movement.

Another enormous anti-aging benefit of exercise is the way it increases your body's population of *mitochondria*. Mitochondria are tiny structures found in most cells, often referred to as the cell's energy powerhouse. The more mitochondria you have, the better able you are to produce energy and burn fat. And exercise is one of the few things that increases the number of mitochondria. In other words, exercise creates more of the cellular structures that will keep you from feeling old and fat. I also see movement as affecting our sense of self. If you feel stuck, what do you do? You sit, because you feel that life has stopped you. If you can find it in yourself to get up and start moving, you feel empowered to move through emotional obstacles as well. This was the sense of empowerment I wanted Aisha to experience, and it was why I was so committed to getting her moving as soon as she was physically able to do so.

Myth: "Your main focus in exercise should be to develop strength and stamina"

When you think about exercise, what first comes to mind?

Most people, I think, start by thinking about the muscles. But what about the parts of our body that lie *between* the muscles, connecting muscle to muscle, muscle to bone, and bone to bone? The *tendons, ligaments,* and particularly the *fascia* are of crucial importance to health and well-being—and yet, they are often ignored, even by physicians, trainers, and exercise gurus.

What's Between Your Muscles?

- **Fascia (pronounced FASH-ya):** bands of soft tissue that are fused with your bones, muscles, tendons, nerves, blood vessels, and organs. Superficial fascia lie close to the surface—just below your skin. Deep fascia lie farther down. You need soft, supple fascia to allow your muscles to move easily, but as you age—and especially if you have had injuries, haven't been active, or haven't stretched properly—your fascia tend to stiffen up. When your fascia aren't doing their job, you can develop *adhesions*: tight places where tissues that should be separated by fascia have fused. Injury can create adhesions. So can inflammation. And so can chronic stress. As a result, you feel stiff, inflexible, off balance, and sometimes in pain. The exercises in your 2-Week Revitalize Program and your lifelong Maintenance Program will help keep your fascia supple.

- **Tendons:** tough cords that attach your muscles to your bones. Your muscles communicate with your brain via your nervous system, so if you want to move, you move your muscles—which then rely on your tendons to transmit power to your bones. Tendons can easily become inflamed, producing the painful condition known as *tendonitis.* The diet, supplement, and lifestyle suggestions described throughout this book can help heal and prevent tendonitis by reducing inflammation. Exercise also has key anti-inflammatory benefits.

- **Ligaments:** tough tissue that connects bones directly to other bones. By holding your bones in place, they support your joints. Healthy ligaments are crucial for preventing sprains, strains, aches, and pains. To prevent straining the ligaments, it's essential to keep the muscles, tendons, and fascia in shape.

Because I know how important these connectors—particularly the fascia—can be, I actually think that *flexibility* is as important as strength, especially as we age. Don't get me wrong: strength is important. When I thought of Aisha, for example, I wanted her to have arms strong enough to lift a suitcase and legs strong enough to carry her body. But I also wanted her to feel supple, flexible, and open to new experiences, because that sense of flexibility and openness is one of our best defenses against feeling old.

Think about what happens when you feel stressed or upset. If you're like most people, you tense up, usually in a characteristic place; you tighten that part of your body over and over and over again. Perhaps when you'd like to snap back at your boss or get into a familiar argument with your spouse, you restrain yourself—and tense your jaw. Perhaps when a family member starts a familiar complaint or round of teasing, you brace yourself—and hunch your shoulders. Perhaps when you think about the long round of errands and obligations that awaits you before you've even gotten out of bed, you try to rouse yourself—and tighten your back. Repeat those movements hundreds and thousands of times over the years, without ever doing yoga, massage, acupuncture, or even gentle stretching to loosen and open the affected areas, and by the time you're in your 40s, 50s, or 60s, you might easily have developed a permanent ache, pain, or stiffness.

These insults to your fascia are exacerbated if you have a job that requires you to sit for long hours at a desk. Your soft tissue realigns to accommodate this habitual posture, sitting slumped and round shouldered. Your hamstrings—the muscles running down the backs of your legs—become shortened, which rounds your *lumbar spine* (your lower back), pulling your pelvis forward. Your shoulders roll forward too, and creep slowly up toward your ears. As you try to focus your eyes, your chin pokes forward, tightening the muscles and fascia at the base of your skull.

By the time you reach middle age, what's the result? You've got a chronically stiff neck, or perhaps a perpetually sore back. Your joints, worn out from the pressure, begin to ache. Your muscles don't respond easily and vigorously—they stiffen as you try to bound up out of your chair, or fight you as you try to sink gracefully back down. Before you know it, you are, as Aisha might put it, "moving like an old person."

As with the other conditions we have considered, stiffness, achiness, and loss of mobility are not the inevitable result of getting older. They result from a way of life, a sedentary life without the movement your body craves. Or, if you have indeed exercised vigorously your entire life, stiffness, aches, and pains are your body's way of telling you that perhaps you neglected to stretch—perhaps you focused on the strength of your muscles, ignoring their flexibility and the suppleness of your fascia.

Making You Feel Old: What Creates
Tension, Adhesions, Aches, and Pains?

- Keeping a muscle in a shortened position for a long time: sleeping in a bad position, sitting at a desk, sitting on a plane
- Repetitive movement: typing, cradling a telephone, running with poor form
- Lack of stretching
- Unhealed or partially healed old injuries
- Adhesions from surgery
- Inflammation
- Air conditioning or cold air
- Viral illness

If stiffness and achiness are, in some sense, things we've done to ourselves, the good news is that we can *undo* them. By choosing to stretch and nurture our fascia, we can regain the youthful openness we might have thought was lost forever.

That's why, in your 2-Week Revitalize exercise program, I have you do a workout that includes some stretching and some fascia exercises. In your Maintenance Program, I show you how to incorporate these going forward, no matter what other types of movement you choose.

If two weeks of the Revitalize Program don't seem to be enough, or if you're feeling so stiff and achy that you can't even engage in the movement I suggest, I strongly recommend bodywork—perhaps acupuncture, Active Release Technique, Rolfing, or deep-tissue massage—along with very gentle restorative yoga. (For more on yoga, see Chapter 6.)

So many of my patients have greatly improved from these simple ways of freeing up the fascia and releasing muscular tension. Once you become aware of how your body holds tension, you can easily learn one of several techniques to release that tension. A habitual practice of releasing tension—through breathing, stretching, and/or yoga—will make a world of difference to your mind, body, and spirit. Your physical flexibility will nurture your mental flexibility so you won't feel so "stiff-necked" and "braced" but will greet the world with more suppleness and grace. Instead of feeling old and stiff, you'll feel vigorous, youthful, and open. That is the gift of movement.

How Stretching Keeps You
from Feeling Old and Fat

- Less soreness because of the decrease in muscular tension: no more back pain, neck pain, or headaches
- Increased flexibility: stretching counters the gradual constriction you can suffer from overuse or underuse of different areas of your body
- Fewer injuries: strains, sprains, tendonitis, muscle spasms
- Faster recovery time from injuries
- Greater body awareness
- Mental and physical relaxation
- Better performance at skilled tasks, including sports
- Better function in the nervous system: less anxiety, depression, brain fog, and fewer memory problems
- Improved circulation: healthier heart and cardiovascular system

Myth: "To exercise optimally, you have to go to the gym"

When Aisha told me life was too short to spend on a treadmill, I saw yet again the power of this particular myth: I tell my patients to move, and they think I'm telling them to "exercise."

I actually would rather not even use the word "exercise," let alone insist that you go to the gym. I'd rather talk about *movement,* because that to me is our birthright. Our bodies were made to move, just as they were made to drink fresh water and eat clean food. When we lack movement, we stagnate, in more ways than one.

I was very much impressed when I read the book *The Blue Zones: 9 Lessons for Living Longer from the People Who've Lived the Longest.* There I found confirmation of what I have long believed and seen in my practice: if you want to live a long and vigorous life, *move.* That's what all the vigorous octagenarians and nonagenarians do in the blue zones—the parts of the world where the longest-lived people reside—and that's what I want you to do too.

Of course, for some people, gyms and home gyms are the perfect way to develop strength and stamina. If you enjoy working out on a treadmill, elliptical, weight machine, or some other piece of gym equipment, or if you like doing a home or gym workout with free weights, you already know the extraordinary physical and mental benefits that such workouts provide. Although I sometimes need my wife's gentle prodding to get me to the gym—otherwise, I admit, I might lose myself in research or get absorbed in listening to music—I am always happy and feel energized after a workout.

This was not always true. Although in my youth I played a lot of sports, my busy schedule after med school put an end to that, and somehow, 20 years passed without my ever being very active.

Luckily, my interest in functional medicine and in non-Western approaches to healing brought me to yoga. Other than the yoga, however, I led a fairly sedentary life.

Then, about 15 years ago, I was invited to give a series of lectures at a spa called Rancho La Puerta. It was sort of a living "blue zone"; I saw so many people in their 60s and 70s who were active, vigorous, and glowing with health. I couldn't help seeing that besides eating clean food and getting enough sleep, these "superpeople" all had one thing in common: they all moved regularly. They each had a routine that combined strength training, core strengthening, aerobics, and stretching—and their bodies showed it. So did their attitudes: optimistic, confident, empowered.

Aha! I thought. *Maybe there is something to this.*

So I asked the trainers at Rancho La Puerta to come up with a gym routine for me, and, somewhat tentatively, I began it.

I was a little bit scared at first that I wouldn't be able to do it, and then I realized how much I enjoyed it. Although I had by that point done yoga for more than a decade, I'd never seen myself as going to a gym and lifting weights or walking on the treadmill. But I discovered that if I put on my headphones and listened to some of my favorite World Beat music, my time at the gym was actually a pleasant and restorative interlude when I had the chance to clear out my mind and reconnect with the rhythms of my body. I began to enjoy the feeling of working my muscles, watching myself grow stronger, and feeling my lungs expand. And afterward, when the workout was over, I felt absolutely terrific! Where else can you get an "up" like that?

The physical benefits were clear. My blood pressure had always been on the highish side, and given my family history of heart disease, this was worrisome. Almost immediately after I started exercising regularly, my numbers improved. My whole body felt more vigorous, stronger, more powerful. The mental and emotional benefits were clear as well. I could see that on the days I'd had a workout, I felt calmer, less reactive, and more able to take a deep breath and really consider what I wanted to do next instead of acting impulsively or feeling overtaken by lethargy or frustration. Yoga had helped a great deal with this already, but moving more built on that foundation in a simply wonderful way.

So I myself am a fan of gym workouts, and if that is something you are willing to experiment with, I encourage you to give it a try. While I want your 2-Week Revitalize Program to be a calmer, gentler time—especially if you find it challenging to give up sugar, caffeine, and some of the other stressors I am having you cut out—I've suggested a more vigorous workout for your Maintenance Program that combines strength training, core support, aerobics, and stretching, along with fascia work and yoga.

Workouts to Keep You from
Feeling Old and Fat

- **Strength training:** to give you stronger muscles. Strength training also challenges your bones, which makes them stronger and helps prevent osteoporosis. It builds your muscles and boosts your metabolism, and you burn more fat even when you are at rest. And since strength training increases your glucose tolerance, you can potentially handle more carbs.

- **Core support:** to support the strength and stability of your abdomen and lower back, which grounds, strengthens, and stabilizes your whole body. Core support is also crucial for *functional movement*—movements that you undertake in daily life, such as lifting a box, bending down to get something from under your chair, or going up and down stairs.

- **Aerobics:** movement that requires your heart and lungs to operate temporarily above normal capacity. Terrific for stress release and to give you that endorphin rush that is even better than a sugar high once you get it going! The best form of aerobic exercise is *interval training:* intense bursts of movement alternating several times with a less intense cooldown period. For a sample recommended interval workout, see www.bewell.com/blog/interval-training-workout.

- **Stretching:** keeping your muscles loose and flexible, with all of the benefits listed on page 75.

- **Fascia work:** releasing and nurturing the bands of tissue that connect your muscles, bones, and organs so you remain supple, open, and pain free.

Now that I've shared with you my own enjoyment of a gym workout, I want to turn around and say the opposite:

You absolutely do not need to ever go to a gym or lift a weight to be healthy.

The most important thing is for you to find a form of movement that you love and to do it for at least 30 minutes a day several times a week.

If, like Aisha, you think you don't like *any* movement, I urge you to experiment until you find something you do like. If you want to avoid getting fat and feeling old, movement is one of your best friends.

Anti-Aging Movement

- Boxing
- Biking or spinning
- Dance: African, ballet, ballroom, jazz, modern, salsa, swing, tango, tap
- Martial arts: aikido, judo, jujitsu
- Sports: basketball, handball, soccer, softball, tennis, squash
- Swimming
- Walking briskly
- Tai chi
- Yoga (see Appendix A)

⬦ THE JOY OF MOVEMENT: 5RHYTHMS ⬦

Sometimes I think that the biggest journey of my medical career has been my slow but steady introduction to different types of movement. One of the most important way stations on that journey was when I encountered 5Rhythms, founded by the extraordinary Gabrielle Roth. I had the privilege of being mentored by Gabrielle before she passed away a few years ago, and it opened me to a new appreciation of what movement can do for both body and soul.

I quote Gabrielle in one of my earlier books, but her words are so eloquent that I'm going to repeat them here: "Movement," she said, "is a way to release the past and become aware of the present. Because change is constant, movement is the only thing we can truthfully rely on."[2]

Gabrielle sought to transform participants by immersing them in five universal rhythms—flowing, staccato, chaos, lyrical, and stillness. Partly, these rhythms give you a chance to connect to your primal physical self. Partly, they release emotional energy—those emotions that you've locked up in the clenched jaw, the hunched shoulders, the tightened back. And partly, they are a form of meditation—the chance to quiet the mind and connect to yourself and the universe around you on a deeper level.

Gabrielle's workshops guide you through the stages of a human life via the five universal rhythms: the flowing rhythms of infancy; the staccato explorations of a child; the explosive movements of puberty; the lyrical movement of maturity; and the ultimate stillness of death. When I tried a 5Rhythms session, I was soon dripping with sweat—and utterly entranced. At the end of the session, I felt profoundly calm.

If you are fortunate to be able to take a 5Rhythms workshop, I urge you to do so. But even if you can't, I share this approach in hopes that you will find your own way toward connecting with the expansive, expressive power of rhythm and movement—your birthright and your way of remaining vital until your very last breath.

⬦—— Enjoy Some Sexercise! ——⬦

One of the best possible exercises you could ever undertake is, believe it or not, sex. Having regular sex is also one of the best ways to feel young and stay slim. It's possible to burn anywhere from 85 to 100 calories by having sex—comparable to a modest workout on a treadmill.[3] And regular sex promotes the release of hormones, including testosterone and estrogen, which can keep you looking young and vital.

Sex is a fabulous way to release tension, and it's even a natural painkiller: it releases endorphins, which are natural analgesics. Sex is also a great resource for happiness; according to a recent study by the National Bureau of Economic Research, a relationship that includes regular sex brings the same levels of happiness as earning an extra $100,000 a year.[4]

What drug can bring all these benefits—without side effects!

Orgasms in particular are a powerful stress reliever. You release loads of oxytocin at climax, a "bonding hormone" that is a natural antidote to stress hormones. Orgasms are also a great anti-aging device. Some experts suggest that if you have 200 orgasms a year, you lower your age by six years.[5] The endorphins released by orgasms will help you sleep better, while three or more orgasms per week reduce your risk of heart attack and stroke by half. Orgasms also boost your levels of immunoglobulin A, which strengthens immunity.

And of course, having sex helps you feel young and vital. It deepens your relationship with your partner and empowers your own sense of being loved, loving, and attractive—a confidence that can carry over into other areas of your life.

Solo sex has all of the same benefits as sex with a partner, although unfortunately, not to the same degree. Being able to give yourself pleasure, however, is also empowering.

One of the great things about the 2-Week Revitalize Program is that by boosting your health, it can also restore your ability to fully enjoy sex. If you feel even after the program that you're not responding at the level you would like—if you're having trouble getting or staying aroused or reaching orgasms—talk to your doctor or find a good functional-medicine practitioner who can help you restore hormonal balance and correct anything that might be going wrong. Sex is too wonderful a part of life to miss out on!

Myth: "The main reason to exercise is to keep your body in shape"

Honestly, folks, as wonderful as exercise is for your body, it is even better for your brain. As we have seen, it literally enables your brain cells to regenerate. By promoting oxygen and blood flow, it keeps you working at peak cognitive function. By combating inflammation, it helps defeat your body's *and* your brain's worst enemy. Studies have shown that for such emotional issues as moderate depression, exercise is even more effective than antidepressants.

Certainly, if your concern is feeling old and getting fat, exercise is crucial. Although my experience has been that exercise doesn't actually help much with losing weight, it is absolutely critical to maintaining a healthy weight, because the higher your proportion of muscle to fat, the more body fat you burn, even when you are at rest.

You know those annoying people who seem to be able to eat whatever they want and never gain an ounce? Those are people who exercise and maintain a high proportion of muscle to fat. You don't need to become a body builder or a marathon runner to achieve that goal. Some form of movement half an hour a day, five days a week, will do it. My Maintenance Program can give you a good start, or you can experiment and design your own program.

That's what Aisha did. For about three months, we worked on reversing her arthritis through a clean diet, restoration of her microbiome, and healing her gut, all of which helped heal her immune system and reduce her inflammation. During that time, I gave her acupuncture, and I also had her doing the exercise plan that I recommend for you on your 2-Week Revitalize Program: stretching, fascia work, and some restorative yoga poses. Although her body wasn't ready for anything more vigorous, I wanted to start healing the fascia and opening up the tense, clenched places while we eased her joint pain.

Then, when Aisha could once again walk comfortably, I invoked our "30-day deal" and challenged her to find *some* type of movement that she enjoyed or was at least willing to do on a regular basis.

After a little experimentation, Aisha discovered a tango class—and suddenly, she was hooked. She loved the sensual and dramatic movements of the tango, and she found that she began relating to her body in a whole new way. Aisha had always shown a lot of courage in her personal life—starting a business, traveling the world—but now she began to feel that courage in her body, feeling sexy, open, calm, energized, and free as she moved across the dance floor, exploring what her body was capable of and discovering a side of herself that she had never really gotten to know.

And so Aisha began to see how the different types of movement I had recommended could actually empower her to make the most of life from her 40s on into her 80s and 90s. The strength training meant she could carry a suitcase or a bag of groceries instead of relying on someone else to do it for her. The aerobics gave her energy to dance, to do errands, to stride through a foreign city without getting tired. The core training kept her feeling grounded and secure, unafraid of sprains or falls. The stretching kept her open, flexible, and free of aches and pains. And the yoga kept her calm, serene, and able to clear her mind at the end of the day so she could wake up ready to face whatever challenges and joys the new day might bring.

What Aisha discovered is what I hope you will discover as well: movement is a big part of who we are. It's not about your pants size or what the scale says or how you look in a photograph. It's not about how many kilos you can bench-press or whom you can beat at squash. It's about using yourself—using all of yourself—and feeling like an active human in the world. And that's when you don't *feel* old, no matter what number your age might be.

Your body was never meant to be tight, cramped, and plagued with mysterious aches. It is designed to be open, flexible, and energetic. Through movement, you can move from feeling old and fat to feeling vigorous, healthy, and empowered.

You Don't Move Enough: Three Quick Fixes

1. Start small: move vigorously or briskly just 5 minutes a day, 5 times a week. Next week, add 5 minutes . . . and continue to do so until you're moving 30 minutes a day, 5 days a week.

2. Take 5 to 10 minutes a day, 3 days a week to do the fascia exercises on page 314. They'll be part of your Revitalize program, but go ahead and start them now—you'll immediately feel as though you just had a terrific massage!

3. Take 5 to 10 minutes every day to do the yoga poses on page 333. They, too, will be part of your Revitalize Program, but the sooner you enjoy their benefit, the better!

REASON #6:

YOU'RE STRESSED!

Callie was a quiet, thoughtful woman in her mid-50s whose life, until recently, had revolved around her job as an architect, her husband, and her three children. Although she had the usual demands of being a working mother, she told me that her life was rewarding and even inspiring most of the time.

Then Callie was struck with one challenge after another. First, her husband of 20 years fell in love with another woman and abruptly ended a marriage that Callie had thought was sound. Then her youngest child was diagnosed with learning disabilities, which sent Callie off on a long odyssey through the public school system trying to get him the help he needed. At around the same time, Callie's widowed mother began to develop Alzheimer's, and Callie—whose two brothers lived thousands of miles away—was left as the primary caretaker with the main responsibility for arranging her mother's care.

"Everything fell apart, and eventually, I did too," was how Callie described the situation. When she came to see me, she was exhausted all the time. Her menopause, which had been proceeding relatively easily, suddenly "turned bad," as Callie put it, and she began having hot flashes and sleepless nights. Her skin broke out. She gained 6 kilos "practically overnight."

Worst of all, Callie—always an upbeat, positive person—began to feel hopeless and helpless, to the point where her previous physician had diagnosed her as suffering from mild depression and had suggested Prozac. Callie hated the idea of being "permanently medicated," as she saw it, so she came to me, hoping for "a natural solution instead of a drug."

Although Callie's stressors had come more quickly and intensely than most, I had seen many patients in their 50s, 40s, and even younger who felt overwhelmed by stress and whose physical health seemed to suffer as a result. There was Dustin, a 35-year-old day trader who had been working 18-hour days to avoid the impending wave of layoffs at his company, and who had come to me with irritable bowel syndrome (IBS), sleep issues, and an extra 4 kilos, as well as a disturbing inability to focus. There was Sasha, a 43-year-old public relations specialist whose spate of difficult clients and demanding deadlines had triggered a series of migraines as well as gas so painful that it woke her up each night. And there was Nell, who at age 23 was so overwhelmed by the challenges of a rocky relationship and a new job that she gained 10 kilos in six months, was stuck with a seemingly perpetual cold, and suffered frequent bouts of crippling anxiety.

Clearly, in all of these cases, the stresses were real. And the emotional stressors were having a significant impact on the health of each person: Callie's exhaustion, hot flashes, and depression; Dustin's IBS, insomnia, and brain fog; Sasha's migraines and indigestion; Nell's perpetual cold and panic attacks, and all four patients' weight gain.

Yet when I considered each of these people, I saw other factors adding to their stress that none of them had taken into account. Each of them ate way more sweets and gluten than their systems could handle, which inflamed their bodies, challenged their guts, and imbalanced their microbiomes. Digestive issues inevitably followed, which in turn caused problems in their immune, endocrine, and nervous systems.

Likewise, none of these people got enough healthy fat, which kept their brains perpetually running on empty. A fat-starved brain can't organize healthy sleep for you. It falls prey to anxiety and depression, as well as to brain fog, forgetfulness, and a general inability to focus.

Although Dustin had once been an active squash player and Nell had been a diligent swimmer in college, both young people had let go of their athletic lives as soon as they got too busy. Callie told me she had never moved regularly; like many suburbanites, she drove everywhere and had no occasion to walk. Sasha described herself as a "gym rat," but I noticed that her routine was a stressful one of hard-driving aerobics or long-distance running, so that while the others were stressed by not enough exercise, Sasha was stressed by too much.

In short, whatever emotional stressors life had thrown at these four people, their level of physical stress was also chronic—and it was making their mental and emotional problems worse. In a truly vicious cycle, their diet and lifestyle were undermining their brains and spirits—which in turn drained them of the resources and resolve to improve their diet and lifestyle!

To make matters worse, if the stress continued—along with the inflammation it provoked— Callie, Dustin, Sasha, and Nell could eventually be facing far more serious chronic illnesses. As we have seen throughout this book, physical stressors on the body provoke inflammation, which creates first symptoms, then disorders. We wrongly attribute this process to aging, but in fact, what we're looking at is loss of function produced by months and then years of physical stress and inflammation.

Symptoms of Physical, Mental, and Emotional Stress

SHORT TERM

General: fatigue, weight gain, weight loss, sleep problems, hair loss

Digestive: gas, bloating, indigestion, constipation, loose stools

Hormonal: PMS, menstrual issues, symptoms of perimenopause and menopause, sexual dysfunction

Immune: perpetual colds and minor illnesses

Dermatological: acne and other skin eruptions

Nervous system: brain fog, anxiety, depression, memory issues, "senior moments"

LONG TERM

Autoimmune disorders, such as Hashimoto's thyroiditis, rheumatoid arthritis, lupus, multiple sclerosis

Depression

Diabetes

Heart disease

Irritable bowel syndrome

Migraine and tension headaches

The good news is that there is a solution—or rather, there are three solutions.

1. **Relieve the physical stressors on your body.** Follow the 2-Week Revitalize Program and the lifelong Maintenance Program so you are eating the foods your body craves, avoiding the foods that provoke problems, and getting the supplements, movement, sleep, and sense of community that you need.

2. **Find ways to relieve your mental and emotional stressors.** Figure out what you might want to change, whether it's a relationship, an aspect of your job, or some other part of your life. Of course, often you *can't* change or remove the stressor, but that brings us to my next suggestion.

3. **Find effective ways to cope with the stressors that you can't change.** Even when you can't change a stressor, you can always change how you respond to it. That doesn't mean you will necessarily like it, but you can find some responses that create less stress. You can also discover the stress busters and stress relievers that are right for you. This process of discovery can sometimes be a challenging journey in itself—but ultimately, a very rewarding one.

Some Effective Ways to Cope with Stress

- Give yourself two hours a week of "me time" to do something you really love or to unwind in a place that brings you peace and fulfillment.

- Take an "electronic sabbath" or at least an "electronic sundown": one day a week with no e-mail, text, or phone, or a time in the evening at which all electronics (including the TV) are turned off.

- Set some limits—find at least one task, obligation, or activity that doesn't inspire you and say no to it.

- Exercise (see Chapter 5).

- Listen to some music (see pages 94–95).

- Do a breathing exercise (see pages 95–96).

- Use guided visualization (see pages 97–99).

- Practice mindfulness (see page 99).

- Meditate (see pages 99–100).

- Do some tapping (see page 101).

- Take up tai chi, yoga, or some other type of "moving meditation" (pages 100–101).

- Renew your commitment to ubuntu (see Chapter 10).

When I laid out this three-pronged approach for Callie, she took a deep breath.

"Honestly?" she said quietly. "It sounds too good to be true. I'd like to believe you, but I just can't. Do you really think giving up sugar and taking a brisk walk is going to make a difference? Or meditating—just sitting in a chair doing nothing? Do you honestly think those things will help?"

"Honestly," I replied, "I do. I don't think those approaches will fix all the problems in your life—how could they? But I have seen it time and time again—if you give your body the support it needs, you immediately feel much, much better.

"Meanwhile, techniques like breathing, yoga, and meditation can make an extraordinary difference when it comes to finding the resources you need and seeing options that right now you can't even imagine. Those activities can make you more *resilient*—better able to handle all the challenges life throws at you and even better at coming up with creative, effective responses."

Callie thought it over and slowly nodded. "It sounds like a leap of faith," she said. "But then, what's my alternative? Nothing else has worked, so I might as well give your way a try."

I admired Callie's courage and openness to change, especially given all that she had been through. And I was excited to get her started on her "stress-busting journey" and see where it took her.

Myths to Break Through

- "Stress is primarily psychological—a matter of the mind and emotions."
- "Stress is generally negative and should be avoided."
- "Managing stress is so difficult that only a few lucky or 'enlightened' people can do it."

Myth: "Stress is primarily psychological—a matter of the mind and emotions"

Many of my patients begin their conversations with me by telling me that they are stressed. When I ask them to explain what kinds of stresses they have, their answers are inevitably about psychological challenges: "I have a difficult boss." "My husband and I aren't getting along." "I'm worried about how to pay my bills."

Those stressors are real, and as we shall see, they can have a significant impact upon your physical health. But I'm struck by the fact that almost none of my patients consider the *physical* stressors that are challenging their bodies, and, as a result, their minds:

- Too many sweets and starches, especially if you're carbohydrate intolerant
- Reactive foods or foods you can't tolerate, especially gluten and dairy
- Ongoing exposure to toxins in your food, water, and personal-care products
- An imbalanced microbiome
- Not enough exercise or, as in Sasha's case, too much
- Not enough sleep
- Too much caffeine
- Deficiency of nutrients
- Too many medications

In my clinical experience, when a patient supports his or her body with the food, supplements, movement, and sleep that it needs, all the other stressors become less severe.

Mind you, they are not necessarily less challenging to the mind and spirit. Eating a healthy diet does not erase the sorrow of losing a marriage or the worry of caring for an aging parent. Getting sufficient sleep does not make it less painful to watch your child struggle with an unsympathetic teacher or eliminate the very real financial challenges that so many of us face.

However, when your body is being supported instead of stressed, you are far better able to find the internal resources to deal with a problem—to be less reactive, braver, more clear headed, and more resilient. You are better able to see and act upon solutions that, in your state of hopelessness or panic, eluded you or seemed out of reach. And you are better able to handle the problems you cannot change with greater courage, determination, and grace.

So if you are feeling stressed, I urge you to begin by giving your body what it needs—especially since you need even *more* physical support when life is throwing emotional challenges at you. Follow the 2-Week Revitalize Program or the lifelong Maintenance Program at stressful times above all others. At the very least, cut back on sweets, starches, excessive caffeine, and unhealthy fats while making sure to take probiotics and a daily dose of healthy fat. Get some exercise, and treat your sleep as sacrosanct.

As I told Dustin, think of yourself as a top athlete preparing for the biggest game of your life. When life is giving you a lot to handle, you need all your physical and mental resources, just as an athlete does. The night before a big game is not the time to eat debilitating foods, skimp on vital nourishment, or short yourself on sleep!

The greater emotional challenges you face, the more physical support you need.

◆ — Stress Can Make You Fat — ◆

As we have seen, physical stressors contribute to weight gain by creating inflammation. Emotional stressors work in a similar way, since any type of emotional stress triggers a surge of cortisol, which, like excess insulin, inflames your body and cues it to retain fat.

This is not a matter of psychology but of biology. Animals, which presumably have only biology and no psychology, also gain weight under stress. Numerous animal studies have shown that when researchers stress lab animals—by crowding them into small cages, putting them on a small platform surrounded by water, or housing them with dominant, aggressive animals—the stressed animals gain weight compared to unstressed animals, even when both groups are given the exact same amount of food.

Animal studies have also shown that when animals feel dominated or powerless, they tend to eat fewer, larger meals, a pattern of consumption that promotes weight gain. By contrast, the dominant animals in the group tend to eat smaller, more frequent meals and to gain less weight.[1]

A fascinating review of both human and animal studies, conducted by social scientist Sally Dickerson and her colleagues, relates weight gain and the suppression of the immune system to both stress and shame. Basically, Dickerson found that if you feel powerless, subordinate, and/or ashamed, you are more likely to gain weight and/or get sick.[2]

This is why I believe so deeply in meditation, yoga, and the other stress-busting techniques I share at the end of this chapter. You can't always change your situation. But if you change your response to that situation—if you can dissipate the stress and regain a sense of power—you can greatly relieve your feelings of helplessness and shame. This can have extraordinary consequences for both your weight and your health.

Myth: "Stress is generally negative and should be avoided"

Now, even though I've just acknowledged all the ways stress can adversely affect your health, I want to be very clear on this point: stress itself is not necessarily a bad thing. In fact, often, stress can be a very good thing.

The stress that has such negative effects on our health is *chronic* stress—the type of stress that is unremitting and constant. Whether chronic stress takes the form of repeatedly eating an inflammatory food or continually facing an upsetting situation, it is taxing on our bodies and, if it continues long enough, can produce exactly the types of problems listed on page 85.

Acute stress, by contrast, is actually good for our bodies, minds, and spirits, as long as it's in proportion to what we can handle. When you challenge your body to climb up a mountain for a summer's hike, that is stressful—but it can also be profoundly satisfying. Your muscles welcome the exertion, while your whole body revels in the chance to move. When you reach the top of the mountain, you feel a profound sense of accomplishment and release. And when you awaken the next day, your muscles have grown stronger from being first stressed by the climb and then repaired during sleep.

Likewise, if you face a challenging project at your job—one that takes every ounce of your creativity and determination—you might emerge from the challenge feeling stronger and more powerful than before. Yes, it was hard work, but now you've learned how much you're capable of and what you can accomplish when you set your mind to it. Because of the way the stress has helped you grow, you become willing to take on even bigger and more demanding projects.

These types of reactions to stress—growth, increased strength, greater power—are called *hormesis* when they occur in the natural world. Hormesis is the process of challenging a plant with low doses of toxins or other stressors. In high doses, the toxins might kill the plant. In low doses, however, the plant "rises to the occasion" and becomes stronger. In fact, through hormesis, a plant creates more antioxidants and healing chemicals to combat the stressor, so the plant actually becomes more nourishing as well as stronger. I believe the same thing happens with humans.

A life without stress, without challenges and opportunities for growth, would be very dull indeed. The right kinds of challenges and stresses make life interesting and, ultimately, fulfilling—even, sometimes, inspiring. Certainly I find it more stressful and challenging to treat patients than to sit on my deck listening to music, but it is also infinitely more satisfying to help my patients find the health and strength they seek, and to solve the mysteries they sometimes present me.

So why are *acute* stressors challenging and exciting, while *chronic* stressors pose a major threat to our health? The answer lies in the structure of the nervous system.

◆——— YOUR NERVOUS SYSTEM: ———◆
TWO HALVES THAT WORK TOGETHER

When we look at how the body responds to stress, we begin with the *autonomic nervous system*. That is the part of our nervous system that regulates "automatic" processes—processes that we don't have to consciously control.

Your breath, for example, is regulated by your autonomic nervous system, which means that you keep breathing even when you aren't consciously thinking about it. Digestion is another function regulated by the autonomic nervous system: once you are done chewing and swallowing, everything your body does to the food happens without your consciously choosing it.

The autonomic nervous system has two halves: the *sympathetic* and the *parasympathetic*. The sympathetic nervous system regulates the stress response. We've nicknamed that response "fight or flight," but as we've seen, it can include any type of unusual exertion: pressing hard to meet a deadline, pushing a boulder out of your path, or any other type of short-term effort, whether mental, physical, or both. Whenever you have to rise to the occasion—to respond to an acute stress—the sympathetic nervous system provides you with the adrenaline and other stress hormones that you need to meet the challenge.

The parasympathetic nervous system regulates the relaxation response. Some people nickname the parasympathetic nervous system as "rest and digest," but this part of your nervous system also includes sexual response and the healing, restorative powers of sleep. When the parasympathetic nervous system is in charge, the stress hormones subside—before they have the chance to inflame your system—and other hormones take over. These other hormones help you digest your food, respond sexually, and heal your body while you rest, recover, and sleep.

So we're back to our old friend *balance*. The stress response is healthy when it is balanced by the relaxation response. You energize your body with a flood of stress hormones . . . and then you calm it down with some "rest, digest, and heal" hormones. You tear down your muscles during exercise . . . and then you build them back up, stronger than ever, while you sleep. You press hard to make a deadline . . . and then you take a nice, relaxing dinner break, eating your food in the calm and peaceful atmosphere that leads to optimal digestion.

When you face an acute stressor—whether it's climbing a mountain or finishing a project at work—the two halves of your nervous system balance each other. Even if it takes you three days to climb the mountain or three months to finish the project, you will find the stress healthy *if it continues to be balanced by rest and relaxation*. You climb for several hours—and then stop, relax, and make camp for the night. You work hard all day—and then stop, come home, and have a pleasant dinner with your family.

Those are the conditions under which stress is healthy. Even if you don't enjoy the stress— even if you have to attend an unpleasant meeting, visit a dying relative, or endure the frustration of a perpetually unsatisfied boss—your body and mind can handle the challenge *if* the stress is followed by a period of relaxation.

Keeping your stress and relaxation responses in balance—using both halves of your autonomic nervous system and not only one—is what keeps you from feeling old and getting fat.

It's what enables you to grow from stress and not be defeated by it.

That is why finding a way to relieve stress is so important. No matter what type of challenges fill your day—pleasant or unpleasant, freely chosen or imposed—you can find a healthy relationship to stress as long as you can let it go at the end of the day.

So how do you let go of stress? There are lots of ways, ranging from a simple shift in attitude to a regular yoga practice. Finding the stress busters that work for you is not always easy, but it can be incredibly rewarding when you do.

Once my patients understand how important it is to balance stress with relaxation, they are able to commit to their own individual forms of stress relief. I hope the same will be true of you. That's why I've devoted the rest of this chapter to sharing a wide variety of stress busters, so you can find the exact types of stress relief that fit your life.

Myth: "Managing stress is so difficult that only a few lucky or 'enlightened' people can do it"

Stress is such a prevalent part of our lives that it can easily seem as though there is absolutely nothing we can do about it. In fact, you have at your disposal a wide variety of ways to relieve stress, and if one doesn't work, another very likely will. You just need to find the approach that works for you.

The basic approach I like to take is embodied in the famous words of the serenity prayer. This three-sentence philosophy has been made popular by 12-step programs to treat addiction and codependence, but it was actually the creation of Reinhold Niebuhr, a German-American theologian, during World War II. Niebuhr was deeply disturbed by the horrors wrought by the Nazis in his ancestral land and found it nearly unbearable that he could do nothing to stop their devastating acts. The original words of the prayer were:

> God give me grace to accept with serenity the things that cannot be changed, courage to change the things which should be changed, and the wisdom to distinguish the one from the other.

Regardless of your religious beliefs or lack thereof, I think the premise of this prayer makes a lot of sense. As you look at the things that disturb you—whether it's the bad behavior of the driver who just cut you off in traffic, the frustrating actions of a colleague or boss, the painful behaviors of a child or spouse, or the policies of a government that you might not agree with—what can you really change? What's worth your energy to try to change? What must you accept? These are not easy questions, and wrestling with them is part of the burden—and the joy—of being human.

However, even asking the question—*"Can I change this, and is it worth my energy to try?"*—can often bring a measure of relief. Instead of feeling helpless, frustrated, or paralyzed with anger, you might find it liberating to simply consider whether the problem you face is within your power to change and worth the energy to try to do so.

Having asked the question, you can then take action. You might make a plan to change the problem that is bothering you: confront the boss, coworker, child, or spouse; leave the relationship; seek a promotion or a transfer to another office. Or you might make a plan for how to cope with it and perhaps even accept it:

- "Next time he does that, I'll take a deep breath, excuse myself to go to the bathroom, and call my friend Suzy, who will help me gain perspective."

- "Tonight, I'd better go for a run to work out all this stress—otherwise, I'll definitely have a tension headache tomorrow!"

- "When this happens again, I'll remind myself that I really love this person, and this is just one really unpleasant thing about her that I cannot change."

Reframing, shifting your focus, and *practicing gratitude* are all useful techniques for those situations in which you choose "acceptance." For example, if a driver cuts you off in traffic, and you find yourself really upset by his rude and dangerous behavior, you might relieve your anger by:

- **Reframing:** Imagine that he had a legitimate reason to hurry, such as getting his injured son to the hospital—since in that case, you would feel not angry but compassionate.

- **Shifting focus:** Praise yourself for your own good driving—"Wow, he came at me out of nowhere! Good for me for being so alert and able to respond so quickly. I'm actually very good at avoiding accidents, even when other drivers are behaving badly. I can really count on myself to stay safe on the highway." Now your focus is on positive qualities in yourself rather than anger against him. The stress hormones that shot up quickly in response to the sudden emergency will subside to a normal level before they have time to stress your body or make you fat.

- **Practicing gratitude:** "I'm so glad I'm okay. I'm lucky to have such good reflexes and such sharp eyes. I'm so glad this car responds quickly. I've got a lot to look forward to today—I'm so glad I'm going to be alive and well to experience it! The sun is shining, and I love the song that's playing on the radio now—I'm going to really enjoy those things for the next few minutes, because if that guy had hit me, I wouldn't be able to enjoy anything!"

A friend of mine, when she encounters coworkers or relatives who get under her skin, will often vent for a few minutes and then say, "Wow, can you imagine being that person? They must be miserable all the time—angry, frustrated, envious, anxious. I'm so glad I'm me and not them!" By summoning compassion, pride in herself, and gratitude, she's able to relieve the stress of feeling victimized or frustrated by someone whose behavior she isn't able to change.

Note that she doesn't excuse the behavior. If there is some action she is able to take, these responses help her do so—but in an empowered and compassionate way where she feels in control of her own behavior, rather than simply losing her temper, lashing out, and perhaps doing something she will regret. Instead of being *under* the situation, she finds a way to get *on top of* it and then choose her response, whether it's action, acceptance, or a combination of both. That is the power of the serenity prayer, which I see as a guide to choosing wisely, tapping into your own power, and, ultimately, relieving stress, even in situations as painful as the ones in which Reinhold Niebuhr—and Callie—found themselves.

⟡ MORE WAYS TO COPE WITH STRESS ⟡

Learn to say no. This can be hard, especially in a corporate culture where you are expected to make yourself available 24/7. I personally find it helpful to set strong limits; for example, I don't answer texts or e-mail after 9 P.M. because that's when I start winding down for the evening. This is certainly easier for me than for some people because I essentially work for myself, but I suggest that you at least explore the possibility that there might be times when you could refuse a task, turn down an invitation, or set a limit that buys you some more time, freedom, and stress relief.

Prioritize what's important. We so often get caught up in an endless round of chores, errands, calls to return, and e-mails to answer that we don't stop and ask ourselves, "What matters to me most?" If you allow yourself to keep asking and answering that question, you might find yourself with more time for the things that nourish and ground you: time with loved ones, a quiet half hour in nature, the chance to read an absorbing book. For most of us, there are always reasons to be busy and seemingly infinite demands on our time, so doing what we truly love rarely comes automatically—it takes work! Being clear about how you *want* to spend your time is at least a first step.

Try to surround yourself with people who don't stress you out! Of course, sometimes you don't have a choice. Still, the less you can be around people who upset you, the less stressful your life will be. If you have to spend time with stressful or upsetting people, try to balance it with time spent with nurturing, supportive, restorative people, whether in person or by phone, Skype, text, or e-mail. Plan a phone date with your best friend in the midst of a stressful family reunion. Make sure to set a date night with your partner at the end of a long, stressful week at work. During a challenging business trip, ask your support network to text or e-mail you once a day so you are in touch with the people who make you feel good about yourself and for whom you are grateful—balancing, once again, stress and recovery.

Don't "should" on yourself! We impose so much stress on ourselves by what we think we *should* do. Try as much as possible to choose what you want and believe in, rather than what you "should" do. When Callie was helping her mother find a live-in aide, for example, she frequently asked herself, "Would you rather *not* do this?" The answer always came to her, "No, even though my mother can sometimes drive me crazy, I want to help her." Of course, Callie would have preferred being able to do something more pleasant, but reminding herself that she was *choosing* to help her mother, rather than being forced to do so, helped relieve the stress.

Focus on what you have and are grateful for. So often, we take the good for granted and focus on the bad. It takes work to refocus your vision, but again, the rewards can be enormous. Recently I treated a patient who was undergoing enormous stress trying to get pregnant for the third time. Finally, I said to her, "Margaret, you have a wonderful husband and two beautiful children. I hope you can have the third child that you want, but even if you can't, you still have a terrific family. Why not focus on them?" Shifting her focus from what wasn't working to what was proved an enormous relief to Margaret, even though she also felt sad. Feeling sad wasn't stressful, however—it was simply sad. The stress had been caused by Margaret feeling powerless and victimized, instead of grateful and proud of the wonderful family she had helped build.

Be willing to believe that your life can get better—or at least, be willing to suspend your belief that it can't! This suspension of belief is what Callie called the "leap of faith," saying "*Maybe* things can get better, even though right now, I don't see how." Just being open to the possibility of a fulfilling future or a change in circumstance gives you the opportunity to see change when it's actually on the horizon and to make the most of it as soon as it appears.

⤙ COPE WITH STRESS THROUGH MUSIC ⤚

One of my most important forms of healing has been music. Growing up in South Africa, I was always angry about the apartheid system. Then, when I was 17, my father died. The loss made my anger even sharper and more painful. My intuitive solution was to listen to hard rock music, which helped me blow off stress, access my grief, and "accept the things I could not change," whether personal or political.

Ever since then, I've turned to music to relieve my stress. For much of my day, I need to be a rational person who takes charge of difficult situations and keeps everything under control. Listening to music allows me to balance rationality and control with emotions and surrender.

Music touches my emotional core in a way that I find to be extremely restorative and healing.

Many scientific studies have shown that music can have powerful stress-relieving effects.[3] It helps lower stress hormones, stimulate digestion, reduce muscle tension, decrease blood pressure, slow down brain waves, and enhance sexuality. In other words, it activates the parasympathetic nervous system: the part of your nervous system responsible for "rest and digest" as well as healing and sexual response. Music also stimulates endorphins, feel-good brain chemicals that produce a profound sense of well-being.

It's hard to believe that something as simple as music can have such important consequences for your health, but I'm here to tell you that both my review of the literature and my clinical experience affirm it's true. Find the music that lifts your spirits and soothes your soul, and figure out when you might like to listen to it: at work, on breaks, at meal times, in your car, as you drift off to sleep, or at other stressful moments. Your mental outlook is likely to improve—and so is your health.

⬥—— COPE WITH STRESS BY BREATHING ——⬥

When we get too busy and flustered we often forget to breathe and just be in the moment. When we stand back and become aware of our breathing, it helps calm the body and mind. This calmness helps us be more aware of our thoughts and feelings and not get swept away by them.

If you make a point of focusing on your breath, that is what we call *mindful breathing*. Mindful breathing helps relieve tension and restore energy. It is the perfect antidote to stress. The breath anchors us, reminds us to get out of our minds/thoughts and tune in to our bodies so we can bring awareness to our experiences. Quiet, mindful breathing helps us connect to every moment, which leads to better health. Most relaxation therapies and meditation techniques focus on the breath as part of the process.

Your first step is to notice how the rhythm of your breathing varies continuously. When you are upset, anxious, or exercising your breathing speeds up; when you are relaxed or sleeping, it slows down. Take a moment as you read these words to practice this form of awareness:

- Breathe shallowly and rapidly and see how you feel.

- Then breathe deeply and slowly and feel the difference.

- As breaths come and go, they teach you to let go and go with the flow.

The same could be said about your life: the events also come and go. Nothing stays constant. Everything is changing. It is not possible to control everything and be perfect. So remember to pay attention to your breath!

Here are a couple of easy breathing exercises you can do anywhere:

Abdominal Breathing

- Find a quiet spot where you won't be disturbed.

- Get into a relaxed position, whether lying down or sitting up.

- Put your hands on your abdomen.

- Close your mouth gently, touch your tongue to your upper palate, and breathe through your nose. If your nose is blocked for any reason, it is fine to breathe through your mouth.

- Inhale deeply and slowly into your abdomen (rather than your chest), being aware of your diaphragm moving downward and your abdomen expanding. Your hands on your abdomen will feel the expansion like a balloon filling.

- At the end of the inhalation, don't hold the breath, but exhale slowly, so your abdomen falls automatically as you exhale.

- Try to get all the breath out of your lungs on the exhalation. The exhalation should normally be about twice as long as the inhalation when you get relaxed.

- Repeat this, keeping your focus on your hands rising on your abdomen with inhalation and falling with exhalation.

Breathing to Release Tension

- Find a comfortable position.

- Do ten abdominal breaths.

- Imagine with your next inhalation that you are breathing into a tense area such as a tight neck, a strained lower back, your head, your buttocks, or wherever you may feel pain or tension.

- With the exhalation, let the tension go out of your nose along with the air.

- Keep repeating this until the pain or tension starts to ease.

Both of these breathing techniques activate the parasympathetic nervous system, so they are a great form of instant stress relief. They are especially good to do when you feel that stress is keeping you from thinking clearly, or just before you begin to eat. Besides being a great stress reliever, they can become one of your best weight-loss aids!

⬦—— COPE WITH STRESS THROUGH ——⬦
GUIDED VISUALIZATION

One of the most powerful resources you have is your own mind. When your mind is ruminating and obsessing over the unpleasant events that have happened in the past or the fearsome events that might happen in the future, it works against you, causing you to feel sad, anxious, and burdened by stress. When your mind is calm and aware, focused on the present moment and your experience of it, it can work for you, helping you relax and release your stress.

Callie liked the idea that her mind was a powerful resource, one that she could train to work for her and not against her. I'd love for you to also experience the power of the mind, so I invite you to try the following exercise.

The Power of Your Mind

1. Find a comfortable, quiet place to sit. Set the timer on your phone for two minutes.

2. Allow yourself to imagine an unpleasant situation, either something that has already happened or something that you fear might happen.

3. When the timer goes off, notice how your body feels. Have your muscles tensed? Are your fists clenched? How does your stomach feel? Your chest? Do you feel heavy or light? Also ask yourself how you feel emotionally—happy, sad, anxious, afraid?

4. Take a moment to realize that your mind has created both your physical and emotional state. Then set your timer for another two minutes.

5. Allow yourself to imagine a sexual situation—a situation in which you feel very attracted to someone and are really enjoying the experience. The situation can be a memory or a fantasy.

6. When the timer goes off, notice how your body feels. Be aware of as many physical details as you can. Then notice how you feel emotionally.

7. Take a moment to realize that your mind has once again created both your physical and emotional state. Then set your timer for the final two minutes.

8. Allow yourself to imagine a situation in which you feel completely content and at peace. It could be in a real place where you feel safe and happy, or a place that you can imagine.

9. Once again, when the timer goes off, notice how your body feels, and how you feel emotionally. Be aware that you have created all three feelings—being upset,

feeling sexual, and experiencing peace—simply through the power of your mind. Be aware also that in each case, your mind has had a powerful effect on your body.

Now that you can see how powerful your mind can be, let me give you some help in harnessing its power. Sometimes simply being aware of your body is enough to dissipate the stresses that life throws at you. The next time you get thrown by an upsetting event—an annoying e-mail, a pressing deadline, an unpleasant conversation—try this exercise in presence and awareness:

Mindfulness Exercise: Be Here Now

- Set a timer for two to five minutes. Commit to this exercise fully for that period of time.

- Ask your mind to focus entirely on your physical sensations.

- As you sit in your chair, feel how your back presses against the chair. Feel the backs of your legs and your buttocks.

- Notice your feet against the ground. Be aware of your heels, your toes. Which bear more weight?

- Bring your awareness to your skin. Feel the air against your bare skin. Feel your clothes as they lie against your covered skin.

- Notice your breath as it falls deep into your chest and as it rises again through your mouth and nose.

- Feel your blood rushing through your veins, and your heart beating in your chest.

- When your mind wanders (and it will), gently bring it back to being aware of your body and to feeling your body.

- Continue to be aware of your body and its sensations until the timer goes off.

The wonderful thing about this exercise is that you can do it at any time, just sitting in your chair—at home, at work, in a doctor's office. If you get an upsetting e-mail, for example, take a minute or two to exhale slowly and focus on your body. You'll see that your anger will dissipate, and you'll have gained a bit of perspective. You'll be able to ask yourself, "Is this his problem or mine?" and to make some space in which you can choose how to respond, not simply react.

I admit that this has not always been so easy for me to do. But as I have practiced slowing down, taking a breath, and tuning in to my body, I have become less reactive and also less stressed.

The key for me, I think, was coming to understand that I can't control other people, and sometimes I can't even control my environment. The one thing I *can* control is the way I respond to an upsetting situation: I can react with anger, or I can stop, breathe, focus, and observe my own reactions. Putting myself in the observer role gives me a measure of power—not necessarily over my circumstances, but over myself. It's a wonderful feeling to discover that you have more control than you think!

⟶ COPE WITH STRESS THROUGH MINDFULNESS ⟵

Mindfulness is an approach to life—an attitude of mind—that can bring profound relief from stress.[4] Most of us can't remain mindful every moment, but striving for mindfuless is surely a worthy goal. I am not always able to be mindful, but trying to be so as often as I can has helped keep every aspect of my life more balanced, rewarding, and sane.

My introduction to mindfulness came nearly twenty years ago when I did a workshop with Jon Kabat-Zinn, Ph.D. I highly recommend his first book, *Full Catastrophe Living*, which has had a lasting influence on me.

If you are intrigued by the possibilities of mindfulness, I have prepared a set of resources for you to explore further. Check out my website to learn more: www.bewell.com/blog/start-meditation.

Cope with Stress Through Meditation

Meditation is a technique that involves quieting your mind so that instead of thinking, recording, judging, reacting, you simply *be*. It is a deeply refreshing, relaxing experience that can bring enormous relief from stress. Although every meditation experience is individual—sometimes you feel peaceful, sometimes you feel angry or sad, sometimes you feel bored, and sometimes you don't feel anything at all—cumulatively, meditation can help bring you a profound sense of peace and acceptance.

This peace often creeps into your life in mysterious ways—one day, you simply notice that something you would once have reacted to with anger doesn't bother you nearly as much, or you see that you have become more resilient, or you start to feel more open and don't know why. I was very interested in getting Callie to meditate because I thought it would bring her relief from some of the tragic and difficult challenges she was facing, at a level that discussion and advice could not reach.

Personally I have always found it difficult to quiet my mind. I got into meditation through yoga, which I see as a moving meditation. If you'd rather meditate while moving, go on to the next section where I talk about yoga, tai chi, and other forms of moving meditation. But if you'd like to learn more about the type of meditation done while sitting still, check out www. bewell.com/blog/start-meditation for some suggestions.

A word of advice as you start your meditation journey: don't imagine that there is any way to get it "wrong." In our busy, overstimulated lives, simply spending 20 minutes sitting still and paying attention to the breath is tremendously beneficial. And the great teachers whose works I have read all agree: whatever experience you have of meditation is the one you needed. Your goal is not to achieve any particular result, but simply to repeat the practice, day after day after day, noticing whatever happens and letting it flow by.

◆——— Moving Meditation: Yoga and Tai Chi ———◆

Yoga is a type of movement developed in India whose goal is to "yoke" the mind and body. Tai chi is a Chinese martial art that also evokes profound mind-body unity. Both forms of movement require such concentration that they are considered forms of moving meditation. Both are also excellent ways to relieve stress, create serenity, and develop a sense of calm and peace.

I have been practicing yoga for the past 20 years. I like it because of its powerful stress-relieving benefits, and because of the way it teaches me to get out of my head and into my body. When I enter a yoga pose, I am reminded of the wise words of one of my wise mentors and teachers, the late Gabrielle Roth: "The quickest way to calm the mind is to move the body."

There are many different types of yoga and tai chi, so you've got lots of choices if you're interested in pursuing either practice. Both have enormous health benefits, over and above their stress-relieving powers: focused concentration, improved flexibility, better balance, increased core strength.

The wonderful thing about both practices is that it's not about being "the best" or doing it "the right way." Whatever you can do begins your experience of a new mind-body relation-ship—*your* mind-body relationship, and no one else's. Your focus is not on some external goal, but on your own ever-deeper connection to yourself. Connecting to your body can be a won-derfully stress-relieving haven in a very stressful world.

Even if you don't develop a full-scale yoga practice, you can benefit from even a single yoga pose, especially from the aspect of yoga known as *restorative yoga:* poses that are intended to restore your depleted energy and enable you to heal from the stresses and strains of daily life. In the Stress Reduction Practices section on page 327, I share with you three of my favorite restorative yoga poses created by yoga teacher, author, and illustrator Bobby Clennell.

Restorative yoga was developed by the late B. K. S. Iyengar, author of the classic book *Light on Yoga* and one of *Time* magazine's 100 most influential people of our time. He created restorative yoga by adapting classic yoga postures using props to help the body maintain the correct position without straining. With this practice, you get the effects of the poses without exerting any energy.

Restorative yoga is particularly helpful when you feel run down, burned out, stressed, or just tired. It's a powerful tool that supports the healing process during and after an illness or injury, when energy must be conserved for the body to heal. These supported poses along with sleep and rest are very important to the healing process. I have found restorative yoga to be both healing and revitalizing.

COPE WITH STRESS BY TAPPING

Tapping is an acupressure-based series of moves known more formally as Emotional Freedom Technique (EFT) that helps release stress quickly and relatively easily. The great thing about tapping is that you can do it just about anywhere. All you have to do is locate the specific points—around your eyes and eyebrows, chin, collarbone, underarms, and on the top of your head—and sharply tap them with your fingertips. The taps activate your body's energy stores and healing powers.

Many of my patients and colleagues have had excellent results with EFT. They tell me that it leaves them feeling empowered, knowing that they have a stress-busting tool that they can always rely on, no matter where they are or what is going on. To find out more about tapping, see Resources.

Relieving Stress in the Midst of Stress

Callie began her "leap of faith" by following my 2-Week Revitalize Program and continuing on to my lifelong Maintenance Program. She also began to explore her own personal journey of awareness and stress relief. She experimented with a variety of the techniques and approaches suggested in this chapter until she finally settled on the practice that was right for her: a quiet ten minutes in the morning when she sat alone in a sunny café near work and slowly sipped a cup of green tea, some abdominal breathing whenever she faced a stressful situation, a twice-weekly class in tai chi, and ten minutes in a restorative yoga pose every night.

When I last saw her, Callie told me frankly that she still felt enormous sorrow about her lost marriage. Watching her mother lose her memory was also "unbelievably painful," and battling her child's school was an ongoing source of frustration and distress. But as she faced all of these challenges, Callie had a quiet assurance, a kind of inner glow, that I hadn't seen before, and she sincerely thanked me for helping her discover these new resources.

"It's still a hard time—the hardest in my life so far," she said. "But before, I felt like I was drowning. Now I have the feeling that I'm swimming toward shore." I thought that image—moving slowly and steadily through pain and turmoil toward a calmer and more peaceful time—was an inspiring way to think about coping with stress and sorrow. I was happy that Callie had found both the physical and the emotional resources to help her on her journey.

You're Stressed!: Three Quick Fixes

1. Practice one of the breathing exercises that I share on pages 95–96.

2. Practice one of the restorative yoga poses that I share on pages 329–332.

3. Give yourself the gift of two hours full of exactly what you want to do: a walk, a concert, a visit to the spa . . .

REASON #7:

YOU'RE NOT GETTING ENOUGH SLEEP

Padma was a dignified, almost regal woman whose calm, authoritative manner seemed to fit her position as chair of the economics department of a local university. When she came to see me, however, she was distraught.

"Ever since I went through menopause, I have been unable to sleep," she told me. "It's driving me frantic! I fall off to sleep as usual, but then, night after night, I wake up. Sometimes I'm sweating or having a hot flash, but sometimes I'm merely—wakeful. If I do fall back asleep, a few hours later I'm up again."

She shook her head. "My last physician told me this is just what I must expect as I get older, but I am not willing to accept that. Nor do I want to rely on the sleeping pills she offered—they leave me feeling groggy and foggy. Please, Doctor, have you a better solution?"

Jerome was a New York–based independent video producer in his mid-30s who thrived on long hours, tight deadlines, and the wide variety of challenges his job threw at him. Then he picked up two new clients, one in San Diego and the other in Paris. Suddenly, he was shuttling between three different time zones and, as he told me, "My sleep has gone completely off the rails."

"Even when I don't travel, I can't fall asleep before two or three A.M.," he told me. "And no matter when I fall asleep, I'm almost always up at sunrise. Every so often, I'll sleep for like, 10 or 12 hours—and then I wake up tired. One of the guys in my company uses Ambien, but frankly, that scares me—I know it has lots of side effects, and when my grandmother used it, she became really confused and disoriented. Is there anything else I can try?"

Gina was a quiet, studious law student who had just landed her first summer internship at an environmental law firm. She loved feeling that she was making a difference in the issues that mattered to her, but she also felt under a great deal of pressure to match the long hours and intense work schedule of her fellow interns. She labored intensely at her computer until midnight each night—and then she couldn't fall asleep.

"This has never happened to me before," she told me. "I just lie there for hours, my mind racing, and then I feel like a zombie the whole next day. I'm mainlining caffeine but now even that is wearing off. Yesterday I almost nodded off at my desk—but then at night, I *still* couldn't fall asleep."

She looked at me with fearful eyes. "The thing is, Doctor, everyone in my office works a sixteen-hour day—at least! But if being a lawyer means never getting any sleep, I don't think I can hack it."

Padma, Jerome, and Gina are far from alone: Many of my patients show up with sleep problems. Indeed, statistics show that between 50 million and 70 million Americans have some type of difficulty sleeping. The market for prescription sleep aids keeps going up and up and up, with 58.5 million prescriptions dispensed in 2012, up 10 percent from 2007. The market for over-the-counter sleeping pills is equally out of control.[1]

The problem isn't even confined to adults: there appears to be an increasing number of teenagers and even children who are unable to fall asleep, stay asleep, or some combination of both. If this keeps up, we'll have to declare sleep an endangered species![2]

To my mind, lack of sleep is one of the most significant health problems we face today. If you are feeling old—senior moments; brain fog; lack of energy; perhaps even a loss of optimism, excitement, or joy—not getting enough good sleep might very well be at the root. If you are gaining weight, sleep problems could be a factor in that as well. Yes, you read that right—not getting enough sleep can literally make you fat!

Yet very few people recognize the serious toll taken by lack of sleep. Although virtually every one of my patients comes in with some kind of sleep deficit, many consider these problems "normal" and would not even mention them if sleep weren't an important section of our patient questionnaire. Padma, Jerome, and Gina were unusual not for having sleep issues but for recognizing that they did.

Do you also struggle to sleep peacefully through the night? If so, take heart: solutions *do* exist. But before we can find solutions, we have to understand the problem. So let me start by asking you a few simple questions about your sleep patterns.

How Well Do You Sleep?

- Do you wake up feeling tired rather than energized?

- Do you often wake up feeling as if you could sleep for hours more?

- Do you find that you don't have enough energy to get through the day comfortably without the use of sugar, caffeine, or other stimulants?

- Do you need coffee or some other form of caffeine to wake up?

- Do you need coffee or some other form of caffeine to stay alert throughout the day?

- Do you need to take long naps during the day?

- Do you feel "wired" instead of naturally tired at night when it's time for bed?

- Do you rely on sleep medications to fall asleep?

- Do you often lie in bed wishing you could fall asleep?

- Do you wake up frequently throughout the night?

If you have answered yes to even one question, you would probably benefit from improving your sleep—and if you answered yes to several, an improvement in sleep quality might significantly improve your health. So take a moment now to think about your overall relationship to sleep:

- Are you getting good, restful sleep each night, waking up energized and refreshed, and drawing on calm, focused energy throughout the entire day without the aid of sugar or caffeine?

- Or does your sleep generally fall short of that optimal level?

If you cannot honestly say that you consistently get great sleep that leaves you full of energy, you run the risk of getting "old and fat before your time"—and perhaps of creating a significant health problem as well.

Here's the type of sleep your body needs to function at its peak:

- You fall asleep easily each night and wake up easily each morning, ideally without relying on an alarm but only on your own natural rhythms.

- You sleep through the entire night, or if you get up to use the bathroom or for any other reason, you fall right back to sleep.

- In the morning, you wake up relaxed, energized, and refreshed.

- You have a sense of calm energy that carries you through the day, so you don't need sugar, caffeine, or other stimulants to keep you awake, alert, and at your peak.

So, is that you? Or does that description sound like an impossible ideal, so far from what your own days and nights are like that it's almost laughable?

Far-fetched as it might seem right now, that type of reliable, restful sleep and calm, sustained energy *is* within your power—and it's exactly what I want for you. As I said at the beginning of this book, I don't want you feeling just okay; I want you feeling terrific! Getting enough good, restful sleep is an absolute precondition for remaining slim, vigorous, and vital.

Lack of sleep contributes to many of the symptoms you might mistakenly attribute to aging: increased weight, slower metabolism, memory issues, and brain fog.

If you want to avoid the chronic diseases we associate with aging—diabetes, heart disease, cancer, memory loss, and dementia—your prescription might be this simple: get good sleep!

Fortunately, if you follow the suggestions in the first six chapters of this book, you're well on your way to sleeping soundly throughout the night. Diet, supporting your microbiome, healing your gut, moving, and finding ways to de-stress will all pay off enormously when you turn out the lights. Addressing any adrenal or other hormonal imbalances will make a huge difference as well.

To fix anything else that's keeping you up at night, read on.

How Lack of Sleep Makes You Feel Old and Fat

- Impaired memory
- Loss of mental clarity
- Low moods: feeling irritable, helpless, easily frustrated, anxious, and/or depressed
- Increased physical and emotional stress
- Decreased ability to tolerate physical and emotional stress
- Decreased immune function
- Tendency to gain weight and difficulty losing it
- Increased tendency to inflammation, increasing the chances of a chronic disease
- Decreased lifespan
- Increased risk of mortality

The Culture of Insomnia

Sometimes as I try to help my patients get more and better sleep, I have the feeling that I am going completely against the grain. Our culture values working hard and being productive, while rest, relaxation, and restoration are held in something very close to contempt.

For example, when I suggested to Jerome that he might consider taking one day every week to do absolutely no work but simply to relax and re-energize, he looked at me as though I'd advised him to run off and join the circus. "I don't have time for that," he said briefly. "I can barely keep my clients happy as it is."

Likewise, when I prescribed for Gina an "electronic sundown"—no electronics of any kind after 10 P.M.—she appeared horrified. "It just doesn't work that way," she said, shaking her head. "Those guys in my office all work around the clock. If they send me a text or an e-mail at midnight, they want an answer by twelve-fifteen."

And when I asked Padma when she had taken her last vacation, she simply seemed bewildered. "When I am not teaching, that is when I have time to do my research," she said seriously. "I enjoy it, but it is not a vacation as such."

Their responses remind me that in our society, we privilege our sympathetic nervous system—the "fight or flight" response—far above our parasympathetic nervous system's "rest and digest." We saw in Chapter 6 how an imbalance between stress and relaxation creates multiple problems for our bodies, minds, and spirits. Such an imbalance also makes it very difficult to get good sleep.

I was reminded of our American overvaluing of work the last time my wife and I went to Spain. There, people work hard—very hard—but they also take a two-hour lunch in the middle of the day, a time when most businesses shut down and the "rest and digest" function is paramount. They take vacations too; almost everyone gets four paid weeks, a full month to refresh, restore, and relax. No wonder their rates of chronic disease are so much lower than ours! No wonder, too, that in their culture, sleep is far from an endangered species.

Of course, we doctors often set the worst example. Many of my colleagues short themselves on sleep, so how can they recognize its importance to their patients? They are far more likely to prescribe a stimulant, a sleep aid, or even an antidepressant than to suggest that their patients commit to good sleep.

Yet sleep is when your body recovers from the stresses of the day. If you're not sleeping properly, all sorts of things go wrong. Even if you have the best diet in the world and are getting ideal amounts of exercise, too much stress and too little sleep will ultimately make you old and fat—no matter what your biological age might be.

Myths to Break Through

- "Sleep isn't so important."

- "Sleep doesn't affect my weight."

- "I can make up for a lack of sleep during the week by getting extra sleep on the weekend."

- "Sleeping pills—either prescription or over the counter—can be effective ways to restore good sleep."

- "What I do during the day does not affect my sleep at night."

Myth: "Sleep isn't so important"

So many of my patients view sleep as a useless endeavor—a waste of time that they might otherwise use to meet a deadline, finish a household task, or watch a favorite TV show. But sleep isn't an empty, unproductive time—your brain and body are actually very active.

One of the most important things that happens while you sleep is that your body secretes human growth hormone (HGH), a natural "fountain of youth." HGH is what your body produced when you were a child and adolescent, helping spur muscle growth and regulate metabolism, among other key functions. The anti-aging effects of human growth hormone are so powerful that some people even inject doses as adults.

While I have some significant concerns about artificially supplementing HGH, I am completely in favor of helping your body's *natural* production of this vital substance. Why pay for an expensive injection and risk dangerous side effects when you can simply turn out the light and crawl into bed?

By the way, the other natural means of boosting HGH is through intense exercise. So, as we saw in Chapter 5, good sleep and lots of movement literally help keep you young!

But secreting HGH is only the beginning of the story. Your body performs a number of other key functions that it can manage only while you are sleeping:

- **Muscle repair.** When you exercise, muscles break down. Then they rebuild, growing larger and stronger—but only during sleep. If you are working out each day but not sleeping at night, you are sabotaging your own efforts.

- **Brain chemistry balance.** When you face a stressful challenge, your brain uses up supplies of key amino acids and other biochemicals. Sleep is when you restore them, preventing you from feeling irritable, overwhelmed, or depressed. That's why you need *more* sleep, not less, when you are working extra hard.

- **Removal of toxic waste from your brain.** A part of our body known as "the glymphatic system" is responsible for clearing toxins from your brain. This system is active only during sleep, so if you don't get enough sleep, your brain suffers.

- **Immune support.** A whole library full of studies links lack of sleep to chronic disease. For example, one group of researchers found that three out of ten healthy young adults in their study became prediabetic after only four days of disturbed sleep.[3] I myself have noticed that if I miss sleep—such as when I travel or have too much going on—I'm more likely to become run down and get a cold.

- **Hormonal balance—including sex hormones.** My female patients tell me that when they're short on sleep, hot flashes and other menopausal symptoms are far more likely to kick in. Lack of sleep can also hurt your sex life: some 26 percent of the people in a National Sleep Foundation poll reported that their sex lives suffer because they're so tired—not surprising when we consider that men who don't get good sleep may be at risk for lower testosterone levels. One high-energy patient, a woman of 42, told me that the only time she and her husband feel like having sex is when they're on vacation. "It's one of the things that makes me feel old," she admitted. I immediately "prescribed" some good sleep for them both—and was rewarded with a grateful call a few weeks later.

- **Pain relief.** If you skimp on sleep, your pain threshold tends to drop, turning minor pains into major ones. Remember: your parasympathetic nervous system helps your body rest, digest—and heal. If you don't give that system "equal time" with your stress-oriented sympathetic nervous system, those aches and pains will have you feeling old before you know it.

- **Memory boosts.** If you're worried about senior moments or memory lapses, a lack of sleep could be to blame. Sleep is when you consolidate your memories, which means that without sleep, your brain has a harder time processing, storing, and, ultimately, retrieving information. Give your brain the sleep it needs—and enjoy the sharp focus and ready memory that you thought were gone forever.

As you can see, sleep is essential for every system in the body. And so, once again, we are back to our old idea of *balance*. During the day, you wear your body out: tearing down your muscles, using up your brain's amino acids and other biochemicals, challenging your immune system, depleting your resources. At night, while you sleep, you build your body back up: repairing and perhaps even growing your muscles, restoring your brain chemistry, supporting your immune system, replenishing your resources. It's fine to exert yourself during the day, but you must balance that exertion with rest—the deep, restorative rest that can happen only while you sleep.

Restoring Your Body Through Balance

Day	Night
Sympathetic nervous system	Parasympathetic nervous system
Stress	Relaxation
Exertion	Rest
Muscle breakdown	Muscle repair
Hormones used up	Hormones restored
Toxins accumulated	Toxins cleared
Brain chemicals depleted	Brain chemicals replenished

◆——— LACK OF SLEEP MIGHT LITERALLY ———◆ SHRINK YOUR BRAIN

I've always known that our brains need sleep to function properly. I was alarmed to discover, however, that lack of sleep might literally shrink and/or atrophy your brain.

A recent study published in *Neurology* involved giving MRI scans to 147 adults. Researchers found that if someone wasn't getting good sleep, portions of his or her frontal cortex tended to be small or atrophied. This is especially disturbing because the frontal cortex is your brain's "executive command center," the portion of your brain where you analyze, evaluate, and decide, suggesting that when you short yourself on sleep, your brain is literally less capable of rational thought. If you're in a job where you need to make logical, intelligent decisions, depriving yourself of sleep is going to hurt your productivity in a big way.

Researchers reported that sleep-related brain shrinkage was especially noticeable among those who were over 60. Clearly, then, brain dysfunction that you might attribute to age is at least partly due to lack of sleep—perhaps even entirely due to it. Some research suggests that poor sleep might also be associated with an earlier onset of Alzheimer's.[4]

Myth: "Sleep doesn't affect my weight"

By this point it should not surprise you to learn that Padma, Jerome, and Gina had all gained considerable weight during their sleepless nights. Lack of good sleep disrupts your metabolism and hormonal balance in a number of ways—each of which tends to reinforce the other:

- **Too much cortisol.** Lack of sleep is a stressor . . . stress stimulates cortisol . . . and cortisol cues your body to retain fat. Excess cortisol also disrupts your insulin response, which further cues your body to retain fat.[5]

- **Insulin resistance.** Excess cortisol can throw your insulin out of whack, so your excess hunger is often a craving for sweet, starchy foods—which can then set off a sugar addiction (see Chapter 1).

- **Not enough glucagon.** Just as insulin cues your body to store fat, glucagon tells your body to burn it. Lack of sleep means you don't have enough glucagon to keep that fat burning.

- **Decreased adiponectin.** Adiponectin is a hormone that promotes insulin sensitivity and helps you break down fat. It also decreases inflammation and supports cardiovascular function. Less sleep means you lose those benefits—and gain weight.

- **Not enough leptin.** Leptin is the hormone that causes you to feel full. When your leptin levels are low, you don't feel full as soon as you should, and as a result, you eat more.

- **Too much ghrelin.** Ghrelin is the hormone that causes you to get hungry. When your ghrelin levels are high, you feel hungrier than you should, and again, as a result, you eat more.

- **Insufficient human growth hormone.** HGH improves your fat metabolism, so when its levels drop, your weight might rise. You make this "fountain of youth" hormone during the deepest stage of sleep. So it's not enough to get sleep; you have to get *deep* sleep, which requires a long, uninterrupted night.

- **Leaky gut.** During sleep, your body rebuilds your gut walls. Lack of sleep brings on leaky gut, inflammation, and an imbalanced microbiome—and all the symptoms that result, including weight gain (see pages 39–40). Moreover, you rely on your gut and microbiome to make the biochemicals that your brain needs to orchestrate sleep. So once again, we're back to balance: you need sleep to heal your gut, and you need a healthy gut to enable sleep.

- **Disrupted body clock.** Researchers working at the University of Manchester have discovered that when your body clock is disrupted, you develop inflammation—which cues your body to hold on to fat.[6] A protein known as *REVERB* is also linked to your body's clock—and REVERB helps regulate both adiponectin and inflammation. As a result, when your body's clock is thrown off—through irregular sleep cycles, changing time zones, or insufficient sleep—a number of interlocking factors keep you holding on to fat.

So here's your takeaway:

Lack of sleep can make you feel old and fat.

Good, restful sleep keeps you vigorous, energized, and at a healthy weight.

Myth: "I can make up for a lack of sleep during the week by getting extra sleep on the weekend"

Many of my patients assure me that while they skimp on sleep all week long, they make up for it on the weekends.

Unfortunately, our bodies don't work that way. So besides *balance,* we also have to look to the concept of *rhythm.*

Our body's most important rhythm is sleep. Like our other rhythms, sleep is meant to be tied to the rhythms of nature. If we are not sleeping when it's dark and waking when it's light, we will soon feel old and get fat—no matter what our biological age.

Sleep begins each night with the secretion of *melatonin,* an essential hormone that tends to make us drowsy and to produce deep, restful sleep. Your body is cued to produce melatonin when your eyes can't see any light, even behind the eyelid, which is why a completely dark bedroom is so essential for good sleep. (If you can't darken your bedroom completely, get an eye mask.)

Even the small amount of light from a laptop or a phone can disrupt your body's production of melatonin, which is why you want to keep all electronics out of the bedroom. And of course, if you stay up late, working on your computer, as Gina did, or watching TV, as Jerome did, your melatonin production doesn't get started early enough, because the blue light from the electronic screens is telling your body, "It's daylight—no need for melatonin yet!" even if it's actually two in the morning.

Remember how in Chapter 4 we saw that optimal cortisol levels fall into a daily rhythm— peaking in the morning to wake you up and then falling gradually, all day long, until it's finally time for sleep. Optimal melatonin levels follow an opposite rhythm, beginning to rise as the sky darkens and falling in response to the light.

Thus your body is keyed to the rhythms of nature—sunrise and sunset. When you break that rhythm, you throw off your production of hormones, particularly cortisol and melatonin, with disastrous consequences for your weight, your energy levels, and your overall health.

This, by the way, is why jet lag is such a potent disrupter of sleep; it throws off your natural rhythms. Your internal clock is designed to be in sync with nature's big clock: melatonin rising when darkness falls, and falling when the sun rises. Break that rhythm—through jet lag, night shifts, or just a late night of TV—and your whole body suffers.

Finally, a great deal of the aging process occurs through *oxidation*—the process that "rusts" your cells and causes them to decay. Not only is melatonin one of your most powerful antioxidants; it also magnifies the effectiveness of other antioxidants. But if you're not shutting down the blue light at night and sleeping in a completely dark bedroom, you're not getting all the melatonin your body needs.

ARE YOU RESPECTING YOUR INTERNAL CLOCK?

One of the most fascinating developments of the past few decades has been the discovery of the suprachiasmatic nuclei (SCN), a group of cells keyed to respond to the light that enters your eye.

If you spend your days indoors and your nights in front of an electronic screen, you never see either natural light *or* natural darkness. Your internal clock has lost its bearings, and your body suffers.

Animal studies suggest that clock disruption might affect sex hormones as well as other aspects of our physiology. According to an article in *Environmental Health News*:

> In the wild, light pollution causes hatchling sea turtles to lose their way from beach to the ocean, and disorients Monarch butterflies searching for migration routes.
>
> In field experiments, Atlantic salmon swim at odd times, and frogs stop mating under skies glowing from stadium lights at football games. Millions of birds die from collisions with brightly lit communication towers, and migratory flocks are confused by signals gone awry.[7]

It's easy to forget that we are animals too—but we are. If turtles, salmons, frogs, and birds are confused by clock disruption, I have to believe that we suffer from it as well.

IN SYNC WITH THE RHYTHMS OF LIFE

Many years ago, my Chinese medicine teachers, Efrem Korngold and Harriet Beinfield, taught me a valuable lesson:

The microcosm mirrors the macrocosm.

That is a powerful notion: each of us individual humans—the microcosm, or "small world"—mirrors the whole planet, the macrocosm, or "big world."

What does this mean? It means that we cannot really achieve optimal health until we see ourselves as part of the larger planet on which we live. The rhythms of our world—sunrise, sunset, and the changing of the seasons—have a profound effect on the rhythms of our bodies. If we ignore those rhythms we compromise our health.

This concept only really sank in about 15 years ago, as more and more patients came to me feeling exhausted, overwhelmed, depressed, achy, run down, and older than their years. These patients were falling through the cracks of Western medicine because they didn't have a recognizable disease. I started calling these patients "spent," because that was how they seemed to me.

I realized that the only time I had *not* seen patients with these symptoms was when I worked "in the bush" 35 years ago, in KwaNdebele, an impoverished rural area in South Africa. There I saw many diseases arising from poverty and malnutrition, but I didn't see anyone who was "spent," as I do today in New York City or as I did when I worked in South African cities.

So what did KwaNdebele have that the urban areas did not? In those days, rural South Africa had no electricity, indoor heating, or refrigeration. People were forced to go to bed when it got dark, to rise with the sun, and to eat whatever foods were available in season. They lived in accordance with the cycles and rhythms of nature—because they had no choice.

Their microcosms were in tune with the macrocosm. Ours are not—and we are paying the price. As part of the natural world, we too must be governed by the global forces of nature. Like the tides and the foliage, our bodies must also change in rhythm with the days and the seasons. When we disrupt that connection, we feel old and get fat.

Of course, I couldn't tell my patients to go live in a hut without electricity. Nor did I want to do so myself! But I began following more regular rhythms in my life—sleeping as soon as possible after it got dark and rising as soon as possible after the sun came up. I observed an "electronic sundown"—no TV, computer, phone, or other electronics for the last two hours before bedtime. I learned to respect the rhythms of nature—and my body began to function better. So did the bodies of my patients who followed my advice.

So now, after more than 35 years of practicing medicine, I am thoroughly convinced of the importance of rhythm to health. The way nature unfolds and evolves is through rhythmic patterns, and our bodies are organized that way as well. Respecting your natural rhythms can keep you from feeling old and getting fat.

Respect Your Natural Rhythms

- As much as possible, go to sleep at the same time each night and wake up at the same time each morning.

- If you're short on sleep one day, try to return to your normal bedtime and wake time as soon as possible, rather than sleeping late or taking a nap.

- Observe an "electronic sundown": avoid all electronic devices for at least two hours before bedtime.

- Keep electronic devices out of the bedroom, including your phone (or put it on airplane mode while you sleep).

- Keep your bedroom as dark as possible, since any amount of light disrupts melatonin production. If you can't manage a completely dark bedroom, wear a sleep mask.

- Try to get some exposure to bright, natural light during the day.

- Avoid fluorescent light, especially at night—it disrupts your body's biological clock.

- If you must fly across time zones, try taking some melatonin when it would be night at your new destination and getting some daylight in the morning of your new destination. If you can tolerate coffee, have some when it is morning in your new destination, so you feel awake and alert. Try your best to get onto a regular schedule in your new time zone as soon as possible.

Myth: "Sleeping pills—either prescription or over the counter—can be effective ways to restore good sleep"

Most Americans are not aware that we are having a sleep crisis—but the numbers tell a different story. Nearly 9 million Americans take prescription sleep aids, pushing the 2011 sales of generic Ambien (zolpidem tartrate) up to $2.8 billion, while in the same year, prescription aid Lunesta sold $912 million.[8]

Side Effects of Zolpidem: Active Ingredient in Ambien and Other Sleep Aids

- Addiction or dependency
- Agitation
- Sleepwalking
- Drowsiness during the day and/or while driving
- Dizziness
- Hallucinations
- Worsening depression
- Alzheimer's

In addition to the side effects associated with normal use, sleep aids can become dangerous when taken with narcotic pain relievers, antianxiety drugs, or sedatives. Combining sleep aids and alcohol—including beer or wine—can also be hazardous.

A disturbing new study came to light as I was preparing this book, associating a class of drugs known as *benzodiazepines* with a significantly increased risk of Alzheimer's and other forms of dementia. Common drugs in this category include Valium (diazepam), Xanax (alprazolam), Klonopin (clonazepam), Ativan (lorazepam), and Ambien (zolpidem). These drugs are often prescribed as antianxiety meds and for some other purposes as well as to promote relaxation and sleep. A large-scale study conducted among Quebec residents over the age of 66 found that long-term use of these medications was closely enough associated with dementia that it "should be considered as a public health concern."[9]

Even when taken alone, sleep aids don't give you such terrific sleep. Many are *anticholinergic,* meaning that they suppress REM (rapid eye movement) sleep, your body's deepest and most restful form of rest.

The real irony is that these expensive and potentially dangerous medications don't actually net you that much more sleep. An NIH analysis of sleep-aid studies found that when compared with placebos, these meds reduce the time it takes you to fall asleep by just under 13 minutes, on average, so that your total sleep time increases by slightly more than 11 minutes.[10] However—perhaps because of the way insufficient sleep can distort your memory—people *believed* they had gotten more than an hour's extra sleep.

Myth: "What I do during the day does not affect my sleep at night"

I hear this myth all the time from my patients who don't understand why a double latte in the morning or a stressful meeting in the afternoon should have any impact on their ability to fall asleep—or stay asleep—at night.

Yet what you do during the day might be the most important factor in your sleep at night. If you want to be sound asleep by 10 or 11 P.M., sleeping deeply all through the night, you might need to make some changes earlier in the day.

Daytime Sleep Disrupters

- Caffeine
- Sugar
- Stress
- Lack of movement
- Too much artificial light/not enough bright daylight
- Evening exposure to electronic light and fluorescent light
- Wine or a drink at dinner or in the evening

Note: These things affect both your ability to *fall* asleep and your ability to *stay* asleep. If you are having sleep problems of any kind, eliminating these sleep disrupters might well be your solution.

◈—— THE CAFFEINE CONNECTION ——◈

Caffeine can be one of the most powerful factors affecting your sleep, altering your body's function for many hours after you consume it. Your liver has to clear caffeine from your body, and some people are fast caffeine metabolizers whose livers get rid of caffeine quickly while others metabolize it more slowly.

To some extent this is genetic. But remember: your liver is also charged with clearing many other substances, including medications, alcohol, and environmental toxins. The harder your liver has to work on those, the less efficiently it can clear caffeine.

Even if your liver is working in peak condition, caffeine might speed up your heart rate, stress your adrenals, and raise your cortisol levels, all of which can have profound effects on your ability to fall asleep, stay asleep, and sleep as deeply as you need. For many of us, myself included, even a morning coffee is enough to throw off an entire sleep cycle.

When I suggested to Jerome and Gina that they cut out the caffeine, they both insisted that their morning and afternoon coffees, sodas, or energy drinks couldn't possibly affect what happened to them after 10 P.M. Yet both of them noticed an immediate improvement when they made the transition to water and herbal tea. Not only were they sleeping longer, but they also began sleeping *better*—more deeply, more restfully, so that they woke up energized and refreshed instead of groggy and fatigued.

Padma, too, insisted that caffeine had no effect on her sleep cycle, pointing out that she could always *fall* asleep—she just couldn't *stay* asleep. But she, too, noticed a significant difference once the caffeine had cleared from her system. "I am sleeping even better than I did as a student," she told me. "I can feel that my sleep is going *deeper* somehow, as though I am really getting an extra layer of rest."

There is actually a great deal of contradictory literature on caffeine, suggesting both that it has some benefits and that it can pose some risks to your health. As with so many health questions, it's an individual matter. However, until you cut out the caffeine completely, you might not realize the subtle or not-so-subtle ways it is affecting your sleep, your energy levels, and your mood.

Is Caffeine Disrupting Your Body?

- Do you have any difficulty falling asleep or staying asleep?
- Do you wake up groggy, foggy, or not fully rested?
- Do you have good, calm energy throughout the day?
- Do you frequently feel anxious?
- Do you frequently feel irritable?
- Do you need a long nap to restore your energy?

- Do you need caffeine, sugar, or another stimulant to restore your energy?
- Do you feel frantic when you haven't had your caffeine "fix"?
- Does even the thought of giving up caffeine make you anxious?

If the answer to any of these questions is *yes,* try this experiment: give up caffeine for four weeks and see if it affects the quality of your sleep and of your daytime energy. (See page 191 for some suggestions on how to let go of caffeine.) Your experience will help you decide whether to add caffeine back into your diet and, if you do, in what amounts.

Because caffeine might be playing a larger role than you think—in disrupting your sleep, affecting your mood, and challenging your adrenals (see Chapter 4)—I encourage you to cut out all sources of caffeine at least for your 2-Week Revitalize Program. That includes coffee, caffeinated tea, sodas, energy drinks, and chocolate. (Don't worry—I help you make the transition and avoid withdrawal symptoms on page 191.)

After you've lived caffeine free, you might find that you really enjoy the deeper sleep and calmer days. Or you might discover that an occasional cup of coffee or tea works well for you. You might also find that you can tolerate caffeine better when you are well rested or relaxed, and that you need to avoid it when you are stressed or tired. Going without caffeine for a while will help you learn what your body needs to function at its peak.

Stress and Sleep

Stress, as we have seen, has profound effects on our entire anatomy, and that includes our ability to fall asleep, to stay asleep, and to sleep deeply.

Gina, for example, had trouble falling asleep—partly because of her late-night exposure to electronic screens, partly because of the stress caused by her job. I, by contrast, can almost always fall asleep, but I notice that when I am under a lot of stress, it will sometimes cause me to wake up earlier than usual, costing me sleep on the other end.

The solution, I believe, is to find effective ways to de-stress, particularly on days that have been more challenging than usual:

- **Exercise** is a great way to blow off steam and set yourself up for healthy sleep.
- **Meditation**—during the day or before bed—can release stress and invoke the healthy balance of the parasympathetic nervous system (see pages 99–100).
- **Breathing exercises**—immediately after a stressful challenge or, again, at the end of the day—can also help release stress and support the parasympathetic nervous system (see pages 95–96).

- **Yoga**—particularly *restorative yoga*—can relieve stress and support healthy sleep. (For some restful yoga poses, see page 329).

Just as a morning coffee can keep you up at night, a morning workout, meditation, breathing exercise, or yoga session can help you sleep at night. As you become more attuned to your body, you will come to know when you need to bring in these de-stressing tools and which ones work best for you.

◆——— WAKEFUL WINE ———◆

Alcohol does help you fall asleep—but then, as your body breaks it down, alcohol can wake you up or cause you to sleep less deeply. The net effect of alcohol is usually sleep loss, which becomes even worse if you make your nighttime drink a habit: the sleep-inducing effect wears off, but the sleep-disrupting effect remains.

So if you can handle an occasional drink, feel free to enjoy—but definitely don't use liquor as a sleep aid. And if you're having trouble sleeping, I'd advise cutting out all alcoholic beverages for a while, since they are very likely part of the problem.

◆——— WATCH OUT FOR BEDTIME SNACKS ———◆

Ideally, you'll stop eating at least three hours before bed so your digestive process doesn't interfere with your sleep. If you must eat later than that, be sure to avoid foods that might make it hard to either fall asleep or stay asleep:

- Sweet and starchy foods, including fruit, bread, crackers, pretzels, and potatoes

- Cereals

- Chocolate

Likewise, stop drinking any type of liquid two to three hours before bedtime so you aren't awakened by having to use the bathroom in the middle of the night.

◆——— HOW MUCH SLEEP DO YOU NEED? ———◆

Patients ask me this question all the time, and I always have the same answer: *it depends.* Research suggests that most of us need seven to nine hours of sleep, though this can vary both by the individual (some people need more, some less) and by the circumstances (during times of stress, intense creativity, or intellectual effort, you might well need more). Generally, you need more sleep when you're younger and less as you age. I have seen people who do very well on six, and people who definitely need at least nine.

Be aware that the amount of sleep you can "get by on" is not necessarily the amount of sleep you *need*. For one thing, unless you fall asleep the moment you turn out the lights, you are likely getting less sleep than you think, since you are probably counting from "lights out" rather than from when you actually fall asleep. Be aware, too, that your need for sleep may vary depending on what you eat, how much you exercise, and how stressed you are by physical, emotional, or intellectual challenges.

If you learn to listen—really listen—to your body, you will discover that it lets you know what it needs, but this listening might take some practice, especially if you are not used to thinking of your body in that way. I myself have had to work on this over the years, especially as it went so counter to the somewhat macho training that we all received in med school and residency, where barreling through on three or four hours of sleep, in complete disregard of our bodies' cries for food, water, and sleep, was an integral part of the medical culture.

What I found, however, was that once I began to listen to my body, I was far better able to avoid illness and achieve genuine, glowing health. And the more I listened to my body, the better able I became to decipher its messages. As you learn how to listen to your body and respect its rhythms, you'll discover for yourself how much sleep your body needs to function optimally so you can restore and recover from the challenges of your day.

SLEEP AND YOUR HORMONES

Sometimes a sleep problem is really a hormone problem. Women facing menopause are particularly prone to sleep problems due to falling hormone levels. Likewise, decreasing levels of testosterone can provoke sleep problems in older men. The resulting lack of sleep can then make these hormonal imbalances worse, and so we have another vicious cycle.

Fortunately, the 2-Week Revitalize Program, the lifelong Maintenance Program, and the additional support in the appendices can both help balance your hormones and improve the quality of your sleep. Just as lack of balance has many ill effects that all make each other worse, restoring balance creates many positive effects that all support each other.

If You Still Have Trouble Sleeping . . .

- **Lower the temperature**—ideally, to 68 degrees or even colder. We sleep best in a warm bed within a cold room.

- **Check your mattress.** Make sure it's firm, supportive, and genuinely comfortable. If your mattress is more than ten years old, it might be time for a change.

- **Take a warm bath.** A hot bath raises your body temperature, which means that once you're out of the bath, your body temperature soon drops. A lowered body temperature helps facilitate sleep.

- **Deprive your senses.** Make sure your room is dark and quiet. Even small light leaks and slight noises can keep you from sleeping as continuously and deeply as possible. If necessary, get some earplugs or maybe a sleep noise machine, which can be set to white noise or some other soothing sound, such as the ocean, the woods at night, or even a low hum of city traffic. A noise machine can be especially useful when you're traveling and want to block out strange sounds that might disturb your rest.

- **Give yourself time to make the transition, perhaps by developing a bedtime ritual.** You can't go 100 miles an hour all day long and then expect yourself to come to a dead stop all at once. Find your own way of slowly winding down.

- **Check for electromagnetic fields (EMFs).** Electromagnetic fields are produced by electrical or electronic activity, so they emanate from any device that you plug in, including a digital clock, smart phone, computer, or TV. Some research suggests that EMFs can disrupt the production of melatonin and serotonin—both essential to prevent inflammation and promote good sleep and a good mood. Other studies indicate that EMFs can disrupt your *pineal gland,* which helps regulate sleep and wakefulness based on your response to light and dark.

- **Try some supplements.** See Appendix D for some natural sleep aids that might help your body and brain relax.

- **If you can't fall or stay asleep, get up.** Give yourself 45 minutes to fall asleep and if that doesn't work, get up and engage in a relaxing, nonscreen activity such as reading or listening to music. After about 60 more minutes, go lie down again. Don't associate your bed with wakefulness; give yourself the chance to create a strong association between bed and sleep.

If You Must Nap, Do It like a Grown-up!

Toddlers need two-hour naps—adults don't. If you must nap during the day, keep it to 20 or 30 minutes at most, preferably before 4 P.M. Long or late afternoon naps damage sleep rhythm and make it tougher to fall asleep at night.

Making Friends with Sleep

Padma, Jerome, and Gina each decided to follow the 2-Week Revitalize Program. Padma also took the supplements I recommended for her hormonal issues (see Appendix C), Jerome followed the suggestions I made for coping with jet lag (see www.bewell.com/blog/end-jet-lag), and Gina took the supplements I recommended for adrenal dysfunction (see Appendix B).

Each of these patients also had to think about the other ways to balance the stress in their lives with relaxation. Padma still chose to spend most of her free time writing and doing research—but she made sure to put aside a portion of time each weekend to read for pleasure, walk in the woods, and have at least one relaxed meal with her loved ones. Jerome cut short his late-night TV, substituting a half hour of yoga or meditation, which he soon discovered vastly increased his productivity the next day. Gina found the courage to set late-night limits on the demands at work, turning off the computer at 9 P.M. She made up for it by getting up earlier the next morning, full of focus and energy.

All three of these hard-driving people also took to heart another message I shared with them: *don't make sleep a performance issue.*

Often just thinking about sleep affects your ability to fall asleep. What happens frequently is that the way you cope with insomnia becomes as much of a problem as the insomnia itself. You can easily fall into a vicious cycle of worrying about not being able to sleep . . . which actually makes your sleep problems worse!

I suggested to my patients that instead of stressing over their lack of sleep, they might be able to use the time productively—but not stressfully. Like so many things in life, getting good sleep is about letting go, going with the flow. Sleep needs to become a natural rhythm like breathing, something that comes automatically and you don't think about.

All three of my patients found ways to make this message their own. If Padma woke during the night, instead of stressing about her lack of sleep, she read a funny novel or an interesting article that had nothing to do with her field. Jerome, as we saw, began to meditate. Gina found breathing and visualization very helpful, both for falling asleep and for generally feeling more confident and clear about her work and her life.

Although every human on the planet needs to sleep, there is still so much about this basic animal function that we do not understand. One thing is clear, though: if you respect your body's rhythms and give your body the right foods and supplements, you can make friends with sleep.

You're Not Getting Enough Sleep:
Three Quick Fixes

1. Darken your room and/or get a sleep mask.

2. Turn off all electronic devices two hours before bed.

3. Stop caffeinated beverages completely, and avoid chocolate after 8 P.M. For help in getting off caffeine, see the protocol on page 191.

REASON #8:

YOU'RE OVERMEDICATED

Leo came to see me because he felt that his current array of doctors—an internist, a cardiologist, a rheumatologist, and a psychiatrist—just weren't making him well. A lawyer in his mid-50s, Leo had gone for a routine physical and was found to have high cholesterol and mildly elevated blood pressure, two conditions that had led to a veritable cascade of medications.

"My internist put me on Lipitor to lower my cholesterol and hydrochlorothiazide to lower my blood pressure. He sent me to a cardiologist, who wasn't really happy with the results, so he switched me from hydrochlorothiazide to Inderal.

"Then my muscles started aching even with minimal exercise, so my internist sent me to a rheumatologist, and she put me on Celebrex. That worked for a while, but eventually it seemed to wear off. I had already been having trouble sleeping, and now the pain kept me up at night, so I went back to my internist for some help, and he gave me Ambien.

"Meanwhile, I was trying to lose weight, but none of my diets were working. I couldn't lose a pound, even though I had given up all my favorite foods. In fact, I was always hungry, and in the past year I've gained at least 10 kilos. I'm tired all the time. And between you and me, my sex life is pretty much over.

"The whole thing has gotten me so discouraged that my doctor sent me to a psychiatrist. He put me on Prozac, which might have helped a little. But most of the time, I feel pretty lousy."

Leo looked at me, trying to seem cheerful, but I could see how disheartened he really was. "Doctor," he said finally, "I'm only fifty-five! Isn't that supposed to be the prime of life? Some days, it seems like my life might as well be over."

Leo's Medications . . . and His Side Effects

Medication	Purpose	Leo's Side Effects*
Lipitor	Lower cholesterol	Confusion, brain fog; memory problems; muscle pain and weakness; fatigue; hunger
Inderal	lower blood pressure	depression sleep problems fatigue decreased sex drive and impotence
Celebrex	Ease muscle pain	Dizziness; nervousness; headache; runny and stuffy nose; weight gain
Ambien	Promote sleep	Daytime drowsiness; confusion; depression
Prozac	Ease depression	Weight gain

* These are only some of the many negative effects possible from the medications listed. Different people respond differently, sometimes with a better overall experience than Leo's and sometimes with an even worse one. In my clinical experience, Leo's experience is not unusual.

Sadly, Leo's situation is all too common. Many patients who first come to me in their 50s or beyond are on two or more medications, as are an increasing number of younger people. Often, as in Leo's case, the negative effects of the first medication lead to the prescription of a second drug . . . whose effects incite the need for a third drug . . . causing the prescription of a fourth drug. On and on it goes, with everyone gaining weight, feeling old, and getting more and more discouraged.

Even if you're only taking one medication, it might be making you feel old and fat. Many common prescription medications create weight gain, brain fog, memory problems, fatigue, joint pain, sleep problems, and other symptoms that we incorrectly associate with the inevitable process of aging, rather than with a very reversible loss of function.

Once again, we think that our symptoms are caused by getting older, when they are actually the result of stressing our body and failing to support it.

How Medications Can Make You Feel Old and Fat

- Weight gain
- Nutrient depletion
- Fatigue
- Muscle aches and pains
- Drowsiness
- Brain fog
- Dizziness
- Memory problems
- Depression
- Dependence and addiction
- Nausea, indigestion, gas, constipation, bloating
- Increased risk of diabetes

The sad thing is that medications are often unnecessary. A great deal of research shows that in many cases, diet, supplements, exercise, stress relief, and improved sleep work better than any medication ever could.

When Diet, Exercise, Stress Relief, Herbs, and Supplements Might Work Better than Drugs

- Moderately high blood pressure (a systolic reading consistently between 140 and 160)
- Coronary artery disease
- Moderately high blood sugar and early-stage Type 2 diabetes
- Arthritis
- Aches and pains
- Viral upper respiratory infections
- Colds and sinusitis
- Prevention and treatment of migraine and chronic headache
- Heartburn and acid reflux (gastroesophageal reflux disease—GERD)
- Irritable bowel syndrome (IBS)
- Acne, psoriasis, eczema, and many other skin conditions
- Mild and moderate depression
- Mild and moderate anxiety
- Many autoimmune diseases

Now, don't get me wrong. Sometimes prescription drugs are lifesavers, helping patients to an almost miraculous degree. I am all for the right medication for the right patient for the right problem. If you have a severe infection, you can give thanks for the antibiotics that keep it at bay. If you have moderate to extremely high blood pressure—a systolic reading consistently above 160—and need to bring it down quickly, a beta blocker or diuretic might well prevent a stroke. If you are severely depressed, suicidal, or disabled by anxiety, the temporary use of an antidepressant or antianxiety medication might give you the breathing room you need to make some new choices. Likewise, if you are in severe pain, suffering from a disabling symptom, or undergoing intense discomfort, the temporary use of a pain reliever or other medication might bring you some much-needed relief.

In all too many cases, though, medications can create more problems than they solve. Often, this is because doctors are focusing on symptoms rather than addressing the underlying cause.

It's as though you were driving your car and the oil light began to flash. Imagine if your mechanic simply put on a Band-Aid to hide the light, rather than seeking out the underlying reason why it went off! You would immediately look for a new mechanic, one with a more sophisticated understanding of how a car actually works. Sadly, we often take better care of our cars than of our bodies.

Worse still, many medications aren't even necessary. Shocking though it seems, doctors frequently prescribe medications to people who won't even benefit from them.

For example, as we shall see, statins have been proven effective only for people who have already had a heart attack (and even so, lifestyle changes might be far more effective than statins). Yet statins are now widely used to *prevent* heart attacks, despite the complete lack of evidence that they do so.

Likewise, as we shall also see, blood pressure medications are effective in lowering blood pressure *numbers*—but, in many cases, they do not lower *risk*. If you have moderately high blood pressure—a systolic reading of 130 through 160—and you take an antihypertensive drug, you can get your numbers down, but *it won't affect your risk of stroke or heart disease.*

That is such a shocking statement that I'll repeat it:

If you have only mild to moderately high blood pressure, medications might change your numbers, but they will not reduce your risk of stroke or heart disease.

Only if you lower your blood pressure through diet, exercise, and stress relief do you experience a reduced risk of heart disease, stroke, and other related problems. (See page 126 for more.)

I'm not saying medications are never necessary. But we need them far, far less often than they are prescribed. Meanwhile, they are a substantial part of the reason why so many of us are feeling old and getting fat.

Do Not Make Decisions about Medications Without Talking to Your Doctor!

Do not—I repeat, DO NOT—change the dosage of any prescription medication you are taking, and NEVER stop taking any medication cold turkey.

If you think you might benefit from reducing or eliminating a medication, DISCUSS IT WITH YOUR DOCTOR.

Many prescription medications have a cumulative effect, and if you reduce or stop them cold turkey, you could be in for painful and even dangerous consequences. If you would like to change your relationship to prescription or even over-the-counter medications, you MUST work with your doctor.

Why Do Doctors Overmedicate?

As a physician, I see it every day—patients like Leo are overmedicated, often with disastrous results. Some problems develop slowly and gradually, such as the Prozac, Lipitor, or many other drugs that led to Leo's weight gain (see page 124). Other issues are more dramatic, such as when statins create muscle pains or brain fog—occasionally to such a degree that patients are wrongly diagnosed with Alzheimer's (see pages 139–140).

A great deal of the problem comes from the way we physicians are trained. Medical school teaches us much that is valuable, but it does not teach us to look at underlying causes, or to focus on such basic solutions as diet, supplements, exercise, stress relief, and sleep. Instead, we're taught to identify symptoms—and then to treat each symptom with its own matching drug.

This is what happened to Leo. Although I saw his problems as all resulting from one main underlying cause—a poor diet causing inflammation—his conventional doctors saw many individual diagnoses: heart disease, arthritis, insomnia, depression. Instead of getting a holistic, integrated view, Leo was treated by several different specialists who didn't even talk to one another. Rather, each prescribed the drugs that his or her specialty demanded, as though Leo's body could be carved up into three separate, independent domains: cardiovascular, rheumatological, and nervous systems.

But Leo didn't have three independent systems—he had one single body. And whenever he took a medication—no matter what it had been prescribed for—his entire body took the hit.

For example, the Lipitor Leo took for his cholesterol caused his muscles to ache. The Celebrex he took to alleviate his muscle aches promoted his weight gain. Meanwhile, the Lipitor and the Ambien, prescribed to help Leo sleep through the muscle pain, contributed to his depression . . . and the Prozac he took in response caused him to gain more weight. The extra weight created more of the inflammation that was the main underlying issue, and it also raised his blood pressure yet again, further stressing his cardiovascular system. Each medication ultimately made Leo's body not better, but worse. And in spite of all these medications, the underlying issue, inflammation, which was caused by his poor diet, was never even addressed.

We physicians aren't the only ones to keep the drugs flowing. Did you know that pharmaceutical companies spend more on marketing than on research? If you watch television, I'm sure you've seen those ads urging you to ask your doctor about prescription drugs for heartburn, psoriasis, joint pain, depression, and anxiety.

Meanwhile, Big Pharma sends its representatives to promote new drugs to doctors, frequently springing for expensive luncheons, dinners, and junkets to sweeten the deal.[1] If you're in a position of power—perhaps on a committee charged with creating guidelines for a new medication—a drug company might very well offer you a speaking gig, a consulting fee, or even a research subsidy, making it awfully tempting for you to support their products.

The result is an economy—and a culture—in which drugs quickly come to seem the only possible response to disease. As the old saying goes, "When the only tool you have is a hammer, every problem looks like a nail." Instead of seeing medications as temporary, limited solutions of last resort, we turn to them first, last, and always.

When I was studying Chinese medicine, I was taught a different approach. My teachers, Harriet Beinfield and Efrem Korngold, urged me to view the human body as I would a plant. When a plant is withering, you look to see what the soil is like and whether it's getting enough sun, enough water, enough nutrients. You don't simply paint the leaves green!

Why don't we do the same thing with our bodies? Instead, we use drugs to "paint the leaves green," changing our patients' numbers without really improving their health. As a result, each time a problem is medicated, a new problem pops up, in an endless game of medical "Whack-A-Mole."

Sometimes, when I look at how our Western medical system works, I get the same feeling I had growing up during apartheid: *This is crazy! Why doesn't everybody else see how crazy it is?* Just as the severe racial segregation of my childhood appeared normal to many of my white neighbors, so does the habitual overmedication of Western medicine appear normal to most patients and doctors. Both systems seem so obviously wrong to me, yet for most people, they are just "the way things are." Because everyone around you is in such complete, unspoken agreement, you sometimes think that *you* must be the crazy one for daring to believe there is a better way.

Fortunately, apartheid eventually came to seem absurd to most South Africans, and the overmedication of Western medication is beginning to seem absurd to many of us Americans as well. A big part of the problem is information. I hope that when you have finished this chapter you feel not discouraged or alarmed but rather empowered, ready to take a more active and informed role in your own health.

Myths to Break Through

- "Properly prescribed or recommended medications are unlikely to have dangerous side effects."
- "Properly prescribed or recommended medications won't make you fat."
- "Properly prescribed or recommended medications won't make you feel old."
- "Drugs are prescribed based on science alone."
- "The more money we spend on health, the healthier we become."
- "You can take several different medications without being concerned about their interactions."
- "When you're sick, a drug is usually the best solution."

Myth: "Properly prescribed or recommended medications are unlikely to have dangerous side effects"

We often like to distinguish between "effects" and "side effects." When a drug has the effect we want, we are satisfied. When it has an effect that we don't like, we call that a "side effect."

Speaking as a physician, this is utter nonsense. The body doesn't distinguish between effects and side effects—it knows only *effects!*

Leo, for example, was feeling old, fat, sluggish, and depressed: that was his condition, not some minor side effect. Perhaps some of his meds were helping him and perhaps they weren't, but meanwhile, he was suffering. I didn't want to trivialize that suffering by calling it a side effect.

The Dangers of Prescription Drugs[2]

- Prescription drugs kill more people than illegal drugs.

- More Americans die because of prescription drugs than because of auto accidents.

- Between 2000 and 2008, drug fatalities more than tripled among people aged 50 to 69.

- In 2009, emergency rooms saw nearly 2.3 million drug-related visits because of adverse reactions to prescription drugs—most of which were being taken exactly as physicians had prescribed.

Many frequently prescribed drugs have dangerous side effects. Let's focus on just a few of the most common:

- Diabetes drugs

- Proton pump inhibitors (PPIs)

- Blood pressure meds

- Antidepressants

- Statins

Diabetes Drugs

If you've got high blood sugar or Type 2 diabetes, you might have been prescribed such medications as DiaBeta, Glucotrol, Micronase, or Tolinase. Although these meds might have some benefit for people whose blood sugar is dangerously high, they will rarely be effective in either preventing or treating diabetes as opposed to just managing it. Because they come with frequent negative effects, they should generally be used only in the short term, until you have a chance to adopt a new diet and lifetyle. By contrast, the "side effects" of switching to a healthier diet are almost always positive.

Potential Negative Effects of Diabetes Drugs

- Hypoglycemia
- Headache
- Gastrointestinal complaints
- Fatigue
- Liver damage
- Increased risk of heart attack and blood vessel disease

⟨— PROTON PUMP INHIBITORS (PPIs) —⟩

If you suffer from acid reflux, you are very often prescribed a PPI such as Nexium, Prilosec, or Prevacid. Acid reflux occurs when some of the acid in your stomach—intended to help digest your food—backs up into your esophagus (the tube connecting your stomach to your throat), where it causes the burning sensation popularly known as heartburn.

PPIs bring temporary relief to acid reflux by inhibiting your stomach's production of acid. However, acid reflux is often not caused by *too much* acid, but rather by *too little*. If your stomach acid is low—as often happens with an altered microbiome, stress, a poor diet, and as we age—your food cannot be properly broken down. As a result, it sits in your stomach too long and might back up into your esophagus, along with some of the acid that accompanies it.

With a healthy level of stomach acid, you could digest your food more efficiently so that it passes down into your intestines rather than refluxing up into your esophagus. So by ending your symptom, that PPI might actually be masking a more serious problem—the medical version of putting a Band-Aid over your car's oil light.

PPIs also alter your microbiome. And they might make it more difficult for you to absorb nutrients. Even if you consume a healthy diet, low stomach acid could prevent you from absorbing it. As a result, you won't get enough calcium, magnesium, iron, or vitamin B12—a type of malnutrition that puts you at risk for a whole new set of negative effects.

Because drugs are often a doctor's first go-to, PPIs are seriously overprescribed, with as many as 69 percent of patients being given PPIs that they don't even need.[3] Meanwhile, PPIs create a kind of physical dependence. Whether or not you needed them to begin with, you might soon find them hard to stop because when you do, you get what's called a *rebound effect*: your body creates *more* acid—and now you really might get reflux from excess acid. That is why you must always taper off PPIs slowly, under a physician's care.

What's the solution? Find natural, healthy ways to increase or decrease your stomach acid as needed. Losing weight might make a difference, as it will reduce the pressure on your stomach that often forces acid upward. Work with a functional-medicine practitioner or see www.bewell.com/blog/halt-heartburn for suggestions on how you may be able to address this problem on your own.

Potential Negative Effects of Proton Pump Inhibitors (PPIs)

- Anemia
- Fatigue
- Seizures
- Kidney disease
- Pneumonia—you need that acid to kill the unfriendly bacteria and viruses you might inhale
- Vulnerability to an infectious bacterium called *Clostridium difficile (C diff)*
- Bone loss and bone fractures—without enough acid, you might not properly absorb the calcium you need
- Abdominal pain
- Headache
- Nutrient deficiencies, especially B12, coenzyme Q10 (CoQ10), glutathione, and magnesium
- Disrupted microbiome

Blood Pressure Medications

As I mentioned earlier, these medications might change your numbers. But unless your blood pressure is very high—with a systolic reading that is consistently 160 or higher—they don't actually reduce your risk of heart attack and stroke.

Bringing your blood pressure numbers down through diet, supplements, exercise, and stress relief will reduce your risk.

Bringing those numbers down through meds will not.

And while these meds are failing to improve your cardiovascular health, they are putting you at further risk for a whole other set of problems.

Potential Negative Effects of Angiotensin II Receptor Blockers (ARBs)

Examples: Cozaar, Avapro, Diovan, Benicar

- Headache
- Dizziness, lightheadedness
- Nasal congestion
- Back and leg pain
- Diarrhea
- Increased risk of cancer

Potential Negative Effects of Beta Blockers

Examples: Inderal, Tenormin, Lopressor, Normodyne

- Fatigue
- Dizziness
- Weakness
- Dry mouth, eyes, or skin
- Diarrhea
- Nausea and vomiting
- Cold hands and feet
- Decreased sex drive
- Shortness of breath
- Sleep disturbances

⬥ ANTIDEPRESSANTS ⬥

Depression is a tricky problem to treat because it involves both physical and psychological factors. Seeing the toll depression takes, I have often wished there *were* a simple medication that could bring my suffering patients some relief.

The problem is that antidepressants are almost never that medication:

- If you have mild depression, they are no better than a placebo.

- If you have moderate depression, they are slightly better than a placebo—but exercise works just as well, and with many more beneficial effects.

- For severe depression, they are effective in one case out of ten.

Although antidepressants don't fit the classical model of "addictive," you do become dependent on them. If you stop taking them cold turkey, without having changed your diet and lifestyle, you are likely to feel more depressed than you did before, which can lead many doctors to put you back on the med or find a new one to prescribe.

You could end up moving from one antidepressant to another for the rest of your life, never really feeling any better—but feeling *worse* when you try to stop.

Meanwhile, as Leo discovered, the negative effects can be highly problematic.

Potential Negative Effects of Antidepressants

- Increased appetite
- Weight gain
- Sexual dysfunction: decreased libido, delayed orgasm/ejaculation, no orgasm/ejaculation, erectile dysfunction
- Nausea
- Constipation
- Fatigue
- Drowsiness
- Insomnia
- Dry mouth
- Blurred vision
- Irritability
- Agitation
- Anxiety
- In people younger than 40, increased suicidal behavior[4]
- In people over 65, increased falls[5]

Many prescription and over-the-counter meds deplete your nutrients

Nutrient depletion is one of the little-known effects of prescription and over-the-counter medications, but it is a very real problem and one that contributes to feeling old and getting fat. Here are just some of the ways common medications both produce negative effects and strip your body of the nutrients that it needs:

Medication	Negative Effects	Vitamin Deficiency
Statins (Lipitor, Crestor, Zocor, Mevacor, Pravachol, etc.)	Muscle and joint aches, nausea, diarrhea, constipation, erectile dysfunction, increased blood sugar, increased risk of dementia, increased risk of diabetes, liver dysfunction, neurological problems, memory loss, Alzheimer's-like symptoms	CoQ10, possibly vitamin D
Proton pump inhibitors (PPI's) (Nexium, Prevacid, Prilosec, Dexilant, Protonix, etc.)	Nutritional deficiencies, constipation, diarrhea, kidney disease, headaches, increased risk of bone fractures	All nutrients because these drugs alter the pH of the gut, especially B12, CoQ10, glutathione, and magnesium
Antidepressants (SSRIs such as Prozac, Zoloft, Paxil, Lexapro, and Celexa. MAO inhibitors such as phenelzine and isocarboxazid. Tricyclics such as doxepin, imipramine, and clomipramine.)	SSRIs: nausea, increased appetite and weight gain, decreased libido, erectile dysfunction, decreased orgasm, insomnia, dry mouth, blurred vision, constipation, dizziness, agitation, irritability, anxiety. MAO inhibitors: nausea, nervousness, headaches, sleepiness, sexual dysfunction, dizziness, stomach upset, weight gain. Tricyclics: blurred vision; constipation; drop in blood pressure when going from sitting to standing, which can result in dizziness; drowsiness; dry mouth; increased appetite often leading to weight gain; increased sweating; rashes; urinary retention.	SSRIs: iodine and selenium, folic acid, vitamins B6 and B12, and melatonin. MAO inhibitors: Vitamin B6. Tricyclics: CoQ10, glutathione, riboflavin, selenium.

Medication	Negative Effects	Vitamin Deficiency
Antianxiety medications (Xanax, Klonopin, Valium, Ativan)	Fatigue, cold hands, dizziness, weakness, sleepiness, brain fog, clumsiness, slow reflexes, slurred speech, confusion and disorientation, depression, lightheadedness, impaired judgment, memory loss, nausea, blurred or double vision	Melatonin
Anti-inflammatory (NSAIDS) (Advil/Motrin, Aleve/ Naprosyn, Celebrex)	Stomach ulcers, nausea, vomiting, diarrhea, constipation, decreased appetite, rash, dizziness, headache, drowsiness, fluid retention, damage to stomach and intestines	Vitamin C, folic acid, iron
Sleep aids (Ambien, Lunesta, Rozerem, Sonata, Silenor, etc.)	Constipation, diarrhea, stomach pains, dizziness, weakness, heartburn, headache, impairment the next day, memory loss	None identified
Biologics (Humira, Enbrel, Remicade)	Increased risk of developing serious infections including viral, bacterial, or fungal infections; increased risk for developing certain types of cancer; reduces your ability to fight infections; fever, sore throat, chills, and other signs of infection; numbness or tingling; swelling of the face, feet, ankles, or lower legs; vision problems; itching and hives; stomach and chest pain; dizziness and fainting; fatigue and weakness; trouble breathing or swallowing; unusual bruising or bleeding	Vitamins B12 and D
Antihypertensive diuretics (Diuril, Dyazide, Lasix, Maxzide)	Diarrhea, dry mouth, fatigue, erectile dysfunction, headache, leg cramps, weakness	Diuretics: calcium, CoQ10, iron, magnesium, potassium, B vitamins, vitamin C, zinc

Medication	Negative Effects	Vitamin Deficiency
Beta blockers (Bystolic, Inderal, Lopressor, Tenormin, Toprol)	Asthma-like symptoms, fatigue, dizziness, depression, sleep problems, erectile dysfunction	CoQ10, melatonin
ACE inhibitors (Capoten, Vasotec, Zestril)	Allergic reactions, diarrhea, dry cough, fever and chills, headache, joint pains, rashes, difficulty breathing, kidney damage	Calcium, magnesium, potassium, zinc
Angiotensin II receptor blockers (Avapro, Benicar, Cozaar, Diovan)	Abnormal taste sensation, diarrhea, dizziness, drowsiness, headache, low blood pressure, rashes	CoQ10, magnesium, zinc
Calcium channel blockers (Norvasc, Procardia, Vasocor)	Dizziness, constipation, headache, palpitations, swollen ankles	Calcium, melatonin, potassium, vitamin D
Steroids (prednisone, methylprednisolone, prednisolone, dexamethasone)	Hormone disruption, baldness, depression, heart problems, acne, high blood pressure, elevated cholesterol, weight gain, mood swings, suppressed immune system	Calcium, folic acid, magnesium, potassium, selenium, vitamin A, vitamin C, vitamin D, vitamin K, and zinc
Antibiotics	Side effects are extremely variable from patient to patient, and from antibiotic to antibiotic. Common ones include weight gain, rashes, diarrhea, abdominal pain, nausea, vomiting, fever, microbiome imbalance, Candida, dizziness, headache, and fatigue. Others include bone loss, IBS, and liver toxicity.	Beneficial bacteria, B vitamins, calcium, magnesium, iron

Myth: "Properly prescribed or recommended medications won't make you fat"

In fact, medications are one of the most common reasons for weight gain, since they cue your body to retain fat through a variety of channels.

How Medications Make You Fat

- Stressing your key fat-metabolizing organ, your liver
- Stressing your gut
- Imbalancing your microbiome
- Slowing your metabolism
- Imbalancing your hormones for hunger and fullness
- Increasing inflammation

Types of Drugs That Might Make You Fat

- Antidepressants
- Antianxiety medications
- Antipsychotics
- Antihistamines
- Blood pressure medications
- Diabetes medications
- Proton pump inhibitors (PPIs)
- Antibiotics
- Birth control pills
- Steroids

Drugs That Make You Fat:
The Top 20 Offenders

1. Allegra
2. Antibiotics
3. Birth control pills
4. Deltasone
5. Depakote
6. DiaBeta, Diabinese, Insulase

7. Elavil, Endep, Vanatrip
8. Inderal
9. Insulin
10. Nexium
11. Paxil
12. Prevacid

13. Prozac
14. Remeron
15. Tenormin
16. Thorazine
17. Tofranil
18. Zoloft
19. Zyprexa

I have seen so many patients who were baffled and distressed about weight gain, only to discover that the culprit was a medication their physician had prescribed or recommended. In virtually all cases, they weren't even warned that weight gain might be one of the side effects. Instead, they found themselves mysteriously gaining weight and unable to lose it, despite their best efforts at diet or exercise. When I told them that their meds might be to blame, they were both angry and relieved.

If you've been gaining weight for no reason you can determine, think back to when your weight gain started. Was it after a medical procedure or an illness that required antibiotics? Was it after you began taking a new medication? Ask your physician whether weight gain is a side effect of any of your prescription or over-the-counter medications, and then look at the "Three Fixes" on page 150 for suggestions on how to respond. Meanwhile, don't stop taking any medication without your doctor's supervision.

Myth: "Properly prescribed or recommended medications won't make you feel old."

As we have seen, many commonly prescribed medications produce symptoms that we associate with feeling old, including brain fog, memory loss, aching muscles, joint pain, fatigue, drowsiness, and depression. Your doctor might downplay these as "side effects," but if you are experiencing them, you could feel old without knowing why.

Dozens of commonly prescribed medications have this "premature aging" effect, so let me zero in on one of the most dramatic: statins. These are prescribed to patients with high cholesterol in the mistaken belief that lowering cholesterol levels helps prevent cardiovascular disease.

Unfortunately, statins *don't* usually decrease your risk of disease. What they might do, meanwhile, is make you feel old.

How Statins Make You Feel Old

One of the most disturbing scientific studies I have read recently involved a 2012 study that first took elderly patients off their statins and then put them back on. While the patients were off their meds, their brain function improved. As soon as they went back on the statins, their brain function declined.

At the same time, I read about an elderly man—formerly a brilliant professor—who had been diagnosed with Alzheimer's and, eventually, was put in a nursing home. As soon as he was taken off his statins, his brain function began to improve, to the point where it soon became clear that he didn't have Alzheimer's after all. Statin free, he went back to his old home and his old life. Chilling.

Now consider that nearly one-fourth of all American adults take statins—perhaps including many who are reading these words.[6] If you have been suffering from muscle pains, brain fog, inability to concentrate, memory problems, and general decline in your ability to think clearly, statins may be at fault.

To make matters worse, statins also increase your risk of diabetes. So three major effects that we commonly attribute to aging—aches and pains, mental decline, and diabetes—might be caused by statins.

These horrifying effects are all the more distressing when we consider that statins are not even an effective approach to reducing cardiovascular disease. True, they do tend to lower cholesterol. But cholesterol itself is not a risk factor for heart disease or stroke. Let's take a closer look.

◇—— WHAT IS CHOLESTEROL? ——◇

Cholesterol is a type of fat that is a vital component of the human body. We need it to think clearly, to remember, to support cell integrity, to enable digestion, and for just about every other bodily function. Although we might ingest some cholesterol from our food, our bodies also make their own cholesterol.

All the parts of your body depend upon cholesterol—but on its own, cholesterol has no way to reach them. If you recall, every part of your body also depends on glucose, and so your bloodstream carries glucose everywhere. But unlike glucose, cholesterol doesn't dissolve in water so it can't travel through the bloodstream on its own. It needs to be transported.

Enter "HDL" and "LDL"—mistakenly called "good" and "bad" cholesterol. In fact, HDL and LDL are not cholesterol at all. They are *lipoproteins*—a combination of fat and protein. "HDL" stands for "high-density lipoprotein," while "LDL" stands for low-density lipoprotein. (There are other types of lipoproteins as well.) All types of lipoproteins carry cholesterol, triglycerides, phospholipids (another type of blood fat), and proteins.

Mind you, we haven't even established that LDL is harmful, although our latest research—which is still evolving—suggests that *one* type of LDL might not be very good for you. Whereas the larger fluffy LDL particles are either neutral or beneficial, the smaller particles tend to invade your artery walls, raising your risk of heart attack and stroke.

However, we don't know this for certain, and even if we did, our standard cholesterol tests don't distinguish between the large and small LDL particles. More sophisticated tests exist, but they don't give us very useful data either, at least not as of this writing.

In other words:

- Cholesterol itself is not harmful, but beneficial. In fact, it's vital to human health.

- LDL (aka the "bad" cholesterol)—which is *not* cholesterol but only carries it—is beneficial in most of its forms but might be harmful in one.

WHAT ARE STATINS?

Statins are medications that reduce cholesterol. They are one of the most profitable medications in human history, netting billions for the drug companies that produce them. And thanks to the latest medical guidelines, their use is likely to expand. Currently, about 25 percent of the adult population takes statins; if the new guidelines are followed, some 44 percent of men over 50 are likely to take them.[7]

Now, given what we've just learned about cholesterol, you might be asking why any doctor would seek to reduce it. After all, cholesterol itself is beneficial. The only harmful substance is—*possibly*—low-density lipoproteins (LDLs), and even then, not *all* LDLs are harmful. So why are you being prescribed statins?

The short answer—and it's an answer that often makes me feel crazy—is *for no really good reason*. That's right: in most cases, there is *no good reason* for you to take statins. When they reviewed the studies, analysts found for every 140 patients treated with statins, only 1 would benefit—and even so, there was no overall reduction in death or life-threatening illness.

The longer answer involves an outdated study that once showed a correlation between high cholesterol and cardiovascular disease. That study has since been shown to be very incomplete and misleading.[8]

True, for men over 50 who have had a heart attack, statins show some ability to lower the chances of a second heart attack. However, this effect doesn't seem to be about lowering cholesterol but rather because statins *might* be able to reduce inflammation. As we have seen repeatedly, inflammation is a major factor in heart disease as well as many other chronic and age-related diseases, and reducing your inflammation should be your primary goal for feeling young, remaining slim, and increasing your vitality and well-being.

However, if reducing inflammation is your goal, there are far better ways to do it than by taking statins. Over and above the statins' negative effects, diet, supplements, and lifestyle are simply more effective.

I should add that a very small number of people—about 1 in 500—have a condition known as *familial hypercholesterolemia,* which means that they have difficulty clearing excess cholesterol from their bodies. If you're in that .2 percent, you might need to lower your cholesterol, and statins might be an appropriate way to help you do it. If you're in the 99.8 percent with the rest of us, you want to focus not on cholesterol, but on inflammation.

So, as far as I can see, there is simply *no* reason for most people to take statins—and yet their use is increasing. The widespread prescription of statins is based on the incorrect application of flawed research—but it is also making an enormous amount of money for many companies. We're not looking at something that betters the human condition; we're looking at something that increases corporate profit. Tragically, both doctors and patients are going along.

Disturbing Facts about Statins

There is no evidence that statins reduce the incidence of first-time heart attack, or that they reduce mortality (the chances of dying).

Three-quarters of first-time heart attacks occur in people whose cholesterol measures low or "normal."

Some tests do give a more nuanced and specific portrait of LDL particles—but there is no research showing that these tests have any ability to predict heart attacks.

According to a recent study of nearly 26,000 people, those taking statins were 87 percent more likely to develop Type 2 diabetes than those who did not.[9]

One in ten people on statins develop muscle pains.

A growing body of research links statins to violent death from suicide, homicide, and accident, probably due to the way that lowering cholesterol affects our *neurotransmitters,* the biochemicals on which our brain depends to process thought and emotion.

Negative Effects of Statins

- Reduced energy
- Lack of interest in activity
- Increased fatigue after exercise
- Muscle pain
- Erectile dysfunction and reduced ability to achieve orgasm
- Memory loss and/or confusion, Alzheimer's-like symptoms
- Liver dysfunction
- Digestive problems: nausea, gas, diarrhea, constipation
- Rash or flushing
- Hunger
- Increased risk of Type 2 diabetes
- Increased risk of cataracts

When I share these facts about statins with my patients, their initial reaction is usually disbelief. Certainly that was Leo's response.

"Every doctor I've ever seen has told me that lowering my cholesterol is vital for my health, and that statins are the only way to get it down," he told me. "It's not just me—many people I know are on statins, and everyone I know is concerned about their cholesterol. Do you mean to tell me that it's all just *wrong?*"

Well, yes. That is what I am saying. A drug with very limited benefit to a very specific population—and many harmful effects to every population—is being prescribed to millions of Americans, and the number is only growing.

As with the apartheid system, it can be hard to credit the way a whole society just buys into a myth that is so palpably untrue. But it does happen—and with statins and cholesterol, it *has* happened. Heart disease is certainly a serious problem. But lowering cholesterol isn't the way to address it, and statins aren't either. The solution—in almost every case—is to follow the suggestions in this book for diet, supplements, and lifestyle, or else to work with a functional-medicine practitioner to address your own individual condition.

Myth: "Drugs are prescribed based on science alone"

By this point, I hope you have begun to see through this myth for yourself! Here are a few more examples of situations in which medications are prescribed based not on science but on some combination of myth and marketing:

- **Prescribing blood pressure drugs to *prevent* hypertension.** If your blood pressure is borderline high—but not yet actually "hypertension"—your physician might prescribe antihypertension drugs to help bring it down.

    Sounds logical, yes? The problem is that there is no good evidence that these drugs have any benefit in preventing hypertension. Meanwhile, they put you at risk for all the negative effects of blood pressure drugs, which you can read about on pages 132–133.

    Now don't misunderstand me. If your blood pressure is borderline high, I very much want you to bring it down. This is a classic example of the "gray area" and the spectrum of illness that we have been talking about throughout this book—and ironically, one of the few times when conventional doctors *do* treat that gray area. But the way to lower borderline high blood pressure is through diet, supplements, exercise, sleep, and stress relief, not with medications that are Band-Aids and often have debilitating side effects.

- **Prescribing blood pressure medications for hypertension.** If you suffer from mild hypertension—between 140/90 to 159/99—you would indeed benefit from bringing your blood pressure down . . . but *only* if you do so through diet and lifestyle. If you take blood pressure meds, your numbers might go down but your risk of heart attack and stroke are not affected.

I realize this is hard to believe, but I assure you that it is true. As with statins, we're looking at a numbers game, a situation in which numbers change but health risks don't. It is the medical equivalent of painting a plant's leaves green; it might look better, but it won't stop dying any faster.

- **Prescribing antidiabetes drugs to prevent or treat diabetes.** If you have high blood sugar levels and particularly if you have Type 2 diabetes, you need to work on reducing inflammation, improving insulin response, balancing your blood sugar, and generally improving your health.

  These are serious concerns, and I urge you to take them seriously. In many cases, these medicines only work to suppress the symptoms without actually treating the cause. And while they may suppress one symptom, they often have side effects, which often leads to new symptoms, which leads to more drugs, and so on and so forth. Instead of taking your chances with risky medications, focus on effective lifestyle changes, in particular exercise and a low-carbohydrate diet.

- **Prescribing antibiotics for upper respiratory infections.** Almost one-fifth of the antibiotics in this country are prescribed for bronchitis and sinusitis. Unfortunately, most of the time these conditions are not caused by bacteria, making antibiotics completely ineffective.

  Meanwhile, our overuse of antibiotics is producing a whole new class of antibiotic-resistant bacteria and an epidemic of *Clostridium difficile* colitis. And, as we saw in Chapter 3, each time you take an antibiotic, you disrupt your microbiome, potentially creating leaky gut and gaining weight that becomes almost impossible to lose.

- **Overprescribing psychiatric drugs.** Danish medical researcher Peter Gøtzsche is the head of the Nordic Cochrane Centre, part of the internationally renowned Cochrane group that reviews medical research. He is also author of the book *Deadly Medicines and Organised Crime: How Big Pharma Has Corrupted Healthcare.* He argues that we are in the midst of what he calls "a psychiatric drug epidemic" in which a class of antidepressants known as SSRIs is being vastly overprescribed.

  Gøtzsche's conclusions are clear: "The way we currently use psychiatric drugs is causing more harm than good." Speaking of the skyrocketing rate at which SSRIs are being prescribed, he continues, "It is hard to believe that so many people have become mentally disturbed and that these prescription increases reflect a genuine need, so we need to look for other explanations." He offers three:

1. Definitions of psychiatric disorders that are so vague that they allow healthy people to be misdiagnosed.

2. Some of the psychiatrists who write the diagnostic manuals get money from the pharmaceutical industry.

3. The portion of the industry that makes psychiatric drugs frequently engages in illegal marketing for its products.[10]

   For more on SSRIs, see page 135.

- **Overprescribing painkillers.** This growing problem has received a lot of coverage from journalists around the country. Two California counties have even brought suit against the companies who manufacture these drugs, accusing them of waging a "campaign of deception."

   Both Orange and Santa Clara counties have seen numerous deaths from overdose and escalating medical costs associated with prescription opioids. In response, they are charging five of the largest drug companies with unfair business practices, creating a public nuisance, and violating California laws against false advertising. The suit accuses companies of advertising the painkillers as safer than they actually are. The suit also charges the companies with claiming unproven benefits for the drugs, such as improved sleep and quality of life.[11]

   Most disturbing is the charge that the drug companies recruit leading physicians to give speeches and write papers that boost the credibility of their products. Likewise, they are charged with creating and co-opting "front groups"—advocacy groups and medical specialty societies—that lend further credibility to their wares.

   In the words of the suit, it was "marketing"—and not any medical breakthrough—that rationalized prescribing opioids for chronic pain and opened the floodgates of opioid use and abuse. Accordingly, the companies promote narcotics despite their claims being "unsupported by competent scientific evidence."

   Previous suits have made similar claims, including a 2007 lawsuit claiming that the maker of OxyContin downplayed the risk of addiction so doctors would be willing to prescribe it. The current plaintiffs claim that the company has continued to market deceptively even after pleading guilty in the previous suit.

   To the shame of my profession, doctors are heavily involved in pushing these dangerous drugs. A 2012 investigation by the *Los Angeles Times* found that between 2006 and 2011, at least one doctor-prescribed drug was involved in nearly half the southern California deaths from prescription drugs.[12]

   As of this writing, the companies have not yet responded to the latest suit. Whatever happens next, the lawsuit has drawn attention to the growing problem of medications that seem to do more harm than good—and that are clearly not prescribed on the basis of science alone.

So why are these expensive and often dangerous medications prescribed? Because U.S. medical training pushes doctors in that direction, so physicians are often afraid to bypass the drugs just in case there is *some* chance that they help. Because U.S. patients are now so used to medications that their doctors risk reproach at best and malpractice suits at worst if they do *not* prescribe the drugs. Plus, pharmaceutical companies spend enormous amounts of money to convince both patients and doctors to use these drugs, sometimes paying doctors huge sums for speakers' fees, research subsidies, and consulting gigs.[13]

Myth: "The more money we spend on health, the healthier we become"

Given how much we in the United States spend each year on health care, I wish this myth were true—but it couldn't be less so. Although we spend almost twice as much per capita as most of the countries in Western Europe, our life span is actually shorter than theirs, by at least a few years.

According to the Institute of Medicine, we spend $210 billion each year on treatments that have at best marginal benefit and often no benefit at all. Most depressing of all, a 2012 study by the Mayo Clinic found that of the tests and procedures reported on in the *New England Journal of Medicine* from 2001 through 2010, a whopping 40 percent turned out to have no value at all.[14]

How can we spend so much money on health care that is worthless nearly half the time? The answer is found in the pages of this chapter, as we consider how expensive—and yet useless—so many medications are, not to mention the costly technologies and surgeries that characterize our medical culture.

As a physician, I am distressed that our current health care system isn't actually making us well. And as a citizen, I am upset about the enormous amount of money we are spending on a dysfunctional system.

Myth: "You can take several different medications without being concerned about their interactions"

As Leo discovered, one medication often leads to another . . . and then another, and then another. Even if the new meds aren't directly caused by the prescription of the previous ones, our symptom-oriented system of treatment increasingly results in multiple prescriptions. Among people over age 65, 44 percent of men and 57 percent of women take at least five medications at any one time.[15]

To be sold, a drug must be tested. But almost always, it is tested alone, not in tandem with other medications. It's only after a significant number of patients have run into trouble that we discover what the problems are.

Ironically, the proponents of conventional medicine frequently criticize those of us who prescribe supplements, saying that there aren't sufficient studies to establish their utility, let alone their safety. But where are the studies demonstrating the safety of multiple interacting drugs? In effect, we have become guinea pigs for the pharmaceutical companies.

I think the problem of multiple drug interactions speaks to a deeper underlying issue in conventional medicine: the tendency to carve patients up into discrete "specialties" while failing to look at the whole person. The cardiologist prescribes statins; the gastrointestinal specialist prescribes a PPI; the ear, nose, and throat specialist prescribes antibiotics; and the psychiatrist prescribes an antianxiety medication. Not only are these specialists failing to look at the root causes of all these disorders, but they are ignoring the problems that might arise when their separately prescribed medications interact. However specialized our knowledge becomes, we must never forget that at the end of the day, we are dealing with one whole body in which all systems, symptoms, and medications are constantly "speaking" to each other. Even when a medication is the best choice, we must always remember to look at it in that larger context.

Myth: "When you're sick, a drug is usually the best solution"

So here's why drugs are rarely the best solution: they usually only hit one metabolic pathway at a time. Being sick, however, usually involves multiple metabolic pathways.

This is why many drugs help *some* people but not *all* people. It all depends on the specific way your body has gone out of balance, and what the particular drug might do to help bring you back into balance.

Scientists and drug companies are very well aware that not everyone benefits equally from all drugs. They even have the term "number needed to treat" (NNT): the number of people who have to take a drug for one person to benefit. When you look at the NNTs, you might be shocked at how few people benefit from commonly prescribed drugs—even by their manufacturers' most optimistic claims.

For example, if a drug's NNT is 50, for every 1 person who gets any benefit from the drug, 50 people have to take it. Put another way, if your doctor prescribes that drug to 50 of her patients, only 1 is likely to benefit. The other 49 will take the drug, pay for the drug, and perhaps experience some negative effects—while getting no positive effects at all. None.

Many widely prescribed drugs have NNTs of 50 or more. Even if a drug has an NNT as low as 5—which is very low—that still means that *only 20 percent* of the patients taking that drug will benefit. The other 80 percent might suffer negative effects. But they won't experience any positive effects.

Statins, for example, have an NNT of 60. That means that if 60 people take statins for five years, 1 prescription might prevent a heart attack among men over the age of 50. The other 59 men taking the drug get no benefit at all. Yet everyone taking the drug has been led to believe that he or she will benefit!

Suppose the drug companies did a test in which, out of 1,000 people, 24 got heart attacks in five years without statins and 16 got heart attacks while taking statins. That doesn't seem like such a big deal, does it? After all, we're talking about a difference of 8 people out of 1,000— only eight-tenths of a percent.

Yet the drug companies can manipulate the statistics to say—accurately—that their meds reduce the risk of heart attack by 33 percent. All of a sudden, those statins start to look pretty good, even though the actual numbers are basically meaningless.

The problem would be bad enough if we had full access to all the data, but disturbingly, we don't. Because 80 percent of all published drug studies are conducted by Big Pharma, they own most of the research—and they are legally free to suppress any studies whose results they don't like. This horrifying point was made in 2005 when Stanford epidemiologist John Ioannidis released an article entitled "Why Most Published Research Findings Are False." Ioannidis revealed that nearly one-third of the studies commissioned by the drug companies are *never published*.

In other words, when the results are positive, we hear about them. When the results are negative—showing either that the drugs are unsafe or that they are ineffective—we don't. So it's very likely that even the benefits of many widely prescribed drugs are inflated, based on a misleading use of statistics and the selective suppression of research results.

What Can You Do?

If you feel discouraged, angry, or frightened by the information in this chapter, you are not alone. I share your responses, and so do many of my functional-medicine colleagues. Overmedication is a horrific problem in modern medicine, and every day I see the destruction it leaves in its wake.

However, I don't want you to feel disempowered, because there is actually quite a bit you can do to make things better, both for yourself and for the system as a whole. Here are some suggestions:

Take Charge of Your Health:
Ten Questions to Ask Your Doctor

- What does this medication do?
- Is this drug intended to cure my underlying condition or is it intended to give me relief from my symptoms?
- What are the potential negative effects? Are they minor or major? Common or rare?

- Have long-term studies been done on this drug? Have studies been done for this drug on people like me—my age, my gender, my specific condition? (Remember, many studies are conducted on young or middle-aged men, who often have different responses to medications and to dosages from other populations. Be especially sure to ask this question if you are going to take the drug long term.)

- Do the benefits outweigh the risks?

- Is this medication intended to *prevent* a problem or *treat* one?

- What is the evidence that it is actually effective?

- What is the "NNT" for this medication? (You can look it up yourself on www.thennt. com, usually by drug category [statins] rather than brand name [Lipitor].)

- Are there natural alternatives I might try first?

- I'd like to try natural alternatives first—would you be willing to let me go that route for three more months and then retest me?

Take Charge of Your Health: Two Possible Solutions

- Try the 2-Week Revitalize Program and the lifetime Maintenance Program in this book. After six weeks, ask your doctor to retest you and redetermine your need for medications. Keep asking to be retested every three months until you have worked your way completely off the meds.

- Find a functional-medicine practitioner: a physician, naturopath, or another skilled provider who will help you employ natural means to heal.

Basically, your goal is to find a doctor who will partner with you on your health journey rather than someone who insists that you have to follow his or her instructions without question. After all, it's your body, your health, and your life. So you need to be part of the decision-making process! The doctor brings his or her knowledge to the table, of course—but *you* need to be at that table too.

Alternatives to Meds

Leo was upset when he realized that each of his medications were just treating his symptoms and not addressing the underlying cause of his problem. To make matters worse, each medication had created an additional set of problems. So he was relieved to hear that he could actually stop all his drugs and I could offer him another solution.

Based on his story and his labs, I determined that Leo was suffering from carbohydrate intolerance. His lab results showed high blood sugars (based on his hemoglobin A1C readings), elevated triglycerides, and decreased levels of vitamin D. Consequently, I believed he would benefit from the Revitalize Program. I also put him on CoQ10, a natural supplement to help with the muscle pains from the statins. After the first two weeks, I encouraged him to go into the Maintenance Program but to stay on a low-carb diet.

As part of his new way of life, Leo began to walk briskly at least 15 minutes a day, as well as doing the Revitalize workout (see page 309). He also began to meditate regularly. And in addition to the CoQ10, he took the nutritional supplements I recommended (see Chapter 9), including a multivitamin, fish oil, vitamin D, and magnesium.

Within the first two weeks of the Revitalize program, Leo began to feel better. His muscle pains went away, his mood improved, and he was sleeping better. These improvements continued into the Maintenance phase, and after about two months, Leo felt better than he had in a long, long time. No more depression, no more insomnia, no more muscle pains—and his lab results all returned to a healthy level.

The sad thing is that Leo didn't have to be on any medication in the first place. His spiral into suffering—into feeling old and tired and fat—was drug induced. Instead of multiple drugs, many treating a side effect of the others, all he needed was to change his diet and start to exercise. As a physician, I am happy to use any means at my disposal to help make my patients well—but the vast majority of the time, food, exercise, and stress relief are truly the best medicine.

You're Overmedicated: Three Fixes

I wanted to give you three *quick* fixes, but for this chapter, I just couldn't. However, here are some steps you can take immediately, even if you might need two or three months to see the benefits.

1. Talk to your doctor and review each one of your meds. Together, make a plan for how you will decrease or eliminate your need for them. If your doctor is not responsive, consider finding a functional-medicine practitioner who will help you reduce your medications. (See Resources.)

2. If you are taking a PPI, try the protocol in www.bewell.com/blog/halt-heartburn.

3. Do the Revitalize Program and begin the Maintenance Program in this book. Six weeks after you begin, ask your doctor to retest you and reevaluate your need for medications.

REASON #9:

YOU'RE NOT GETTING ENOUGH NUTRIENTS

When I first met Bethany, I was struck by how much effort she had already put into improving her health. She carefully explained what she ate, how she exercised, and the commitment she had developed to a daily yoga practice. Hearing her describe her routine, I would have expected her to be in peak condition, glowing with vitality and health.

Yet although she was only 38, Bethany was exhausted, had problems falling asleep, and was irritable much of the time, which suggested to me that her adrenals might not be getting the support they needed. She frequently came down with colds and flu, and that made me think that her immune system also lacked support or perhaps that she was deficient in Vitamin D. Her dry and rough skin made me believe she might need more omega-3 fatty acids, while her frequent bouts of gas, bloating, and constipation made me think that her gut and microbiome were not functioning well either.

I asked Bethany whether she was currently taking a multivitamin, probiotics, vitamin D, fish oils, or any other supplements, and she shook her head vigorously.

"I don't believe in them," she said bluntly. "After all, people have lived on this planet for generations without ever taking pills to be healthy. Don't you think we should be able to get everything we need from our food?"

"We *should*—but in most cases, unfortunately, we *can't*," I replied. "Even if you're eating a healthy, clean, organic diet, in our modern world, there are many reasons why you might still be undernourished and why your body might need more support. The best way I know how to ensure good nutrition and optimal function—to keep you from feeling old and getting fat—is to combine a healthy diet with a few key supplements."

Myths to Break Through about Supplements

- "I should be able to get all the nutrients I need from diet alone."
- "Supplements can be dangerous because they stress my liver."
- "Most supplements are not even absorbed by my body and just end up making 'expensive urine.'"

Myth: "I should be able to get all the nutrients I need from diet alone"

I love the idea of getting all the nutrients you need from a great diet, but I do believe that is wishful thinking. Yes, if you are eating a clean, organic diet, full of vegetables, proteins from good sources, healthy fats, and perhaps some fruit, you *should* be getting all the nutrients you need. You should be—but you're not. Sadly, I believe that very few of us living in our modern era can expect to get enough nourishment for optimal function without the aid of supplements.

Why not? There are several reasons why even whole, organic foods are less nutritious than they used to be:

- **Soil depletion:** Our depleted soil contains less phosphorus and fewer trace minerals, which means that we're not getting those key nutrients in our foods.

- **Toxins:** Foods certified as organic might have been raised or grown without toxic fertilizer, pesticides, or feed—but they still live on the same planet as the rest of us. Our air, water, and soil are all affected by an enormous toxic burden from industrial chemicals, heavy metals, and other pollutants, and all of these affect even the cleanest foods.

- **Nonlocal foods:** Most foods are transported long distances, and this means they are days or even weeks away from being picked or killed. A lot of nutrients are lost even from organic foods as a result.

- **Transport and storage time:** Even local organic foods have probably been picked at least a day or two before you bought them and might well sit in your refrigerator for another day or even longer.

- **Cooking and heating:** We cook many foods, causing us to lose some heat-sensitive nutrients.

We're looking at another double whammy here, because it's not just that our food lacks some essential nutrients. We also *need* more nutrients than previous generations because of the ways our bodies and minds are being stressed. Our 24/7 work schedules, "culture of insomnia," industrialized food system, fast food culture, and enormous toxic burden are stressing our bodies in ways unknown to previous generations.

Why We Need More Nutrients than Prior Generations

- **Physical stress:** Since the 1940s, industrial chemicals and synthetic products have flooded our environment. We are the first few generations of humans to be exposed to so many chemicals—and the number continues to grow. While our bodies are equipped to deal with low levels of some toxins, this explosion of toxins in our air, food, and water has significantly overtaxed our natural cleansing systems. Thus the toxins accumulate in our bodies, preventing our systems from operating at optimal strength and efficiency. In a natural environment, the nutrients in food would be enough. In our current environment, our bodies need some extra help.

- **Mental stress:** The stress of our fast-paced lives, multitasking, overcommitting, and trying to combine working long hours with intensive parenting takes a toll on all of us.

- **Emotional stress:** Lack of community, pressures on family life, and economic uncertainty put us all under an extreme amount of stress—and that stress both depletes our body's nutrients and increases our need for more nutrients.

- **Overmedication:** As you saw in the chart on pages 135–137, many common medications strip the nutrients from our bodies—and many people are on lifelong regimens of five or more medications.

- **Prepared foods:** Even if you cook only clean, organic foods, chances are that you are more likely to buy prepared foods or eat in restaurants a greater proportion of the time than your grandparents' or even your parents' generation. Consequently, a greater proportion of your food lacks nutrients and contains toxins, antibiotics, and other harmful substances that rob your body of key vitamins, minerals, and other important ingredients.

- **Aging:** The older we get, the harder it becomes for our bodies to absorb nutrients. Since our life expectancy is longer than previous generations, we need more nutrients.

- **Loss of microbial diversity:** According to the pioneering work of researcher Martin J. Blaser, people living in developing countries enjoy robust microbiomes populated by a wide variety of species. By contrast, the diversity of the Western microbiome has been shrinking since the early 20th century as stress, toxins, antibiotics, and an unhealthy diet combine to sabotage our friendly bacteria. Yet we depend on those bacteria to absorb the nutrients in our food—which means that sometimes we have to compensate by consuming more nutrients.

As a result, even those of us who don't have a vitamin *deficiency* still might not be getting enough vitamins for *optimal* functioning. If you don't want your function to decrease as you get older, supporting optimal functioning with nutrients is key. Why wait until you are actually nutrient deficient before you start taking supplements? Once again, we shouldn't look at this issue as black and white, but rather should focus on getting out of the "gray zone."

Think for a moment about what supplements are and why I am recommending that you take them. Just as your body needs *macronutrients*—"big" nutrients, such as protein, healthy fats, and carbohydrates—so does your body need *micronutrients:* "small" nutrients, such as vitamins, minerals, and other biochemicals. Our metabolic processes require an intricate balance of biochemicals to operate optimally. Until you've taken the supplements I recommend, you might not even realize how good it's possible to feel—how easy it is to feel vigorous, sharp, and focused and how simple it is to maintain a healthy weight when your body gets what it needs to function optimally.

There is one other reason to take supplements, and that has to do with supporting your *telomeres.* Telomeres are the protective "caps" at the tip of every one of your chromosomes. They naturally get shorter as we age, but there's a lot we can do to slow and even reverse their erosion. Research has found that supplements can help with this process, which addresses aging at our body's most fundamental level.

Myth: "Supplements can be dangerous because they stress my liver"

The week before I saw Bethany, a couple of articles had run in major magazines on the alleged dangers of supplements. Bethany asked me about the possibility that, as she had read, supplements might stress her liver.

I had seen these reports as well. However, after decades of clinical experience, of taking supplements myself, and of prescribing them for patients and my family, I had never observed any problems with them. Basically, most supplements are benign if used appropriately, and it is extremely rare for anyone to have a problem taking too many supplements, or too high a dose of a particular supplement.

Sometimes people have a problem with the cheaper supplements because they use poor-quality ingredients for both the primary ingredients and for the fillers used to create pills, powders, or capsules. That's why it's essential to purchase supplements from reliable sources. But I stand 100 percent behind good-quality supplements such as the ones I recommend in the Appendices.

Having said that, here are a few cautions. I don't want these cautions to keep you from taking supplements in the appropriate doses—just to keep you from going "mega" in certain cases.

- Vitamins A, D, E, and K are fat soluble. That means your body takes what it can use and stores the rest in fat. You don't want stores of these vitamins building up in your body, so be sure to take only the appropriate doses. *Do* take them, however, as these vitamins are vital for your health and will help keep you feeling young and slim.

- Vitamin B3 can create some problems in too-high doses, so again, make sure you're taking a recommended amount.

- While virtually all other vitamins and minerals are safe, I do suggest being careful with herbs and herbal mixtures, which function more like medicine. Except for the antimicrobial herbs I recommend to kill the bad guys in the gut, I suggest taking herbal supplements only under the guidance of an experienced practitioner.

Most of the other vitamins are water soluble and safe. That means your body takes what it needs and then excretes the rest. Stick to the recommended dosage and you should be fine.

Myth: "Most supplements are not even absorbed by my body and just end up making 'expensive urine'"

Bethany raised this concern too. I explained that if her body genuinely didn't need a particular supplement, yes, it would be excreted. And yes, sometimes with cheaper supplements, fillers and other materials used to make the product might keep some micronutrients from being properly absorbed.

However, a high-quality supplement is produced in such a way as to allow for maximum absorption. And I can tell you as a physician using and prescribing these supplements for more than 25 years that virtually everyone I see—including myself—has a need for at least the four key supplements I have recommended in this chapter. I consider them baseline anti-aging supplements for people of all ages—anti-aging in the sense that they promote optimal function and help our bodies repair the wear and tear of daily life.

These days, we are all assaulted by an ever-growing toxic burden, while even organic foods are stored and transported in ways that deplete their nutrients. I wish we didn't need the supplements I'm recommending; I wish we *could* feel certain that they were simply giving us "expensive urine" so we could afford to pass them by.

Sadly, in my clinical experience, that is not the case. When my patients support a healthy diet and lifestyle with these supplements, they feel younger and find it easier to lose weight. Their skin clears up and takes on a healthy glow. Their hair gets thicker and stronger. They feel more energized and their digestion improves. They feel clearer, sharper, more alert and focused. They feel calmer and more optimistic, less prone to anxiety or depression, and able to get good sleep. I notice these effects myself, and if for some reason I miss my supplements for a week or two, I begin to feel the loss.

But, as with everything in this book, you don't have to take my word for it. Give the supplements in this chapter a try for a couple of months and see how you respond. Your body will let you know what it needs.

Can Supplements Substitute for Diet?

Once Bethany knew that I recommended supplements, she wondered whether supplements could actually *substitute* for a healthy diet. If she took enough supplements, she asked me, could she take less care about what she ate?

My answer is an unequivocal *no*. Supplements can help fill in nutritional gaps and protect your body against the occasional slip-up, but they won't make up for a consistently bad diet. The vast majority of your nutrients should come from what you eat.

There are several reasons why this is so. First, whole, natural foods contain many ingredients that we have not yet identified, so we haven't yet isolated them in supplement form. The best way to ensure that you are well nourished is to build a lot of variety into your diet, especially by eating lots of different-colored vegetables, raw or lightly cooked. The colors represent different "non-nutrients"—elements that contain no calories but have a biochemical effect.

Second, the sensory experience of food is an important component—for pleasure, of course, but also for our health. The smells of food help trigger the enzymes, acids, and other biochemicals that we need for optimal digestion. "Mouth-watering" is not just a figure of speech; when you smell a delicious aroma, the saliva in your mouth begins to flow—and that saliva contains key enzymes that help break down your food and that in turn trigger a whole cascade of biochemical responses.

The texture of food plays a significant role in our health as well. It's part of *satiety:* the sensation of feeling full. You also need lots of fiber in your diet—to feed your microbiome and to facilitate digestion—and you can't really get enough fiber from supplements.

Finally, the cultural and social experience of food is important too. Enjoying the foods of your family traditions, sharing a meal with people you love, preparing foods for a holiday celebration or a romantic dinner—these are all part of the fabric of human life and have been since we have been on this planet. I could get all scientific and tell you that nonstressful eating triggers the parasympathetic nervous system and supports healthy digestion, or that it reduces cortisol and other stress hormones, thereby decreasing inflammation and promoting a healthy weight. But I'd rather just encourage you to enjoy your human birthright: delicious foods, social meals, holidays, and family traditions.

In sum, supplements can support your health—but food is the cornerstone of your health. Supplements are just what the name suggests: a *supplement* to a healthy diet.

Which Supplements Should I Take?

So, now that you are ready to take some supplements, which ones should you take?

Go to any nutrition store, drugstore, or supermarket and you can easily feel overwhelmed by the long shelves full of competing products. And if you're even a casual reader of health articles or blogs, you'll notice that every few weeks there's a new "miracle supplement" touted as being the latest weight-loss wonder or magical panacea.

But you can't take hundreds of pills a day, so it's important to prioritize. For my Revitalize Program, the supplements focus on balancing the microbiome and improving liver function to help reset and jump-start your body. For my Maintenance Program, I've chosen four key supplements that I believe everybody needs to take, and added seven supportive supplements that are particularly useful to promote anti-aging.

If you can only take a few supplements, focus on the basic four. If you are looking for the best possible anti-aging program, broaden out to the "supportive seven."

In my practice, I often prescribe additional supplements targeted to specific needs. In the Appendices, you'll find recommendations for supplements that can support your adrenals, balance your hormones, and improve your sleep. If you want to go further, addressing specific conditions with a targeted set of supplements, I strongly recommend working with a functional-medicine practitioner—a physician or a naturopath—who has experience with supplements and can monitor your progress. That's the best way to ensure that you get all the supplements you need—and no more.

Finally, I want to encourage you to stick to the recommended doses, whether that recommendation comes from this chapter, a practitioner, or the bottle itself. I've noticed that some people seem to have the philosophy that "if one is good, five is better," routinely taking more supplements than recommended. At best, you're creating more expensive urine; at worst, you're risking some negative effects. Treat supplements with respect and don't overdose!

Your Four Key Supplements

- Multivitamin that includes methylated B12 and folic acid
- Vitamin D: 2,000–5,000 IU of vitamin D3
- Fish oils: one to three grams of EPA/DHA
- Probiotics: powders, pills, or capsules containing at least 10 billion to 50 billion live bacteria each day

⟶ MULTIVITAMIN: A GOOD MULTIVITAMIN THAT ⟵ INCLUDES METHYLATED B12 AND FOLIC ACID

As I see it, a good multivitamin is your insurance policy—the assurance that every day, you're getting certain baseline nutrients, protecting your body against the vitamin and mineral shortfalls that can occur even in healthy diets. By supporting optimal function, a daily multivitamin helps keep you from feeling old and getting fat.

I specify B12 as a key ingredient in your multivitamin because I want to make absolutely sure that you are getting enough of this nutritional powerhouse. B12 is crucial to the proper functioning of your brain and nervous system, which means it plays a vital role in mental clarity, sharpness, and focus, as well as emotional balance and calm. Lack of B12 makes your body more vulnerable to physical and emotional stress—to the wear and tear that we usually associate with aging, but which I see more as lack of proper function.

Folic acid—also known as *folate* and as vitamin B9—is another crucial B vitamin. Because folic acid helps you to repair DNA, it has significant anti-aging benefits. Folic acid is another key defense against brain fog, irritability, depression, and other responses to physical and emotional stress.

⬦— WHY DO YOU NEED "METHYLATED" —⬦ FOLIC ACID AND VITAMIN B12?

Methylation is a process that your cells perform billions of times each second. If your cells are not methylating properly, you will likely have trouble with one or more of the following bodily functions:

- Detoxification

- Inflammation control

- Immune function

- Mood balancing

- Energy production

- DNA maintenance

Many of us have minor genetic defects that interfere with methylation, which means we don't properly absorb our nutrients. Imperfect methylation is another reason you might be *consuming* a lot of healthy nutrients without fully *absorbing* them.

Without proper methylation, your body will not be able to respond properly to stress—either to physical stressors, such as toxins and challenging foods, or to psychological stressors, such as life challenges and pressures. As a result, you'll be more vulnerable to chronic diseases, including cardiovascular disease, diabetes, chronic fatigue syndrome, autoimmune conditions, and Alzheimer's and other neurological problems. Improper methylation also makes you more vulnerable to the decline in function that we usually associate with aging.

You can get genetic testing (the MTHFR gene test) to find out whether you have one of these defective genes. Or you can simply play it safe and get a multivitamin that includes *methylated* forms of vitamin B12 (as methylcobalamin) and/or folic acid (as L-5-methyltetrahydrofolate), which helps your body respond to stress. When you take methylated vitamins, you don't need to worry about whether your own body is able to methylate them properly, and you can be sure that you are giving your body extra support in its fight against stress.

How to Choose a Multivitamin

- Look for multis in capsule form with an easily absorbed enteric coating. The tablet versions are harder to digest.

- Avoid brands that include other ingredients, especially sugar, lactose (derived from milk products), artificial colors, or other unnatural substances.

- If you are still on medications, review your multi's contents with your physician to make sure there aren't any contraindications.

- Because there is currently little regulation of supplements in the U.S., be sure to buy from a reputable company. (See Resources for some recommendations.)

- Make sure the B12 and folic acid are the methylated forms (B12 as methylcobalamin and folic acid as L-5-methyltetrahydrofolate).

How to Take a Multivitamin

- **With food, to support absorption.** Some vitamins—such as vitamins A, D, E, and K—require fat for full absorption. Minerals are also better absorbed with food.

- **Two to three times a day.** It's impossible to make one pill big enough to contain all the vitamins you need in your daily supplement. And a divided dose means that you are less likely to excrete your vitamins and are more likely to absorb them.

⬥—— 2,000–4,000 IU of Vitamin D3 ——⬥

Despite the name, vitamin D is actually a prehormone: an essential precursor to hundreds of disease-preventing proteins and enzymes. And since every cell in your body has vitamin D receptors, we can conclude that vitamin D is an essential support for every one of your cells.

When you look at the numerous benefits vitamin D offers, you feel as though you are seeing an offer to turn back the clock, with such anti-aging functions as

- Weight management
- Better sleep
- Healthier skin
- Stronger hair
- Improved hearing

- Better absorption of nutrients
- Immune support
- Anti-inflammatory effects
- Enhanced muscle strength
- Bone building
- Improved cardiovascular health
- Anti-cancer actions
- Reduced risk of multiple sclerosis

By the same token, a long-term shortage of vitamin D can leave you vulnerable to such chronic "diseases of old age" as heart disease, diabetes, and at least 16 types of cancer, including breast, colon, lung, ovarian, pancreatic, and prostate.

Vitamin D is also a key regulator of genetic expression. We are still learning more about the 30,000 genes in our bodies, but so far we know that vitamin D influences at least 2,000 of them.

Considering all of these reasons, it's not surprising to learn that in 2007, a new European meta-analysis published in the prestigious *Archives of Internal Medicine* reported that vitamin D can help lower your risk of dying from any cause.[1]

Unfortunately, it's virtually impossible to get adequate amounts of vitamin D from food alone. You need daily exposure to the sun; or, if you're not getting enough vitamin D that way, you need a daily supplement.

When I suggested to Bethany that she make sure to spend some time each day in the bright sunlight without sunscreen, she looked at me in surprise. "But I thought that could give me skin cancer," she said. "Not to mention the way it ages my skin."

I explained to Bethany that the amount of sun you need depends on the season, the time of day, where you live, and your particular skin pigmentation, among other factors. As a general rule, though, 20 to 30 minutes a day of sun on your face and arms *without sunscreen* is a good rule of thumb. Remember: even a mild sunscreen shuts down your body's production of vitamin D from the sun, so apply the sunscreen only after you've had some sun exposure.

Another good rule of thumb is to stay in the sun just long enough for a tiny response: pale pink, if you're naturally fair, or just a hint of red if you are darker. Or you can download the app "dminder," which tracks the amount of vitamin D you get from the sun based on your age, location, body type, and time of day, and even includes a timer.

Your goal is never to burn—which, besides being uncomfortable, can increase your risk of melanoma. Instead, keep building up your tolerance slowly over the summer or when in a sunnier climate than you are used to. And please avoid tanning booths!

By the way, sitting by a sunny window won't get you the D you need, even if it feels as though the sun is coming through. The UVB rays that you need to get your vitamin D production going are absorbed by the glass.

To me, our fear of sun is a perfect example of the lack of balance that Western medicine seems to be so good at. Yes, too much sun is bad, and if Bethany were living in a desert climate, or if she were living by the ocean, which magnifies the sun's reflective powers, I would urge her to use sunscreen and to avoid overexposure.

But the fact that *too much* exposure to the sun is bad doesn't mean we want no exposure at all! In what human society have humans ever had *no* exposure to the sun? It seems to me that we've been scared by doctors and dermatologists into avoiding the sun completely. It's simply crazy.

The key is balance. Too much sun exposure can cause melanoma and skin aging, while without *enough* sun, you risk vitamin D deficiency as well as sleep problems and depression.

Even with exposure to the sun, most people seem to be deficient in vitamin D and need supplementation. The only problem is that vitamin D3 is fat soluble, which means that when you take more than you need, the excess gets stored in your fat and can be toxic. However, most people's levels of vitamin D are much too low, and far from prescribing too much supplementation, physicians tend not to prescribe *enough*.

So here's what I recommend. First, ask your physician to test your blood levels of this crucial vitamin (the official name is the 25-hydroxy vitamin D (25-OH-VitD) level). Optimal levels are 50 to 80 nanograms/milliliter (ng/ml), so if your levels are within that range, you don't need to supplement. If you test lower, see Appendix E for my recommendations, which are based on specific blood results. You usually can't get enough vitamin D in a multivitamin, so expect to take a separate daily dose.

Fish Oils: One to Three Grams of EPA and DHA Combined Each Day

Fish oil supplements are rich in the essential omega-3 fatty acids EPA and DHA, which are vital to good health. As we saw in Chapter 1, our modern diets tend to give us way more omega-6 fats relative to omega-3s. Taking fish oil is one way to help restore the balance.

Omega-3s are a terrific support for your body's efforts to prevent chronic diseases and reduce inflammation. They also provide a number of other benefits:

- A stronger immune system
- Cardiovascular support
- Improved joint health
- Better vision
- Stronger, healthier skin, hair, and nails
- Enhanced nutrient absorption
- Better metabolic function

- Improved attention, mood, and memory
- Enhanced fertility

If you're already focused on a healthy diet, fish oil can seem like an "extra," but remember: your body can't make its own fatty acids—you have to get them from outside sources. And the fatty acids in fish oil aren't called "essential" for nothing. Taking a daily dose is a great defense against feeling old and getting fat.

Of course, if you are eating a lot of fatty fish, you might not need to supplement; the fat in your diet should be enough. But with great sorrow, I can't recommend eating a lot of fatty fish because they're so full of mercury and other toxins. It's really a tragedy: fish *was* one of our healthiest foods—but not really, not any more. If you buy a high-quality fish oil, you can count on them filtering out the toxins and/or choosing safer fish.

How to Choose a Good Fish Oil

Make sure to choose a high-quality brand. Since many fish carry a significant toxic burden of pesticides, PCBs, and heavy metals, you want to be sure that these contaminants have been filtered out.

Probiotics: Powders, Pills, or Capsules Containing at Least 10 Billion to 50 Billion Live Bacteria Each Day

Probiotics are powders, pills, or capsules that contain the naturally occurring "friendly" bacteria that live in your gut and play a significant role in your ability to stay vigorous and slim.

As we saw in Chapter 3, your microbiome is a crucial part of your overall health. Yet every day it takes multiple hits from toxins, challenging foods, and stress. A daily probiotic helps support your microbiome, which in turn promotes good gut health, a strong immune system, and support for your entire body.

When I prescribed probiotics for Bethany, I also urged her to begin eating more fermented foods. These healthy choices are natural probiotics because they, too, contain live bacteria. However, in our toxic, stressful world, it's difficult to give enough support to your microbiome through food alone. Please do eat more fermented foods—but also, please, take a daily probiotic. (For more on fermented foods, see page 41 in Chapter 3.) Be especially sure to take probiotics if you are taking antibiotics, or if you consume industrially raised animal products, including milk—in restaurants, for example—that are not certified as "antibiotic free."

How to Choose a Good Probiotic

Our understanding of the microbiome is still in its infancy. There are thousands of different strains of bacteria, which makes choosing the right probiotic a bit of a crapshoot—we don't really know the most optimal formula. The good news is that all of the probiotic bacteria are friendly, so you can't go far wrong. Here are some recommendations based on what we currently know:

- Look for probiotic capsules or powders with the two most researched and effective beneficial bacteria, *Lactobacillus* and *Bifidobacterium;* ideally with the following four strains: *Lactobacillus plantarum, Lactobacillus acidophilus, Bifidobacterium longum, Bifidobacterium lactis.*

- Choose probiotics with the widest possible variety of bacteria. The more diverse your microbiome, the healthier you are likely to be.

- Change them up every three to six months.

The Supportive Seven

In addition to the basic four, I generally recommend an additional seven supplements for optimal aging. If you want to feel young, sharp, and vigorous, and if you want to maintain a healthy weight, these seven will support you!

Your Supportive Seven Supplements

- S-acetyl glutathione: 100–300 mg/day
- Magnesium: 300–600 mg/day of magnesium glycinate or 2 gm/day of magesium l-threonate
- CoQ10: 200–400 mg/day of the ubiquinol form
- Alpha-lipoic acid (ALA): 300–600 mg/day
- Turmeric: 400–600 mg/day of turmeric extract
- Mitochondrial formula (which also contains many of the B vitamins)
- Powdered greens

⟡ —— S-Acetyl Glutathione: 100–300 mg/Day —— ⟡

I've known about the wonders of glutathione for a long time, but only recently have I been able to recommend taking it as a supplement. That's because until recently, it was impossible to find a form of glutathione that could be absorbed orally. If you wanted to supplement with it, you either needed to take it intravenously or load up on supplements that converted to glutathione within your body.

Now, finally, there is a form of glutathione (s-*acetyl glutathione),* that you can take orally, and I am delighted to recommend it to you. Glutathione is one of the best detoxifiers that I know. It is absolutely your best protection against the toxins that abound in food, air, and water, and it has remarkable anti-aging properties as well.

Composed of three amino acids, glutathione is the single most powerful antioxidant that your body produces. It's made in the liver, so if your liver isn't functioning optimally, you are even more in need of supplementation.

How Glutathione Keeps You from Feeling Old and Getting Fat

- DNA protection
- Immune support
- Mitochondrial support (*mitochondria* are the portions of your cells that pump out energy, so mitochrondial support both gives you more energy and boosts your metabolism to maintain a healthy weight)
- Reduction of inflammation
- Protection against heart disease, cancer, neurological decline, dementia, and other chronic diseases

---

Glutathione is known as an anti-aging supplement, since low glutathione levels have been linked to every major aging process in the human body. After the age of 20, your natural production of glutathione slows down, dropping about 10 percent with every passing decade. By the time you reach age 60, you're making only about half as much glutathione as you did in your teens, which contributes to flagging energy, lowered immunity, and many of the minor and major ailments that we frequently associate with aging. Taking glutathione supplements can turn this process around, keeping you vital and fit no matter how old you are.

By the way, there are some other ways to boost your body's supply of glutathione in addition to taking the supplement. You won't be surprised to learn that many of these ways are already part of my Revitalize and Maintenance programs: exercise, stress relief, and the avoidance of toxins through eating organic foods and drinking filtered water as well as wise choices in personal-care products. You can also increase your natural supply of glutathione through diet.

Foods That Boost Glutathione

- Garlic
- Onions
- Asparagus
- Avocado
- Sprouts
- Cabbage
- Cauliflower

- Kale
- Parsley
- Watercress
- Cinnamon
- Cardamom
- Curcumin

◈—— MAGNESIUM ——◈

Magnesium is a mineral found in your blood, bones, tissues, and organs. It's crucial for the optimal functioning of your heart, brain, and musculoskeletal, digestive, and circulatory systems, and it's responsible for the correct metabolic function of more than 350 enzymes in your body. Magnesium helps regulate blood pressure, strengthens muscles and bones, and keeps the immune system strong.

Many people are aware of the importance of calcium to maintaining adequate bone health. But if you want your bones to be able to absorb calcium, you need sufficient supplies of magnesium.

Magnesium is a powerful muscle relaxant which can ease constipation (as your intestinal walls relax) and lower blood pressure (as your arterial walls relax). The relaxation that magnesium engenders can also help you fall asleep more easily. And if you're prone to muscle cramping, that's often a sign that you're short of magnesium—and it's a problem that additional magnesium can remedy.

Magnesium also helps your body detox. It helps clear both toxins and heavy metals.

As with other key nutrients, it can be hard to get enough magnesium just from diet. Some studies estimate that up to 80 percent of us are deficient in magnesium.[2] And the costs for shorting yourself on magnesium are high.

So the form of magnesium is important. Magnesium oxide and citrate are a great laxatives and stool softeners, but if you want to support your body's stores of magnesium, you need to use other forms. I recommend two forms of magnesium that do not have a major laxative effect, and therefore enable you to take more of it, if needed: magnesium glycinate and l-threonate. Magnesium l-threonate is supposedly able to get through the blood-brain barrier—your body's natural protection against elements in your blood reaching your brain—so it can be more helpful for an "aging" brain.

Possible Results of Insufficient Magnesium

- Allergies
- Anxiety and panic attacks
- Asthma
- Blood clots
- Bowel disease
- Depression
- Diabetes
- Fatigue
- Heart disease
- Hormonal symptoms: PMS, cramps during menstruation, infertility, various pregnancy and birth complications
- Hypertension
- Hypoglycemia

- Insomnia
- Memory problems
- Migraine
- Musculoskeletal conditions, including fibrositis, fibromyalgia, muscle spasms, eye twitches, cramps, and chronic neck and back pain
- Nerve problems, including muscle contractions; gastro-intestinal spasms; calf, foot, and toe cramps; vertigo; and confusion
- Osteoporosis
- Raynaud's syndrome
- Tooth decay

In addition to taking a supplement, I advise you to load up on dietary sources of magnesium. You can focus on whole foods and green drinks—drinks made from leafy greens and spinach, both of which are rich in magnesium.

Foods That Contain Magnesium

- Wild-caught Pacific halibut
- Leafy greens
- Spinach

- Black beans
- Pumpkin seeds
- Squash seeds
- Green drinks

⟶ CoQ10: 200–400 MGS/DAY ⟵
OF THE UBIQUINOL FORM

This remarkable antioxidant is a powerful anti-aging supplement that will boost your energy, protect your heart, and support your cellular health. If you have any concerns about aging, fatigue, or heart disease, take CoQ10, especially if you are over 40. If you take statins, CoQ10 supplements are even more important, since statins can lower your CoQ10 levels by as much as 40 percent because they inhibit your body's synthesis of it. This is not a "side effect" of statins but a direct inherent function of these drugs.

How to Choose the Right Form of CoQ10

- Look for the ubiquinol form of CoQ10. It's more easily used by the body than the more commonly available ubiquinone form.

Foods That Contain CoQ10

- Grass-fed red meat
- Organ meats
- Broccoli
- Spinach

⟶ ALPHA-LIPOIC ACID: 300–600 MG/DAY ⟵

Alpha-lipoic acid is found in every cell of your body. It's a potent, versatile antioxidant that fights inflammation, balances blood sugar, and protects your skin. Its effect is magnified by the way it boosts the effectiveness of other antioxidants in your body. ALA also promotes nerve health, helps remove heavy metals from the body, and purifies the liver.

Although your body does produce ALA, it often doesn't make as much as you need, so you have to look to outside sources—both through supplements and in your diet. Because insulin resistance and dysfunctional sugar metabolism is such a common underlying issue when we get old and fat (see Chapters 1 and 2), ALA is one of my go-to supplements for virtually all of my over-40 patients as well as an increasing number of younger ones.

Foods That Contain Alpha-Lipoic Acid

- Organ meats
- Broccoli

- Spinach

TURMERIC: 400–600 MG/DAY OF TURMERIC EXTRACT

This delicious spice contains curcumin, an anti-inflammatory powerhouse that offers numerous health benefits. It takes about four to six weeks to start seeing results, but when you do, they are considerable. Because inflammation is such a common underlying mechanism for making us old and fat, I almost always recommend this supplement to my patients.

How Turmeric Keeps You from Feeling Old and Getting Fat

- Reduces pain
- Decreases fatigue
- Boosts mood

- Sharpens mental focus
- Improves cognition
- Helps protect against cancer

MITOCHRONDIAL FORMULA

As you will recall from earlier chapters, mitochondria are the powerhouses of the cells. They produce energy, which translates into *you* having energy and also into you remaining at a healthy weight.

As we age, our mitochondria decrease in both numbers and in function, which is one of the reasons we associate age with slowing down. A supplement can slow or even reverse this process, so you continue to look and feel young.

Exercise is a great way to boost your mitochondria, so when you make movement a regular part of your life, you're well on your way to supporting these energy powerhouses. If you want to take further steps to protect and improve mitochondrial function, I highly recommend supporting your mitochondria with nutrients they need to function optimally. By improving mitochondrial function, you can tune up your metabolism, increase your energy, think more clearly, feel less achy, and prevent all sorts of age-related diseases—and who can say *no* to that?

Nutrients to Look for in a Mitochondrial Formula

- B Vitamins, including B-1 (thiamine), B-2 (riboflavin), B-3 (as niacinamide), and B-6 (as pyridoxal-5-phosphate)
- Vitamin C
- CoQ10

- Alpha-lipoic acid
- Magnesium
- Manganese
- D-ribose
- L-carnitine
- Resveratrol

POWDERED GREENS

If you're not loading up each day on fresh leafy greens, a powdered green drink can be an effective way to pick up the slack. A green drink nourishes every system in your body, with numerous health benefits. These drinks are full of vitamins and minerals, antioxidants, enzymes, phytonutrients, and other health-enhancing nutrients. One of them provides the same antioxidant support of three to five servings of fruit and vegetables.

How Powdered Greens Keep You from Feeling Old and Getting Fat

- Enhanced immunity
- Boosted energy levels

- Better digestion

How to Choose the Right Form of Powdered Greens

- Make sure they're made with organic fruits and vegetables.
- Avoid the products with those all-too-common fillers and bulking agents, which greatly diminish the nutritional value of the drink.

Shooting for "Terrific"

Even after we spoke, Bethany was a little skeptical about taking the supplements I recommended. But she agreed to give them a try and see how she felt.

At our next appointment, she couldn't wait to tell me about all the changes she had noticed. "I was so cranky and irritable with everyone, but now . . . I don't know, I just feel calmer," she said. "I haven't had that awful feeling of a cold coming on—I can tell that I'm just stronger. I've still got some of that bloating that used to drive me crazy, but much, much less. And look! My skin is *way* better!"

Bethany agreed that the supplements had indeed made a difference. She added, "It really makes me wonder about all those years I wasn't taking them, even when I wasn't feeling bad or when my skin was okay. Because maybe, if I had been taking them, I would have felt even better, and my skin would have been even better. I feel like these supplements make the difference between feeling good—and feeling *terrific.*"

You're Not Getting Enough Nutrients: A Quick Fix

This one is simple: start taking the nutrients I recommend in this chapter! In some cases you'll notice a difference within just a few days. Certainly, within a month, you should be feeling their effects, especially if you complete the 2-Week Revitalize Program and go on to the lifelong Maintenance Program. Supplements are no substitute for a healthy diet, enough movement, good sleep, and other types of stress relief. But they definitely *supplement* those aspects of your life, and help you move from "good" to "terrific."

REASON #10:

YOU'RE NOT GETTING ENOUGH "UBUNTU"

My patient Miriam, a striking, rather glamorous woman in her mid-50s, was having a tough time. Miriam's youngest child had just left for college. All three of her children were doing well—two in colleges on the West Coast and one teaching English in Korea. Her marriage was "in good shape," as she put it, and her work as a financial analyst in a midtown New York City firm was going well. As Miriam herself expressed it, "I have nothing to complain about!"

And yet, Miriam told me, she was—not sick, exactly, but not really well either. She had frequent bouts of indigestion. She had put on an extra 6 kilos, "almost overnight." Her muscles and joints had started to ache. Many nights out of the week, she woke up at 2 or 3 A.M., unable to get back to sleep for several hours. As she entered menopause, she suffered from uncomfortable hot flashes. She felt that her sex drive—and indeed, her sexuality itself—were drying up.

Worse, Miriam went on, she felt flat and empty.

"I don't think I'm depressed in the traditional sense," she explained. "I'm not crying all the time—I'm not even particularly sad. I just feel . . . stale. Like, what's the point? I know I should be grateful for my job, my husband, my beautiful children—and I am! But right now, none of that seems like enough."

Passion, Meaning, Community

As we have seen throughout this book, the kinds of symptoms Miriam was experiencing might have many causes. Diet, gut health, the microbiome, hormonal imbalances, lack of exercise, stress, sleep issues, medications, and a lack of key nutrients might all be playing a role.

In addition to the physical issues, however, I thought that Miriam was suffering from some deeper concerns:

- **Passion.** When Miriam was younger, she had taken a great deal of pleasure in building a family and becoming proficient at her career. She was one of those lucky people who had been passionate about both her personal life and her work life. Now, however, her work had ceased to interest her very much, while her home life had changed drastically: she no longer had children to care for, and she wasn't at that exciting (if challenging) stage of building a new marriage. Without the concerns that had shaped her 20s, 30s, and 40s, Miriam felt that the passion had gone out of her life.

- **Meaning.** If *passion* speaks to how deeply we care for something, *meaning* speaks to how a person or an activity connects us to something larger than ourselves. Caring for her children had given Miriam a deep sense of meaning—the feeling that what she did *mattered*. Above and beyond caring for them physically, Miriam had found meaning in helping her children grow up: teaching her son and two daughters to be strong, adventurous, caring, and ethical; helping them discover their true interests and develop their true potential; and modeling for them how to become successful adults. Now that her children no longer needed this kind of day-to-day care, Miriam felt that her life had lost its meaning.

- **Community.** When Miriam's children were at home, Miriam had two communities: colleagues at work, and other parents in her children's schools. Now that her children were gone, Miriam had lost that second community, and as work ceased to engage her, she felt she didn't really belong in the first. Like meaning, *community* connects us to something larger. Without access to this larger dimension, Miriam's health was suffering.

Myths to Break Through

- "Health is primarily a matter of our physical state."
- "Passion is not an important factor in our health."
- "Meaning has no impact on our health."
- "Community is not important for our well-being."

Myth: "Health is primarily a matter of our physical state"

When I discussed this myth with Miriam, I introduced her to a new concept: *ubuntu*. Ubuntu is a Xhosa word that means "what makes us human is the humanity we show each other."

I first became aware of this concept while I was growing up in South Africa. I came to realize its importance when I lived and worked in KwaNdebele among the Ndebele people, for whom it was a central part of their culture. Someone who values ubuntu knows that you can't be fully human thinking only of yourself: your job, your home, your new car, your pension plan. You need to discover your own humanity by connection to the humanity of others.

I think this concept of ubuntu has enormous significance for us here in America. Most of us live in cultures where the focus is solely on the individual. Indeed, there is a great deal of pressure on each of us to ensure that we have the job and home and health care that we need to feel safe and healthy; that our children have access to good schools and good opportunities; that our parents and, eventually, we ourselves are protected in old age.

These economic pressures are real—but they are not the whole story. Being part of a larger community is an important dimension in each of us, even if we aren't always so aware of it. Just as we might not realize that we need vitamin D or probiotics to support the optimal function of our bodies, we might not realize that we also need ubuntu: the chance to express our humanity through the humanity we show to others.

I want all of you who are reading this book to take care of your bodies and promote optimal function. I also want you to realize that finding passion, meaning, and community—ubuntu—is just as important to your health as whole, fresh foods, healthy exercise, and good sleep.

Myth: "Passion is not an important factor in our health"

Some of us, like Miriam, have been lucky enough to feel a great deal of passion in our 20s, 30s, and 40s. Some of us have never quite found the activities or relationships that spoke to our deepest passions. Either way, it's quite common to feel a lack of passion as you approach your 50s and beyond—a sense that life has become somewhat stale and flat.

This lack of passion is a huge part of why so many of us feel old. It's passion—a deep, strong excitement about a person or activity—that makes us feel young and vital. Passion is sexy, whether we're turned on by a new love, international travel, or a newfound interest in some activity.

I've often noticed that when my patients take up a new interest (or fall in love!), they lose weight, seemingly without trying. There are many reasons for this, including the way *dopamine,* the deeply pleasurable "excitement" biochemical, affects our appetite and metabolism.

━━◈ DOPAMINE: THE PASSION CHEMICAL ◈━━

You feel a dopamine rush when you first fall in love, whether that excitement is generated by a person, a place, or an activity. Dopamine is also frequently associated with novelty—the thrill of the new. In fact, one of the standard suggestions for a couple who feels that the passion has gone out of their relationship is that they find new things to share. Going to a new city, hiking together up a mountain, even taking a thrilling ride on a roller coaster stimulates your dopamine. The thrill of a "dopamine experience" extends to the person you share it with, making an old, familiar relationship seem new and thrilling once again.

So you have two ways to stimulate passion in your life, alone or with a partner:

1. **Find something you absolutely love—something that turns you on.** Learn how to tango. Start playing poker. Take a jewelry-making class. Find out how to give a great massage. Enroll in a workshop for standup comedy or clowning. Study a martial art. If your first effort doesn't really click, try something else. It might take a while to find your passion, especially if you haven't felt excited about anything for the past few years. But the quest for a new passion can help you feel young and vital, even before you actually find it.

2. **Look for new experiences.** One of the reasons many of us feel old at 50 and 60 is because so much of our lives seems familiar. In our 20s and 30s, so many experiences are new. After that, novelty can be harder to come by. However, if you're willing to seek out the new, you can also regain your youthful sense of openness and excitement. Learn a new language. Visit a foreign city. Take an unusual trip—one of those sailboat voyages where you can crew on the boat and see the world from the deck of a ship, or a volunteer stint on an organic farm, or an Elderhostel where you combine tourism with study. Or look for new experiences closer to home: Find a new neighborhood of your town or city and spend some time walking or biking through it. Visit an unfamiliar house of worship in your community and spend some time sitting there quietly or perhaps attend a service. Seek out a historic building or museum that you have never visited. Go to a lecture at the local historical society, or walk through a nearby botanical garden. Get out of your comfort zone, challenge yourself, and explore something new. This can take a bit of courage, but that in itself will help you feel young.

━━◈ "AM I BEING SELFISH?" ◈━━

When I suggested to Miriam that she needed more passion in her life, one of her first responses was to feel "selfish."

"I have so much already," she told me. "Do I really need to spend more time thinking about myself?"

Now, as we'll see in the rest of this chapter, I'm all for extending yourself and focusing on ways to give to others. I believe that by giving to others, we enrich our own lives immeasurably, and that, ultimately, is the true meaning of ubuntu. So if you are hungering to find meaning and community through volunteering to help others, joining a community action group, or some other type of outward-directed activity, that, too, will make you feel young and vital.

I also know that for many people, it can be hard to give yourself permission to put yourself first. Women in particular are socialized to put other people first. "We're not used to putting ourselves first," Miriam agreed when I raised this point with her. So when the opportunity comes—when the space finally opens up to think of yourself rather than of your spouse, children, parents, or friends—putting yourself first might not come so easily.

However, if you don't have passion in your life—if you have never really focused on yourself—it can be hard to give to others. I see many women in their 50s and 60s who seem absolutely drained and spent. Some of that comes from the physical factors we have discussed throughout this book, and some of it comes from a lack of meaning and community. But some of it comes from a lifelong pattern of looking after others with no real focus on what *they* need and want.

So, I told Miriam, "selfish" doesn't have to be miserly in spirit. It can simply mean "someone who gives to themselves." You don't have to give to yourself to the exclusion of others. In fact, you can be more comforting and generous to others when you feel terrific about yourself.

I told you when I began this book that I want you feeling *great!* Part of that is finding something that ignites your passions, so you can feel truly great about something you do. I invite you to go on your own "passion quest" because passion is part of what keeps us young.

Myth: "Meaning has no impact on our health"

Miriam was very struck when I pointed out how much meaning she had gotten from raising her children and, consequently, what a great hole that had left in her life. At first, it was difficult for her to even consider other ways of finding meaning. "I've always just focused on my family," she kept saying. But together we made a list of ways she might find more meaning in her life:

- **Spiritual and religious activities.** You might find meaning through meditation, prayer, religious study, or attending services and participating in a congregation. You might also connect to your spirituality in more individual ways, such as yoga; spending time in nature, by the ocean, or in beautiful surroundings; walking through the streets of a beloved city; or keeping a journal focusing on your spiritual journey. If you are "spiritual but not religious," you might consider the communities around such denominations as Unitarian Universalists, Friends

(Quakers), or Reconstructionist Jews, all of whom focus less on a particular religious doctrine and more on a personal connection to the divine or to your fellow humans.

- **Artistic activities.** Self-expression and creativity are hugely important sources of meaning. Whether or not you consider yourself "an artist," giving some space to your creative side can be an extraordinarily powerful way of feeling vital and open—which is another way of feeling young. Here is something I wrote about creative expression in my first book, *Total Renewal:*

  > Creative expression is something most of us pursued joyfully as children but which too many of us give up for so many reasons as adults. We become achievement oriented and fear failure or criticism. Or we are afraid to appear frivolous or silly. Or we simply do not allow ourselves the time that it takes to imagine and create. In the process, we deprive ourselves of one of the most fertile opportunities to reconnect to our emotional landscape. By journaling, painting, drawing, sculpting, dancing, making music, cooking, knitting, taking photographs, or any other activity that enables us to express and create, we can regain a sense of childlike enthusiasm and individuality and reconnect with our emotional self.

  Creativity and the arts are yet another road to self-knowledge and freedom. Remember, creativity is an act that can be purely of and for yourself, although you may also enjoy sharing the fruits of your creativity with others. It is about unleashing your spirit, ideas, and emotions in any form that brings you pleasure and satisfaction. You cannot do it "wrong." Read *The Artist's Way* by Julia Cameron to explore what the act of creation means to you. Take a workshop or class through a local adult learning center, Y, or institute. Then dream, play, and create.

- **Mentoring.** One of the greatest gifts of age is having wisdom to share with the young. Paradoxically, this sharing process helps us feel young because it connects us with the generations that come after and reminds us how valuable our experience, knowledge, and insight still are. Feeling useless and isolated makes us feel old; feeling useful and connected makes us feel vital. There are many options for mentoring. Here are a few suggestions—perhaps you can think of more:

  - Informal mentoring at your job or in an organization to which you already belong
  - A formal mentoring program in your community

- Becoming a Big Brother or Big Sister

- Getting involved in a mentoring organization, such as Girls Write Now, which pairs girls who like writing with older writer-mentors

- **Volunteering.** Sometimes what you really want is to know that you've made someone's life better. Serving in a soup kitchen, reading to residents of a nursing home, or volunteering through a local social service organization or school can all be profoundly satisfying. Although your goal is to help, you might well find that you get at least as much from the interaction as the people you serve.

  If you want to feel better, helping others will probably help you as much as whomever you are helping—and maybe even more! Giving without receiving or expecting anything in return is extremely uplifting. I believe what it does physiologically to you is the opposite of the stress response: it stimulates the parasympathetic system. Lowering the stress response decreases cortisol, and as we have seen, cortisol cues your body to retain fat.

  In addition, when we stop focusing on ourselves and when we are sharing or being compassionate to others, we let go of a lot of unnecessary anxiety about our own dilemmas. And letting go of anxiety can help you feel energized, liberated—young.

  So, helping others can help *you* to feel young and stay slim!

❖ How I Gave . . . and Received ❖

My wife and I both grew up in South Africa. We were unwilling to live with the injustices of apartheid, so we left our home country soon after I finished my medical training. But we never stopped loving South Africa and wanting to somehow give back to the country that had given us so much.

When apartheid ended, we had our chance. We became involved in an organization called the Ubuntu Education Fund as well as a second nonprofit in South Africa, Monkeybiz.

I never would have imagined how much meaning Janice and I have gotten from this connection to our country and its people. By giving, we're receiving so much more than we ever might have dreamed. I can't even really express what we get, except perhaps the feeling of a deep connection that somehow is very healing.

I wouldn't exactly call that connection "happy." The nonprofits help families and children living in incredible poverty—children who are HIV positive and live in communities that have been devastated by AIDS. When I read correspondence from the fund, or when I visit that community, I frequently find myself moved to tears. Yet somehow it's a privilege to share in its remarkable resilience and accomplishments in spite of the severe hardships of people's daily lives. When I see how others are living—how happy they often are even when they have very few material possessions—that helps me shift my own perspective and stay in touch with what really matters. It is a way both to stay grounded and feel inspired.

Myth: "Community is not important for our well-being"

One of the things that makes us feel old fast—and which undoubtedly causes us to gain weight as well—is feeling isolated. An enormous body of research supports the notion that a key to aging well is not growing old alone but rather doing so as part of a larger community.[1]

Of course, at any age, we need to find our "tribe"—the people who value what we value and who make us feel recognized and valued. Connecting to our tribe might be easier in this age of the Internet and the cell phone, but I also worry that the rapid spread of technology means that each of us functions far more in isolation. No need to visit a library or bookstore—you can buy any book you want online. Why go out to a movie or play or sporting event when you can stay home and watch television, download a movie, or rely on pay-per-view? Tweeting, texting, and e-mail keep us connected to individuals and to our tribe, but it can also promote the feeling that no one is available for more than 140 characters worth of sharing. The happy-face photos on Facebook can easily lead you to feel that everyone is out there having a good time but you.

So I think that in these days of technology and social media, creating a tribe is more important than ever. Finding or creating your tribe lets you feel that you belong to something; you're not alone; it's not only *you* who has this problem or that fear. I think that's very comforting and helps in the healing, while being isolated does the opposite. I'm very struck that the longest-lived and most vital people in the world—the people who live in the so-called "blue zones" (see page 75)—all feel that they are part of a tribe, whether it's the Seventh-Day Adventist community of Loma Linda, California, or the Okinawan island society in Japan.

Your tribe might be your coworkers, your family, or the members of your church, synagogue, mosque, or zendo. It might be a political or community group, or a group of friends who frequently socialize together. (The power of the tribe can be seen in the many television programs about just such groups of friends, who seem to spend every night and weekend doing things together.)

If, like Miriam, you feel that you've had a community and lost it, you might need to put some extra effort into finding or building a community that suits your current time of life. This can be a long, slow, and perhaps discouraging process, much like dating after a divorce or breakup. But like finding a new relationship, finding a new tribe can give you a new burst of energy, a new sense of groundedness—and a very welcome sense of feeling young and vital.

✦ —— THE HEALING POWER OF COMMUNITY —— ✦

My patient Zee was only 19 years old, but he was suffering greatly from not having found his tribe. Zee had been diagnosed with depression but was unwilling to take the meds that had been prescribed for him, so his parents sent him to me. I immediately diagnosed his problem not as a biochemical imbalance but as a lack of community.

The problem for Zee was that he had grown up in a wealthy and rather complacent suburban community where he didn't fit in at all. Passionate about community activism and environmentalism, Zee felt thoroughly alienated from his classmates' focus on cars, dates, and the latest fashions. His parents didn't understand him and neither did his friends.

One of my health coaches worked with Zee to help him identify some places in New York City where he might find people who shared his interests and his values. Already a vegetarian—for which he was frequently mocked both at home and at school—Zee simply lit up with recognition when he took his first yoga class at a local studio. Finally, he had found people who understood him—even some people who could guide him.

Zee's depressive symptoms immediately vanished. He became lively, open, engaged. No one who saw him would have recognized the young man who just a few months ago looked mopey, sullen, and shut down. For Zee, the greatest healing was finding his tribe.

LONGING TO BELONG

As you can see, I think that a sense of belonging is really important—in fact, it's essential. Being isolated is stressful; knowing you're not alone is a profound version of stress relief. If you feel crazy because you're isolated and you visit a conventional doctor who confirms that you're crazy—as Zee's first doctor did with him—it can be devastating.

I'll never forget finding my tribe as a young student in South Africa. Although the apartheid system left me feeling profoundly alienated and somewhat crazy—how could everybody act as though such an oppressive system were normal?!—joining an antiapartheid youth group let me feel that I belonged. I'll never forget going to the protest rallies with my friends and fellow activists. Frightened but determined, we'd carry picket signs, knowing that every rally would inevitably end the same way—with the police chasing us with bats. It was scary, but it was also exhilarating, because we believed in what we were doing and we had each other. This early experience gave me a vision not only of the fight for justice, but also of an important component of health. You feel empowered when you belong to something greater than yourself, and that empowerment helps make you healthy. You feel a sense of self-worth and security when you're part of a community because your fellows are endorsing the way you think and react. That self-worth also helps keep you healthy.

Are You Looking for Your Tribe?

Here are some suggestions to support your search:

- **Start with the relationships you already have.** Is anyone you know already in your tribe? Are there people you would like to know better who seem to be in your tribe? Figure out how to spend more time with these people and, perhaps, to become friends with their friends as well. Possibly these relationships will enable you to create a tribe or even join a readymade one.

- **Look for organizations and activities.** Zee found a yoga studio. I found an antiapartheid activist group. Where might your tribe be found? Make a list of likely places and then start checking them out. Be patient, and don't give up. It can take time to find your tribe, but the results are more than worth it.

- **Start your own group.** What about a study group or reading group about topics you're interested in? A political action group or community organization that speaks to an issue you care about? An artistic or performance group, such as a band or string quartet? A committee at your church or in a political party you belong to? If you define what matters most to you, you might well attract others who feel the same way.

- **Look online.** These days, there are online support groups, forums, blogs, and websites for just about every group and subgroup you can imagine. For many people, these provide a sense of community and a tribe with whom they can share opinions. Be careful, though. Sometimes an online group—while useful for getting information or ideas—doesn't really provide the sense of connectedness and being "seen" that are what you need to overcome isolation.

Miriam Finds Her Tribe

Miriam very much liked the idea of ubuntu, and she loved the idea of finding her tribe—of breaking the isolation that was making her feel "old before her time." After so many years focused on family and career, it took her a while to discover other sources for passion, meaning, and connection, but she was inspired to begin the journey.

At first, Miriam asked herself what she might enjoy. She tried a few different activities—a dance class, a hiking club, a book group—but nothing really clicked.

Then Miriam got involved with a program in her community that paired adults with young people who were trying to start their own businesses and needed mentors. "I didn't just want to do the Big Sister program because I've already had children," Miriam told me. "I wanted it to be a little different from that." The program she found enabled her to translate her skills and life experience into another arena, one where the focus was not on her personal advancement but on helping someone else. Sharing what she knew made Miriam feel valued and vital—no longer "old and irrelevant," but part of the flow of life.

Through the mentoring program, Miriam met a whole new set of people engaged in a wide range of innovative businesses. She also felt inspired to think of other ways to experience ubuntu. She began volunteering at a local women's shelter, where she found herself moved by the courage of the women she met, as well as by the dedication of the staff people at the shelter.

"I feel almost as though I'm getting a second chance at life—as though I'm starting a whole new chapter," Miriam told me on her last visit. By becoming part of a larger world, Miriam had transformed herself as well: a true example of how the microcosm mirrors the macrocosm!

You're Not Getting Enough "Ubuntu": Three Quick Fixes

These are not necessarily *quick* fixes, but they will make a big difference in your life:

1. Discover your passion

2. Look for opportunities to create meaning in your life

3. Find your tribe

YOUR 2-WEEK REVITALIZE PROGRAM:

GETTING READY

by Kerry Bajaj, Health Coach

Okay, so now that you're getting ready to start your 2-Week Revitalize Program, how do you feel? Are you psyched to get started with the diet and lifestyle changes that are going to have you feeling terrific? Are you looking at the list of all the foods you'll be avoiding on this two-week program and wondering what in the world you *will* be able to eat? Or maybe you're asking yourself when you'll find time for your daily exercise, or how you'll ever get yourself to bed by our recommended bedtime of 10 P.M.

Whatever you're feeling, I can promise you I've heard it all before, and probably more. As one of Dr. Lipman's health coaches, my job is to work with individual patients and help them figure out exactly how to implement their own versions of the Revitalize and Maintenance programs. I'm going to try to reach out through the pages of this book and do the same for you—although you are also very welcome to call 888-434-9483 and work with me or one of the other health coaches by phone. Sometimes that personal touch is just what you need!

Meanwhile, we've done everything we can to make this program clear and easy to implement. Tricia Williams, our fabulous chef, has created two weeks of delicious meal plans for you—it won't feel anything like a diet, I promise! Because we know you're busy, no recipe will take more than about half an hour to prepare. To further streamline the work process, Chef Williams has organized everything so that you're making a bit extra and using the leftovers for a later meal, so you can save yourself as much time as possible.

Although we'd love you to cook for yourself, we get it: sometimes, for business or pleasure, you just have to eat in a restaurant. For those times, we've provided you with some suggestions so you know exactly what to order (see pages 194–195).

Jim Clarry is a personal trainer to whom we often refer people, and he's come up with a wonderful, gentle two-week workout for your Revitalize Program and a more vigorous work-out for your Maintenance Program. The workout is designed to be useful both for people who haven't been moving much in a while, and for those who are more active. It combines cardio, strength training, core strength, flexibility, and fascia release exercises from Dr. Keren Day, an Active Release Technique practitioner who works with us at the wellness center. All you need are two inexpensive and portable pieces of equipment: a large rubber band (the kind big enough to go around your ankles) and a foam roller, which you can use to give yourself a fascia-opening massage that will have you feeling as though you've just taken a trip to the spa. Again, we know you're busy, so Jim and Keren have made sure you can finish the workout in less than 30 minutes. You'll be amazed at how good it makes you feel.

So you can see how committed we are to making this program as easy and doable as possible for you, whether you're working a demanding job with lots of overtime, running a home with three kids, or just feeling intimidated by cooking, exercising, and committing to an early bedtime. Like I said, we get it: Making a lot of changes in a short time can sometimes feel as though the rug is being pulled out from under you. And to be honest, we want this first two weeks to be dramatic—not because we want to make your life difficult, but because we want you to get the most bang for your buck.

So let me offer you a deal.

Let's Make a Deal

Here's what you get:

- You'll make a significant start to bringing down your inflammation, healing your gut, replenishing your microbiome, and balancing your hormones.

- If you have symptoms—achy joints, headache, indigestion, and the like—they will more than likely start to disappear and might even vanish completely.

- Your skin will start to glow.

- Your brain will feel sharper.

- Your emotions will feel calmer.

- Without ever feeling hungry or deprived, you will very likely lose some weight.

And here's what *you* have to do: follow this 2-Week Revitalize Program with 100 percent commitment.

Now, if you only take the program 90 percent of the way, will you still get results?

Yes, almost certainly. But they won't be the *same* results.

What about 80 percent? Or 70 percent? What if you just make a few of the changes we suggest?

Look: making even a single positive change can often make a difference. The problem is that it won't make *enough* of a difference to really change your life. As Dr. Lipman says to all his patients, "Feeling just a little bit better is not enough. I want you feeling *terrific*." And if you want to feel terrific—if you don't want to keep feeling old and fat—you need to make some dramatic changes just to get the ball rolling.

As you'll see, the initial 2-Week Program is considerably stricter than the Maintenance Program. We want to be sure that you clear out all the foods that might be causing you problems. We want to give your gut and your microbiome a break from stressors and make sure they get the healing, replenishing support they need. If you are carbohydrate intolerant, we want to cut your intake of grains, beans, starchy vegetables, and fruits far enough to show you how terrific you can feel when you're not eating more carbs than your body can handle.

As you've seen throughout this book, these types of changes have a cumulative effect. There is an amazing synergy that can really build when you give your body *everything* it needs: food, exercise, sleep, and stress relief. All of us here in Dr. Lipman's office want you to give yourself the chance to support your body at full speed so you can get the full benefit of that synergy.

So that's our deal: you give us 14 days of following the Revitalize Program, and we give you *terrific*. We also give you a lot of new knowledge about what your body wants and needs. After the two weeks are up, you can decide for yourself whether you want to add some foods back in or modify the program in other ways. We're betting that once you know how great you can feel, you'll naturally want to keep doing whatever it takes to keep feeling that way.

The Revitalize Program: Time to Stop Feeling Old and Fat!

You're reading this book because you're tired of feeling old and fat, right? And because you want to start feeling vigorous, clearheaded, and optimistic, all while achieving a healthy weight?

Great—that's what we want for you too. Here's how we're going to get you there:

- **Clean up your diet.** You'll stop eating the inflammatory foods that make you feel old and fat and replace them with nourishing foods that will balance your blood sugar and your hormones while freeing you from cravings.

- **Heal your gut.** You'll take out the gut-irritating foods, use specific herbs to kill your "bad" bacteria, and start taking *probiotics*—friendly bacteria—to replenish your microbiome.

- **Detox your system.** You'll have some shakes with gut-scrubbing fiber, which will bind with toxins and help pull them out of your system by supporting elimination. The shakes also have nutrients to support the liver's detoxification functions.

- **Keep you energetic and flexible.** You'll start a workout that includes cardio, core strengthening, stretching, and fascia release.

- **Reduce your stress.** Each day you'll meditate, practice mindfulness, engage in relaxing types of breathing techniques, and/or practice restorative yoga.

- **Improve your sleep.** You'll maintain a healthy early bedtime with the help of a supportive sleep routine.

Make This Program Your Own

Now, we want you to follow this program 100 percent. And we want to give you lots of support as you do. So we've laid out every single day for you: what you'll eat, how you'll work out, when you'll start your bedtime routine. If you want to simply put yourself in our hands, that's great—just lean on us.

What if you'd like a little latitude? Well, we don't want you to violate any of our core principles. You'll get optimum results if you avoid all the foods on our list on page 189, exercise and practice stress relief every day, and commit to getting good sleep. So those points are non-negotiable. But you *can* customize your program in other ways:

- Switch any of the meals around to suit your taste—just switch dinners with dinners, lunches with lunches, and so on.

- Feel free to make a big batch of delicious and nourishing bone broth (see page 192 and the recipe on page 226) and add a cup of it to any meal or enjoy it as a snack.

- If you'd rather follow Jim's guidelines for getting exercise rather than do his workout—or if you've been exercising for a while and have a routine that works for you—feel free to go with your own plan, so long as you're moving at least 30 minutes each day.

- If you want to experiment with different types of stress relief from the ones we suggest, go right ahead. Just make sure you get at least ten minutes of stress relief every single one of your 14 days.

Again, the effects of all these practices are cumulative, and we want you feeling terrific! One of the best things about my job is watching patients do their 2-Week Program and seeing the weight come off, the energy come flooding back, and a whole new sense of well-being emerge. One of my patients told me she was sleeping so well that she started waking up without an alarm clock. Another said his pants were loose for the first time since he left college. People even tell me that their wedding rings finally fit again!

As you come to the end of your two weeks, you'll discover a new awareness of how the foods you eat are affecting your health. This knowledge will prove invaluable as you go forward: you'll always know which foods work for you and which do not. As your body changes, you may be able to tolerate different foods, or some foods might stop working for you. At that point, you'll be creating your own program—and you'll have the tools to figure that out.

What to Expect

Because we start with a big leap, you might need some time to adjust. Some people start feeling terrific right away—but some of our patients do have a challenging three or four days at first. You might experience some headaches, cravings, fatigue, constipation, or a general feeling of grumpiness. Try to plan for this and allow time for plenty of sleep, possibly a nap, and lighter exercise if you're used to strenuous workouts.

However, before the first week is over, these symptoms should disappear. You'll start feeling more energetic, focused, and alert. Your stress-relief practices will help you feel more calm and collected amid the chaos of your day. Your body will become more flexible, your thoughts will be clearer, and your cravings will subside. You'll probably start losing some weight. And don't be surprised if you start to get compliments about how good you're looking!

The Revitalize Program: Eating Plan

So here is where the rubber meets the road. Thanks to our fabulous chef Tricia Williams, you're going to be loading up on delicious, energizing foods that leave you feeling full and satisfied. Each day is packed with tons of vegetables; nourishing protein sources like free-range chicken, wild-caught fish, and grass-fed beef; and healthy fats like avocado, coconut oil, nuts, and olives.

You'll also notice that this plan calls for a "beverage makeover," taking out the drinks that are messing with your health: coffee, tea, booze, fruit juices, and brown bubbly sugar water (aka soda). Instead you will be hydrating with lots of water, herbal tea, and fresh vegetable juices.

Meanwhile, you'll completely eliminate the foods that stress your system, create inflammation, and challenge your gut, including grains, beans, dried pulses, dairy, corn, soy, processed foods, natural and artificial sweeteners, and alcohol. As we've seen throughout the first three chapters of this book, these foods can negatively affect your body in various ways. You might be able to add some of them back after your two weeks on the Revitalize Program, but first give yourself a chance to see how your body functions without them.

I know this way of eating might seem odd at first, but by cutting out sugar cold turkey, you stop cravings dead in their tracks. And as you give up junk food, your taste buds will come alive, allowing you to notice the subtle tastes of whole foods—the sweetness of a dish of fresh berries or the earthy, juicy richness of some grass-fed beef. You'll soon effortlessly start to prefer the foods that keep you young and slim.

Revitalize: The Overview

Foods to Embrace:

- Nonstarchy vegetables, except for the nightshades (aubergine, peppers of all types, and tomatoes, which are potentially reactive)
- Organic or free-range lamb, chicken, turkey, duck, wild game, and grass-fed beef
- Wild-caught fish and seafood/shellfish
- Small fish, such as black cod, herring, sardines, and trout
- Nuts and seeds (raw almonds, cashews, walnuts, hazelnuts, Brazil nuts, sesame seeds, and pumpkin seeds)
- Healthy fats, such as coconut, avocado, sesame, flaxseed, and extra virgin olive oil
- Almond and cashew butter
- Unsweetened almond, rice, hemp, and coconut milk
- Gut-healing and fermented foods, including bone broth, sauerkraut, and kimchi
- Noncaffeinated green or herbal teas, spring or sparkling water, fresh vegetable juices
- Vinegar (apple cider, white wine, red wine, and balsamic)
- Herbs and spices
- Cacao nibs, unsweetened cocoa powder, raw cacao

Foods to Enjoy No More than Once a Day

- Low-sugar fruits such as berries of all types, green apples, and citrus fruits, with a focus on berries
- Starchy vegetables: squash of all types, sweet potatoes, yams, turnips, swedes, beetroot (but no white potatoes, which are nightshades)
- A little butter from grass-fed cows
- *At most,* one daily cup of coffee or caffeinated tea (see pages 190–191)

Foods to Eliminate:

- Gluten
- All grains, including brown rice, oats, and quinoa
- Soy (tofu, tempeh, miso, edamame, soy milk)
- Corn
- Eggs
- Dairy
- Beans and pulses (split peas, lentils, dried pulses)
- Nightshade vegetables (tomatoes, potatoes, aubergines, peppers)
- High-sugar fruits, such as bananas, cherries, figs, grapes, lychees, mangoes, pineapples, pears, watermelon
- Dried fruits
- Factory-farmed meats
- Farmed fish and high-mercury fish (tuna, swordfish)
- Processed foods
- Alcohol
- Salted and roasted nuts and all peanut products
- Added sugars and natural sweeteners, including agave, honey, and maple syrup
- Artificial sweeteners
- Fruit juices and energy drinks
- Processed seed and vegetable oils, such as canola, sunflower, safflower, corn, soy, margarine, and shortening
- Commercial salad dressings, ketchup, relish, barbecue sauce, mayonnaise
- Candy, energy bars, and protein bars

If you would like to use a sweetener, you can enjoy small amounts of stevia.

Stay Hydrated

During the Revitalize Program, we'll have you drinking 1.8 litres of water each day. This is going to help you out in lots of ways:

- If you're like most people, you aren't drinking nearly enough water each day, and you've gotten used to being chronically dehydrated. We want to give you the chance to experience what good hydration feels like so you've got a good solid baseline going forward.

- If you drink enough water, you'll feel less hungry.

- You're trying to get rid of toxins, and all that water will help you flush them out.

If plain water doesn't appeal to you, add a slice of fresh lemon and, if you like, a pinch of Himalayan sea salt.

If you have trouble fulfilling your 1.8 litre quota, do what I do: get yourself a 450ml water bottle and make it your mission to fill it four times each day. I personally love the BKR brand of glass water bottles. If you use a plastic water bottle, please make sure it's BPA free.

Start with a big glass of water first thing in the morning, as we often wake up dehydrated. Drink more throughout the morning and afternoon. Slow down your water consumption by early evening so you don't wake up in the middle of the night needing to use the bathroom.

Ideally, you won't drink much *while* you're eating, as too much water can wash away the enzymes you need for optimal digestion. Here's a sample schedule:

Sample Water-Drinking Schedule

7 A.M.: Wake and drink 450ml of water
11 A.M.: Drink 450ml of water
3 P.M.: Drink 450ml of water
6 P.M.: Drink 450ml of water

However, don't stress too much about *when* you drink. Customize as you like, and of course, if you want to, drink *more*. Remember: if you're feeling thirsty, that means you're *already* dehydrated. Drink up!

Coffee, Tea, and Caffeine

Okay, if your heart has been sinking at the thought of giving up caffeine, I have some good news for you: you don't necessarily have to.

Yes, in the ideal world, you'd probably get the most benefit from the program by cutting out caffeine 100 percent for two weeks or even four weeks. Once you experience the effects of being caffeine free—the deeper sleep, the greater calm, the overall balance—you can decide whether you want to reintroduce caffeine and if so, how much and at what time of day.

However, for many people caffeine isn't really such a big problem. Certainly, sugar is far worse for you, and if you can't give up both, Dr. Lipman would rather have you focus on the sugar. If you just can't bear the thought of giving up your caffeinated coffee or tea, go ahead and have one 250ml cup each day. Just be sure to have it in the morning so it doesn't interfere with your early bedtime.

Certainly, coffee is by far the hardest substance for our patients to cut out. So as you cut it out or cut it back, we don't want you going "cold turkey"—you'll probably get headaches and other withdrawal symptoms. Here's how you can taper off over several days:

5 Days to Cut Out Caffeine

Day 1	¾ regular, ¼ decaf
Day 2	½ regular, ½ decaf
Day 3	¼ regular, ¾ decaf
Day 4	All decaf
Day 5	Herbal tea

Getting Ready to Cook

I'm so excited for you: 14 days of real food! Your body recognizes real food, packed with vitamins and minerals, and very soon you'll notice the difference. If you've been plagued with constant cravings, you'll notice how quickly they simmer down on this program.

We'd like you cooking at home as much as possible because otherwise, it can be awfully hard to get healthy. The more you can get comfortable in the kitchen, the better off you'll be. But you don't have to make cooking a major focus. As this book was going to press, I was just coming back to work after having my first child, and I can promise you that I didn't want to spend a minute longer in the kitchen than I had to. On the other hand, I did want my family to eat a healthy meal every night. This is a dilemma all of us health coaches share: most of us aren't cooking as an art or a hobby—we just want to prepare nourishing, delicious, and *quick* meals.

Chef Tricia is going to help you all she can, and I'm going to share some tips with you too. Before you get started on your program, invest a little in some prep:

- Cleanse your pantry of unhealthy temptations before your start the program.

- Take advantage of the way Chef Tricia has saved you time by having you cook extra food so you can use the leftovers soon after.

- After your first two weeks, plan ahead. Knowing what you'll eat a few days at a time makes for a smooth experience.

Equipment List

- Blender or food processor
- Muffin pan for 12 muffins
- Cast-iron frying pan, 25 to 30 cm

Portion Sizes and Calorie Counting

No calorie counting for you! Your body is counting nutrients, not calories, so just focus on the foods to enjoy and the foods to eat in moderation.

As for portion sizes, we'd rather you go by how you feel than by what you measure. Your goal is to eat until you are 80 percent full: that is, satiated, not stuffed. However, if you'd like some rough guidelines, use these:

- Salads: about the size of two open hands
- Vegetables: about the size of one open hand
- High-quality carbohydrate, such as a sweet potato: about the size of your fist
- High-quality protein: about the size of your palm
- High-quality fats such as coconut oil: one to two tablespoons

The Revitalize Program: Gut-Healing Plan

The Revitalize Program includes foods and supplements to heal your gut and replenish your microbiome with friendly bacteria. Supporting your gut and microbiome is one of the fastest ways to stop feeling old and fat and start feeling young and slim.

Enjoy Gut-Healing Bone Broth

A staple of the human diet for thousands of years, bone broth is enjoying a resurgence of interest due to its powerful health benefits. Bone broth is full of gelatin and collagen, which soothes the intestinal tract and helps heal leaky gut. Bone broth supports your immune system and reduces inflammation throughout the body. To supplement your 2-Week meal plan, feel free to enjoy bone broth with any meal or as a snack.

The Revitalize Program: Cleanse Shakes

You'll get by far the best results from the Revitalize Program if you stick to the recommended meal plans, including our recommendations for consuming shakes—rather than whole foods—for breakfast, mid-morning snack, and mid-afternoon snacks.

Some of my patients are a bit surprised by this recommendation at first, especially because, in most cases, whole organic foods are so good for you. However, when you are trying to cleanse your system of the excess fats, sugars, and preservatives you might have consumed— the types of foods that make you feel old and fat—you will find it useful to focus on healthy shakes that are full of healthy gut-scrubbing fiber that can promote weight loss, improve digestion, and help heal your intestinal tract. In addition, the shakes we recommend are rich in the very nutrients your liver needs to detoxify your system. They are healthy, filling, and delicious, providing you with a terrific boost on your way to becoming slim and feeling young.

When we started recommending shakes several years ago, we wanted to make things as easy as possible for our patients, so we developed the Be Well Cleanse shakes in packets, which include all the protein, fiber, and nutrients you need. However, if you don't want to buy the packets, you can substitute pea protein and fiber powder—just make sure to get the highest-quality ingredients. Whether you use the Be Well packets or make up your shakes from scratch, you can follow Chef Tricia's scrumptious recipes, which will speed you on your way to optimal health.

Our patients have seen tremendous success with these shakes, improving gut health and liver function as they lose weight, gain energy, boost mood, and regain focus, concentration, and mental clarity. We consider them to be an essential element of the Revitalize Program, and we're thrilled to share them with you.

The Revitalize Program: Supplements

Throughout your 2-Week Revitalize Program, you will be taking the supplements that Dr. Lipman recommends to his patients for overall vitality as well as for gut healing. Because gut problems are such a big part of feeling old and getting fat, these gut-healing supplements, which include antimicrobial herbs to kill the bad guys and digestive enzymes to help with digestion, are a crucial part of the program. You might be tempted to skip the supplements and focus only on the foods. However, you will get the best results if you follow *all* parts of the program, including the supplements.

If you choose not to follow the supplement protocol exactly, I urge you to find a digestive enzyme formula to improve digestion and an antimicrobial formula to wipe out bad bacteria from the gut. The antimicrobial formula should include as many as possible of the following herbs:

- Sweet wormwood extract

- Berberine sulfate

- Caprylic acid

- Grapefruit seed extract

- Barberry extract

- Bearberry extract

- Black walnut hull

By the time you get to the Maintenance Program, your gut health will have improved and your overall vitality will have increased, making supplements more of an optional choice. At that point you can decide whether you want to keep taking them, using the information in Chapter 9 to decide which supplements are right for you. But for the first two weeks, please follow the program, including the supplements. I promise—you'll be glad you did!

What about Restaurants During Revitalize?

Many of my clients ask me whether they'll be able to eat in a restaurant—or whether they'll turn into that annoying dinner date who asks for lots of modifications on their order. Not true! You will, however, have to skip the bread basket; ask for a dish of marinated olives and have a few of those instead. Otherwise, follow the same principles as when you're eating at home: fill up your plate with lots of vegetables and protein from good sources. Here are some ideas for what to look for when you're scanning a menu:

Lunch Option #1:
Main course: Entreé salad with protein such as roasted chicken, wild salmon, or shrimp

Lunch Option #2:
Appetizer: Seaweed salad
Main course: Sashimi

Dinner Option #1:
Side: Roasted vegetables, such as Brussels sprouts
Main course: Wild salmon

Dinner Option #2:
Side: Sautéed greens, such as broccoli rabe
Main course: Grass-fed steak

Dinner Option #3:
Appetizer: Butternut squash soup
Main course: Roasted chicken with vegetables

Getting Ready to Move

Of course, if you have any concerns at all about exercising—even the relatively gentle program that we have provided—make sure you check with your physician. Other than that, the only prep you need is to purchase two inexpensive pieces of equipment: a rubber band large enough to fit around your ankles and a foam roller, which you'll use for fascia release. Both are available online or at any store that sells exercise equipment.

The Revitalize Program: Stress-Reduction Plan

One of your most powerful tools to revitalize is stress reduction. We'd like you to get in the habit of doing ten minutes of stress relief each day: 4–7–8 Breathing plus either Mindful Breathing Practice or meditation. Or you can sub in a restorative yoga pose (page 329). Pick your own time of day for stress relief—or break it into two five-minute sessions—but ideally, do your stress relief at the same time each day. You'll be surprised at how consistency multiplies the effects.

The Revitalize Program: Your Sleep Plan

- By 9 P.M., start your electronic sundown by turning off all devices: TV, computer, phone, and anything else with a screen.

- By 9:30 P.M., start your wind-down routine.

- By 10 P.M., lights out.

Does this seem extreme? I totally get it. But if you don't give yourself the chance to restore your circadian rhythms and get deep, restful sleep, you'll never know how big a difference it can make—to your mood, your mental function, and even your weight. Sleep is what you need, not doing more work, answering e-mails, watching TV, or late-night snacking.

Create Your Wind-Down Routine

As a new mother, I have recently gotten a crash course in how to get a baby to sleep, and it all boils down to one thing: *consistent routine*. Every single night, we follow the exact same steps in the exact same order: bath, pajamas, bottle, pull the shades, turn on the white-noise machine, swaddle, sleep. Following the same steps in the same order every night signals to the baby that it is time for sleep. By the time the white noise machine goes on, she is rubbing her eyes and knows what's coming next.

I would never put the baby in the crib without those preparatory steps, yet as adults we go-go-go all evening and then are surprised when we can't fall asleep. Following a consistent sleepy-time routine is a powerful tool for adults as well. That's why we encourage you to create your own wind-down routine during the Revitalize Program.

Sample Wind-Down Routine
9:30 P.M.: Brush teeth and wash up
9:40 P.M.: Read in bed
9:55 P.M.: Mindful breathing for five minutes
10:00 P.M.: Lights out

Customize that routine as you please. Here are some elements you might want to include:

- Evening prayers

- Meditation

- A bath

- A restorative yoga pose (see page 329)

- Dabbing some restful essential oils on your wrists and breathing in the scent

The choice is yours—just make sure you allocate 30 minutes to winding down. And by the way, keep all activities out of the bedroom except sleep and sex (and maybe some restful reading). All work-related and electronic activities belong in another room, keeping your bedroom as a peaceful, distraction-free oasis.

Get Ready to Feel Young and Slim!

My favorite part of my job is seeing people come back to the office after their 2-Week Revitalize Program. I love seeing their energy—their glow—and hearing about their weight loss. I love learning about the symptoms they no longer suffer from, how two weeks have made such a big difference in reducing or even eliminating their headaches, aching joints, indigestion, acne, or sleep difficulties.

I wish I could be there when *you* finish the Revitalize Program, because I know it's going to make a big difference in your life too. Get ready to enjoy a whole new burst of vitality along with some healthy weight loss—the first few steps toward feeling young and slim!

REVITALIZE:
WEEK ONE

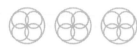

DAY 1
Breakfast: Shake of your choice (pages 211–213)
Mid-Morning Snack: Shake of your choice (pages 211–213)
Lunch: Smoked Salmon Salad (page 213)
Mid-Afternoon Snack: Shake of your choice (pages 211–213)
Dinner: Ginger Miso Halibut Stir Fry (pages 215–216)
Beverages: 1.8 litres filtered water
Supplements: Take the antimicrobial formula and digestive enzymes twice a day with lunch and dinner
Exercise: Routine A (pages 309–317) at any time of your choosing
De-stress: 4–7–8 Breathing + Meditation Practice, in the morning or evening, or, alternatively, a restorative yoga pose in the morning and/or evening
Sleep: 9 P.M.–10 P.M.: Electronic sundown, wind-down, and lights out

DAY 2
Breakfast: Shake of your choice (pages 211–213)
Mid-Morning Snack: Shake of your choice (pages 211–213)
Lunch: Ginger Miso Halibut Filet with Mixed Greens (pages 215–216)
Mid-Afternoon Snack: Shake of your choice (pages 211–213)
Dinner: Cauliflower Soup (page 230) + side salad
Beverages: 1.8 litres filtered water
Supplements: Take the antimicrobial formula and digestive enzymes twice a day with lunch and dinner
Exercise: Routine A (pages 309–317) at any time of your choosing
De-stress: 4–7–8 Breathing + Meditation Practice, in the morning or evening, or, alternatively, a restorative yoga pose in the morning and/or evening
Sleep: 9 P.M.–10 P.M.: Electronic sundown, wind-down, and lights out
DAY 3
Breakfast: Shake of your choice (pages 211–213)
Mid-Morning Snack: Shake of your choice (pages 211–213)
Lunch: Cauliflower Soup (page 230) + side salad
Mid-Afternoon Snack: Shake of your choice (pages 211–213)
Dinner: Lamb Chops with Stir-Fry Greens (page 222)
Beverages: 1.8 litres filtered water
Supplements: Take the antimicrobial formula and digestive enzymes twice a day with lunch and dinner
Exercise: Routine A (pages 309–317) at any time of your choosing
De-stress: 4–7–8 Breathing + Meditation Practice, in the morning or evening, or, alternatively, a restorative yoga pose in the morning and/or evening
Sleep: 9 P.M.–10 P.M.: Electronic sundown, wind-down, and lights out

DAY 4
Breakfast: Shake of your choice (pages 211–213)
Mid-Morning Snack: Shake of your choice (pages 211–213)
Lunch: Lamb Chops with Greens, Pomegranate, Mint, Apple Cider Vinaigrette (pages 222–223)
Mid-Afternoon Snack: Shake of your choice (pages 211–213)
Dinner: Mediterranean Vegetable Paella (pages 224–225)
Beverages: 1.8 litres filtered water
Supplements: Take the antimicrobial formula and digestive enzymes twice a day with lunch and dinner
Exercise: Routine A (pages 309–317) at any time of your choosing
De-stress: 4–7–8 Breathing + Meditation Practice, in the morning or evening, or, alternatively, a restorative yoga pose in the morning and/or evening
Sleep: 9 P.M.–10 P.M.: Electronic sundown, wind-down, and lights out
DAY 5
Breakfast: Shake of your choice (pages 211–213)
Mid-Morning Snack: Shake of your choice (pages 211–213)
Lunch: Mediterranean Vegetable Paella (pages 224–225)
Mid-Afternoon Snack: Shake of your choice (pages 211–213)
Dinner: Roasted Chicken Breast with Root Vegetables (pages 219–220)
Beverages: 1.8 litres filtered water
Supplements: Take the antimicrobial formula and digestive enzymes twice a day with lunch and dinner
Exercise: Routine A (pages 309–317) at any time of your choosing
De-stress: 4–7–8 Breathing + Meditation Practice, in the morning or evening, or, alternatively, a restorative yoga pose in the morning and/or evening
Sleep: 9 P.M.–10 P.M.: Electronic sundown, wind-down, and lights out

DAY 6
Breakfast: Shake of your choice (pages 211–213)
Mid-Morning Snack: Shake of your choice (pages 211–213)
Lunch: Asian Chicken in Lettuce Cups (pages 219–220)
Mid-Afternoon Snack: Shake of your choice (pages 211–213)
Dinner: Sesame Shrimp and Broccoli (page 218)
Beverages: 1.8 litres filtered water
Supplements: Take the antimicrobial formula and digestive enzymes twice a day with lunch and dinner
Exercise: Routine A (pages 309–317) at any time of your choosing
De-stress: 4–7–8 Breathing + Meditation Practice, in the morning or evening, or, alternatively, a restorative yoga pose in the morning and/or evening
Sleep: 9 P.M.–10 P.M.: Electronic sundown, wind-down, and lights out
DAY 7
Breakfast: Shake of your choice (pages 211–213)
Mid-Morning Snack: Shake of your choice (pages 211–213)
Lunch: Sesame Shrimp Salad (pages 218–219)
Mid-Afternoon Snack: Shake of your choice (pages 211–213)
Dinner: Carrot Ginger Soup (page 229) + side salad
Beverages: 1.8 litres filtered water
Supplements: Take the antimicrobial formula and digestive enzymes twice a day with lunch and dinner
Exercise: Routine A (pages 309–317) at any time of your choosing
De-stress: 4–7–8 Breathing + Meditation Practice, in the morning or evening, or, alternatively, a restorative yoga pose in the morning and/or evening
Sleep: 9 P.M.–10 P.M.: Electronic sundown, wind-down, and lights out

REVITALIZE
WEEK ONE
SHOPPING LIST

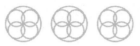

Dry Goods
  almond milk, unsweetened
  apple cider vinegar
  1 jar artichokes
  avocado oil
  Be Well Cleanse kit (www.bewell.com/cleanse)
  black peppercorns
  chicken or vegetable broth
  ground cinnamon
  cocoa powder, unsweetened
  coconut milk, unsweetened
  coconut oil
  Dijon mustard
  2 large bottles extra virgin olive oil
  fiber powder
  kalamata olives, pitted
  pea protein powder, non-GMO
  1 box peppermint tea
  sea salt
  sesame seeds
  tamari, wheat free
  toasted sesame oil
  turmeric
  white miso
  za'atar

Meat, Poultry, and Seafood
  2 boneless skinless chicken breasts
  Two 30g halibut filets
  4 to 6 medium lamb chops, about 570g

450g medium wild shrimp, cleaned
One 115g package wild smoked salmon

Produce
  Fruit:
  1 avocado
  7 lemons
  9 limes
  1 pack pomegranate seeds

  Greens:
  1 bunch rocket
  450g baby spinach
  1 head butter lettuce
  450g mixed greens
  1 head watercress

  Vegetables:
  6 pieces baby bok choy
  2 heads broccoli or 1kg broccoli florets
  4 large carrots
  2 heads cauliflower
  1 medium celeriac
  1 cucumber
  2 heads garlic or 1 jar minced garlic
  1 ginger root
  2 parsnips
  1 head red cabbage or 1 pack sliced red cabbage
  1 red onion
  4 shallots
  1 medium turnip
  1 white onion

  Herbs:
  2 bunches chives
  1 bunch coriander
  1 bunch Italian parsley
  1 bunch mint
  fresh thyme sprigs

Storage Tips
  Keep herbs in a jar with an inch of water in the bottom.

REVITALIZE:
WEEK TWO

DAY 8
Breakfast: Shake of your choice (pages 211–213)
Mid-Morning Snack: Shake of your choice (pages 211–213)
Lunch: Carrot Ginger Soup (page 229) + side salad
Mid-Afternoon Snack: Shake of your choice (pages 211–213)
Dinner: Za'atar-Crusted Grass-Fed Flank Steak with Parsnip Fries and Broccoli (pages 223–224)
Beverages: 1.8 litres filtered water
Supplements: Take the antimicrobial formula and digestive enzymes twice a day with lunch and dinner
Exercise: Routine A (pages 309–317) at any time of your choosing
De-stress: 4–7–8 Breathing + Meditation Practice, in the morning or evening, or, alternatively, a restorative yoga pose in the morning and/or evening
Sleep: 9 P.M.–10 P.M.: Electronic sundown, wind-down, and lights out

DAY 9
Breakfast: Shake of your choice (pages 211–213)
Mid-Morning Snack: Shake of your choice (pages 211–213)
Lunch: Za'atar-Crusted Grass-Fed Flank Steak with Baby Spinach Salad and Tahini Dressing (pages 223–224)
Mid-Afternoon Snack: Shake of your choice (pages 211–213)
Dinner: Asparagus Soup (page 228) + side salad
Beverages: 1.8 litres filtered water
Supplements: Take the antimicrobial formula and digestive enzymes twice a day with lunch and dinner
Exercise: Routine A (pages 309–317) at any time of your choosing
De-stress: 4–7–8 Breathing + Meditation Practice, in the morning or evening, or, alternatively, a restorative yoga pose in the morning and/or evening
Sleep: 9 P.M.–10 P.M.: Electronic sundown, wind-down, and lights out
DAY 10
Breakfast: Shake of your choice (pages 211–213)
Mid-Morning Snack: Shake of your choice (pages 211–213)
Lunch: Asparagus Soup (page 228) + side salad
Mid-Afternoon Snack: Shake of your choice (pages 211–213)
Dinner: Seared Salmon Filet with Coconut Oil Stir-Fry Vegetables (page 214)
Beverages: 1.8 litres filtered water
Supplements: Take the antimicrobial formula and digestive enzymes twice a day with lunch and dinner
Exercise: Routine A (pages 309–317) at any time of your choosing
De-stress: 4–7–8 Breathing + Meditation Practice, in the morning or evening, or, alternatively, a restorative yoga pose in the morning and/or evening
Sleep: 9 P.M.–10 P.M.: Electronic sundown, wind-down, and lights out

DAY 11
Breakfast: Shake of your choice (pages 211–213)
Mid-Morning Snack: Shake of your choice (pages 211–213)
Lunch: Salmon Kale Salad (pages 214–215)
Mid-Afternoon Snack: Shake of your choice (pages 211–213)
Dinner: Roasted Spaghetti Squash with Kale Miso Almond Pesto (page 225)
Beverages: 1.8 litres filtered water
Supplements: Take the antimicrobial formula and digestive enzymes twice a day with lunch and dinner
Exercise: Routine A (pages 309–317) at any time of your choosing
De-stress: 4–7–8 Breathing + Meditation Practice, in the morning or evening, or, alternatively, a restorative yoga pose in the morning and/or evening
Sleep: 9 P.M.–10 P.M.: Electronic sundown, wind-down, and lights out
DAY 12
Breakfast: Shake of your choice (pages 211–213)
Mid-Morning Snack: Shake of your choice (pages 211–213)
Lunch: Roasted Spaghetti Squash with Kale Miso Almond Pesto (page 225)
Mid-Afternoon Snack: Shake of your choice (pages 211–213)
Dinner: Turkey Shepherd's Pie (page 221)
Beverages: 1.8 litres filtered water
Supplements: Take the antimicroblal formula and digestive enzymes twice a day with lunch and dinner
Exercise: Routine A (pages 309–317) at any time of your choosing
De-stress: 4–7–8 Breathing + Meditation Practice, in the morning or evening, or, alternatively, a restorative yoga pose in the morning and/or evening
Sleep: 9 P.M.–10 P.M.: Electronic sundown, wind-down, and lights out

DAY 13
Breakfast: Shake of your choice (pages 211–213)
Mid-Morning Snack: Shake of your choice (pages 211–213)
Lunch: Turkey Shepherd's Pie (page 221)
Mid-Afternoon Snack: Shake of your choice (pages 211–213)
Dinner: Get Your Greens On Soup (pages 230–231) + side salad
Beverages: 1.8 litres filtered water
Supplements: Take the antimicrobial formula and digestive enzymes twice a day with lunch and dinner
Exercise: Routine A (pages 309–317) at any time of your choosing
De-stress: 4–7–8 Breathing + Meditation Practice, in the morning or evening, or, alternatively, a restorative yoga pose in the morning and/or evening
Sleep: 9 P.M.–10 P.M.: Electronic sundown, wind-down, and lights out
DAY 14
Breakfast: Shake of your choice (pages 211–213)
Mid-Morning Snack: Shake of your choice (pages 211–213)
Lunch: Get Your Greens On Soup (pages 230–231) + side salad
Mid-Afternoon Snack: Shake of your choice (pages 211–213)
Dinner: Pan-Seared Scallops and Wilted Rocket (pages 216–217)
Beverages: 1.8 litres filtered water
Supplements: Take the antimicrobial formula and digestive enzymes twice a day with lunch and dinner
Exercise: Routine A (pages 309–317) at any time of your choosing
De-stress: 4–7–8 Breathing + Meditation Practice, in the morning or evening, or, alternatively, a restorative yoga pose in the morning and/or evening
Sleep: 9 P.M.–10 P.M.: Electronic sundown, wind-down, and lights out

REVITALIZE
WEEK TWO
SHOPPING LIST

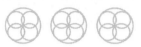

Dairy
    grass-fed butter

Dry Goods
    almond milk, unsweetened
    1 bag raw almonds
    avocado oil
    Be Well Cleanse kit (www.bewell.com/cleanse)
    50g cashews
    chicken or vegetable broth
    ground cinnamon
    cocoa powder, unsweetened
    coconut milk, unsweetened
    ground cumin
    fiber powder
    liquid stevia
    pea protein powder, non-GMO
    ground black pepper
    1 box peppermint tea
    sea salt
    tahini
    za'atar spice

Meat, Poultry, and Seafood
    450g grass-fed flank steak
    450g ground turkey, dark or white meat
    Two 200g wild salmon filets
    450g sea scallops

Produce
> *Fruit:*
> 1 avocado
> 4 lemons
> 2 limes
>
> *Greens:*
> 1 bunch rocket
> 450g baby spinach
> 2 bunches kale
> 450g mixed greens
>
> *Vegetables:*
> 450g asparagus
> 2 baby bok choy
> 1 bunch broccoli
> 1 carrot
> 1 head cauliflower
> 1 leek
> 2 medium parsnips
> 1 red onion
> 1 shallot
> 1 medium spaghetti squash
> 1 white onion
>
> *Herbs:*
> 1 bunch chives
> 1 bunch coriander

Storage Tips
> Keep herbs in a jar with an inch of water in the bottom.

REVITALIZE RECIPES

by Chef Tricia Williams

As we explained on page 193, you can make these shakes either with the Be Well Cleanse shake packets or with high-quality pea protein and fiber powder. You can prepare these shakes in a blender, or, for added convenience, get a portable blender bottle and shake them up by hand. Either way, you'll find them filling, energizing, and delicious.

COCONUT CINNAMON SHAKE

Makes 1 Serving

240ml coconut milk, chilled
¼ teaspoon cinnamon
1 Be Well Cleanse shake packet or 1 serving pea protein powder + 1 serving fiber powder

Place all ingredients in a shaker or blender. Mix well until powder is fully dissolved. Enjoy over ice.

ROYAL FLUSH SHAKE

Makes 1 Serving

Juice of 1 lime
1 teaspoon white miso
1 teaspoon turmeric
360ml coconut milk, chilled
1 Be Well Cleanse shake packet or 1 serving pea protein powder + 1 serving fiber powder
Liquid stevia to taste

Place all ingredients in a shaker or blender. Mix well until powder is fully dissolved. Enjoy over ice.

GINGERSNAP SHAKE

Makes 1 Serving

360ml almond milk, chilled
½ teaspoon cinnamon
¾ teaspoon minced ginger
1 Be Well Cleanse shake packet or 1 serving pea protein powder + 1 serving fiber powder
Liquid stevia to taste

Place all ingredients in a shaker or blender. Mix well until powder is fully dissolved. Enjoy over ice.

LEMONADE SHAKE

Makes 1 Serving

360ml coconut milk, chilled
Juice of 1 lemon
1 Be Well Cleanse shake packet or 1 serving pea protein powder + 1 serving fiber powder
Liquid stevia to taste

Place all ingredients in a shaker or blender. Mix well until powder is fully dissolved. Enjoy over ice.

CHOCOLATE SHAKE

Makes 1 Serving

360ml unsweetened coconut or almond milk, chilled
1 tablespoon unsweetened cocoa powder
Dash cinnamon
1 Be Well Cleanse shake packet or 1 serving pea protein powder + 1 serving fiber powder
Liquid stevia to taste

Place all ingredients in a shaker or blender. Mix well until powder is fully dissolved. Enjoy over ice.

PEPPERMINT STICK SHAKE

Makes 1 Serving

240ml strong chilled peppermint tea
120ml almond or coconut milk, chilled
1 Be Well Cleanse shake packet or 1 serving pea protein powder + 1 serving fiber powder
Liquid stevia to taste

Place all ingredients in a shaker or blender. Mix well until powder is fully dissolved. Enjoy over ice.

SMOKED SALMON SALAD

Makes 2 servings

200g mixed greens
¼ red onion, sliced
¼ avocado, sliced
1 tablespoon Lemon Vinaigrette (page 231)
One 115g package smoked wild salmon

Place the mixed greens, onion, and avocado in a medium bowl. Toss with the Lemon Vinaigrette. Place the smoked salmon over the salad.

⇨——— Day 1 Revitalize

SEARED SALMON FILETS

Makes 2 servings

Two 200g salmon filets
Sea salt and pepper to taste
1 tablespoon avocado oil

Pat the salmon filets dry with a paper towel. Season with sea salt and pepper.

Heat the avocado oil in a cast iron frying pan over high heat. Place the salmon filets skin side down and reduce heat to medium low. Cook about 7 minutes or until browned. Turn the fillet and cook for 4 more minutes.

> Store 1 Seared Salmon Filet in an airtight container in the refrigerator for lunch.

 ### DINNER:
SEARED SALMON FILET WITH COCONUT OIL STIR-FRY VEGETABLES

1 tablespoon coconut oil
1 teaspoon minced garlic
1 teaspoon grated ginger
35g sliced red onions
40g sliced baby bok choy
165g cauliflower florets, blanched
75g sliced carrots
Sea salt and pepper to taste
Juice of 1 lime
1 teaspoon chopped coriander
1 Seared Salmon Filet

Heat the coconut oil in a cast iron frying pan over medium heat. Add the garlic, ginger, onions, bok choy, cauliflower, and carrots. Season with sea salt and pepper. Sauté for 8 minutes. Remove from heat and add the lime juice and coriander.

Plate the vegetables and top with the Seared Salmon Filet.

Lunch:
SALMON KALE SALAD

200g stemmed kale

1 tablespoon Lemon Vinaigrette (page 231)

6 kalamata olives, pitted

25g thinly sliced red onion

1 Seared Salmon Filet

Mix the kale in a medium bowl with the Lemon Vinaigrette. Massage the dressing into the kale. Plate the kale and top with the olives, onions, and Seared Salmon Filet.

———— Days 10 and 11 Revitalize

GINGER MISO HALIBUT FILETS

Makes 2 servings

2 tablespoons white miso

Juice of 1 lime

½ teaspoon grated ginger

1 teaspoon wheat-free tamari

1 teaspoon chopped coriander

Sea salt to taste

Two 200g halibut filets

Preheat the oven to 375 degrees Fahrenheit.

Mix together the miso, lime juice, ginger, tamari, coriander, and sea salt in a bowl. Set aside.

Place the halibut filets in a baking pan and bake for 12 to 14 minutes, depending on the thickness of the fish. Remove from the oven and spread the miso mixture evenly over the filets.

> Store 1 Ginger Miso Halibut Filet in an airtight container in the refrigerator for lunch.

DINNER:
GINGER MISO HALIBUT STIR-FRY

1½ tablespoons coconut oil

130g small broccoli florets

55g sliced baby bok choy

Sea salt to taste

1 Ginger Miso Halibut Filet

Heat the coconut oil in a cast iron frying pan over medium heat. Add the broccoli, bok choy, and sea salt to frying pan. Sauté for ten minutes or until vegetables are soft. Plate the vegetables and top with the Ginger Miso Halibut Filet.

LUNCH:
GINGER MISO HALIBUT FILET WITH MIXED GREENS

200g mixed greens

15g sliced red onion

1 tablespoon Asian Vinaigrette (page 233)

1 cold Ginger Miso Halibut Filet

Place the mixed greens and red onion in a bowl and toss with the Asian Vinaigrette. Serve with the Ginger Miso Halibut Filet.

———— Days 1 and 2 Revitalize

PAN-SEARED SEA SCALLOPS

Makes 2 servings

350g sea scallops

Sea salt and pepper to taste

1 tablespoon avocado oil

Clean the scallops and pat dry on paper towels. Season with sea salt and pepper.

Heat the avocado oil in a cast iron frying pan on high heat. Once the pan is hot, sear the scallops on each side for two minutes or until well caramelized.

> Store half of the scallops in an airtight container in the refrigerator for lunch.

DINNER:
PAN-SEARED SCALLOPS AND WILTED ROCKET

50g rocket
40g sliced avocado
200g Pan-Seared Sea Scallops
1 lemon wedge

Plate the rocket and avocado slices. Place the Pan-Seared Sea Scallops on top of the rocket (this will cause the rocket to wilt). Squeeze lemon onto the scallops and salad.

LUNCH:
SCALLOP ROCKET SALAD

50g rocket
15g sliced red onion
¼ avocado, diced
1 tablespoon Lemon Vinaigrette (page 231)
200g Pan-Seared Sea Scallops

Place the rocket, onion, and avocado in a medium bowl and toss with the Lemon Vinaigrette. Top with the Pan-Seared Sea Scallops.

—•—— Day 14 Revitalize; Day 1 Maintenance

SESAME SHRIMP

Makes 2 servings

1 tablespoon coconut oil
450g medium shrimp, cleaned
1 teaspoon minced garlic
1 teaspoon minced ginger
1 teaspoon sesame seeds
Sea salt to taste

Heat the coconut oil in a cast iron frying pan over medium-high heat. Toss the shrimp with the garlic, ginger, sesame seeds, and sea salt in a medium bowl. Place evenly in the frying pan. Cook on each side for 90 seconds or until done. Remove from heat and let cool.

> Store half of the shrimp in an airtight container in the refrigerator for lunch.

DINNER:
SESAME SHRIMP AND BROCCOLI

2 teaspoons coconut oil
525g small broccoli florets
Sea salt to taste
225g Sesame Shrimp

Heat the coconut oil in a cast iron frying pan over medium heat. Add the broccoli and sea salt. Sauté for 1 minute and then add 120ml water. Continue cooking until the broccoli is soft, about 6 minutes. Serve 350g of the broccoli with the Sesame Shrimp.

> Store 175g broccoli in an airtight container in the refrigerator for lunch.

LUNCH:
SESAME SHRIMP SALAD

200g watercress

75g sliced carrots

15g sliced red onion

175g broccoli florets

1 tablespoon Asian Vinaigrette (page 233)

225g Sesame Shrimp

Place the watercress, carrots, red onion, and broccoli in a medium bowl and toss with the Asian Vinaigrette. Place the Sesame Shrimp on top of the salad and serve.

⬥—— Days 6 and 7 Revitalize

ROASTED CHICKEN BREASTS

Makes 2 servings

1 tablespoon avocado oil

2 boneless skinless chicken breasts, patted dry

Sea salt and pepper to taste

Preheat the oven to 375 degrees Fahrenheit.

Heat the avocado oil in a cast iron frying pan on medium-high heat.

Season the chicken breasts with salt and pepper. Add the chicken to the frying pan. Sear on each side for about 2 minutes. Place the pan in the oven and allow to cook for 10 minutes. Remove from heat and let cool.

> Store 1 chicken breast in an airtight container in the refrigerator for lunch.

DINNER:
ROASTED CHICKEN BREAST WITH ROOT VEGETABLES

1 medium celeriac, diced

2 medium parsnips, diced

1 medium turnip, diced

2 tablespoons avocado oil

Sea salt and pepper to taste

4 thyme sprigs

1 Roasted Chicken Breast

Preheat the oven to 400 degrees Fahrenheit.

Place the celeriac, parsnips, and turnip in a medium bowl. Coat with the avocado oil and season with sea salt and pepper.

Spread the vegetables evenly on a roasting tray. Top with thyme sprigs and roast for 18 to 20 minutes or until soft and slightly caramelized. Remove from heat and discard the thyme sprigs. Top with the Roasted Chicken Breast.

 LUNCH:
ASIAN CHICKEN IN LETTUCE CUPS

100g thinly sliced cabbage

2 tablespoon Asian Vinaigrette (page 233)

1 Roasted Chicken Breast, shredded

4 large butter lettuce leaves

1 teaspoon sesame seeds

Toss the cabbage with the Asian Vinaigrette in a small bowl until the cabbage is well coated. Place the shredded Roasted Chicken Breast evenly in the 4 lettuce cups. Top each lettuce cup with the cabbage. Sprinkle the sesame seeds on top.

———— Day 5 and 6 Revitalize

TURKEY SHEPHERD'S PIE

Makes 3 servings

2 teaspoons sea salt

1.3kg cauliflower florets

1 tablespoon avocado oil

450g ground turkey, dark or light meat

50g finely diced white onion

½ teaspoon ground cumin

1 teaspoon minced garlic

120g baby spinach

Boil 1.9 litres water and sea salt in a medium pot over high heat. Add the cauliflower florets. Cook for 8 minutes or until the cauliflower is soft. Remove from heat and drain. Place the cauliflower in a blender and purée until smooth.

Heat the avocado oil in a large frying pan over medium-high heat. Add the ground turkey and onions to the frying pan. Mix in the cumin and garlic. Cook, stirring frequently until the meat is browned. Remove from heat.

Transfer the turkey to a large pie pan or baking dish. Spread the spinach on top of the turkey and allow it to wilt. Spread the cauliflower purée evenly over the spinach.

Broil the turkey shepherd's pie until the cauliflower has a golden-brown color, about 6 to 8 minutes. Allow to cool.

> Store ⅓ of the turkey shepherd's pie in an airtight container in the refrigerator for lunch.

> Store the other ⅓ of turkey shepherd's pie in an airtight container in the freezer for Day 28 Maintenance dinner.

—◇— Days 12 and 13 Revitalize; Day 28 Maintenance

LAMB CHOPS

Makes 2 servings

4 medium-large lamb chops (about 565g total)

Sea salt to taste

1 tablespoon avocado oil

Pat the lamb chops dry on both sides with a paper towel. Season with sea salt.

Heat the avocado oil in a cast iron frying pan over high heat. Once pan is hot, sear the lamb chops on each side for 2 minutes. Stand the chops on their fatty side and brown for an additional minute.

> Store 2 chops in an airtight container in the refrigerator for lunch.

 ### DINNER:
LAMB CHOPS WITH STIR-FRY GREENS

1 tablespoon avocado oil

25g thinly sliced white onions

150g chopped baby bok choy

1 teaspoon garlic, minced

60g baby spinach

Sea salt to taste

2 Lamb Chops

Heat the avocado oil in a cast iron frying pan over medium-low heat. Add the onions and cook until translucent, about 2 minutes. Add the bok choy and sauté for 2 minutes. Add the garlic and baby spinach and sauté for 1 minute. Season with sea salt. Remove from heat, and plate. Top with the Lamb Chops.

 ### LUNCH:
LAMB CHOPS WITH GREENS, POMEGRANATE, MINT, APPLE CIDER VINAIGRETTE

25g rocket

75g thinly sliced baby bok choy

75g sliced cucumber

10 mint leaves, chopped

85g pomegranate seeds

1 tablespoon Apple Cider Vinaigrette (page 232)

2 Lamb Chops

Place the rocket, baby bok choy, cucumbers, mint leaves, and pomegranate seeds in a bowl and toss with the Apple Cider Vinaigrette. Plate, and top with Lamb Chops.

—⬦—— Days 3 and 4 Revitalize

ZA'ATAR-CRUSTED GRASS-FED FLANK STEAK

Makes 2 servings

2 tablespoons avocado oil

2 tablespoons za'atar spice

Sea salt and pepper to taste

450g grass-fed flank steak

Heat the avocado oil and spices in a cast iron pan over high heat. When the pan is hot, sear the flank steak until well caramelized, about 4 minutes on each side. If the flank steak is too long for the pan, cut it in half and repeat the cooking process. Remove the meat from the heat and let rest on a cutting board for at least 10 minutes. Slice and let cool.

> Store half in an airtight container in the refrigerator for lunch.

DINNER:
ZA'ATAR-CRUSTED GRASS-FED FLANK STEAK WITH PARSNIP FRIES AND BROCCOLI

2 parsnips

2 tablespoons avocado oil

Sea salt to taste

175g broccoli florets

½ recipe Za'atar-Crusted Grass-Fed Flank Steak

Preheat the oven to 375 degrees Fahrenheit.

Peel the parsnips and cut lengthwise into french fries. Place on half of a roasting tray and brush with 1 tablespoon avocado oil. Season with sea salt.

On the other half of roasting tray, coat the broccoli florets with the remaining tablespoon of avocado oil and season with sea salt. Roast for 12 to 15 minutes.

Plate, and serve with Za'atar-Crusted Grass-Fed Flank Steak.

LUNCH:
ZA'ATAR-CRUSTED GRASS-FED FLANK STEAK WITH BABY SPINACH SALAD AND TAHINI DRESSING

60g baby spinach

35g thinly sliced red onion

165g shaved cauliflower florets

1 tablespoon Tahini Dressing (page 232)

½ recipe Za'atar-Crusted Grass-Fed Flank Steak

Toss together the spinach, onion, cauliflower, and Tahini Dressing in a medium bowl. Mix well until the salad is evenly coated. Top with the Za'atar-Crusted Grass-Fed Flank Steak.

——— Days 8 and 9 Revitalize

MEDITERRANEAN VEGETABLE PAELLA

Makes 2 servings

1 teaspoon sea salt

2 teaspoons turmeric

1.6kg cauliflower florets

70g pitted kalamata olives, sliced

170g halved jarred artichokes

4 tablespoons chopped parsley

1 teaspoon lemon zest

1 tablespoon extra virgin olive oil

Sea salt and pepper to taste

Boil 1.9 litres of water, sea salt, and turmeric in a large pot over high heat. Add cauliflower florets and cook for 4 minutes. Strain cauliflower and pat dry.

Finely chop the cauliflower until it resembles rice. Place it in a large bowl. Add the olives, artichokes, parsley, lemon zest, and olive oil and mix well. Season with sea salt and pepper and serve warm.

> Store half in an airtight container in the refrigerator for lunch.

◆——— Days 4 and 5 Revitalize

ROASTED SPAGHETTI SQUASH WITH KALE MISO ALMOND PESTO

Makes 2 servings

1 medium spaghetti squash
200g kale, stemmed
2 garlic cloves
120ml extra virgin olive oil
50g raw almonds
1 tablespoon white miso
Pinch sea salt

Preheat the oven to 350 degrees Fahrenheit.

Cut the spaghetti squash in half lengthwise. Scrape out all of the seeds.

Pour 240ml water on a roasting tray. Place the spaghetti squash on the sheet skin side up. Roast for 25 minutes or until soft. Remove from the oven and allow to cool for 10 minutes.

Meanwhile, blend the kale, garlic, olive oil, almonds, miso, sea salt, and 2 tablespoons water in a blender or food processor until smooth. Add water as needed.

Using a fork, gently flake the squash out of the skin. As you do this, you will notice it starting to look like spaghetti.

Spread 6 tablespoons of the kale-miso-almond paste on top of the spaghetti squash and serve.

> Store half in an airtight container in the refrigerator for lunch.

◆——— Days 11 and 12 Revitalize

BEEF BONE BROTH

Makes 2.4 litres

1.8kg beef knuckle bones
3 celery stalks, sliced
3 carrots, sliced
2 onions, quartered
1 head garlic, halved
1 bunch thyme
120ml apple cider vinegar
Sea salt to taste

Place the bones in a large pot. Add the celery, carrots, onions, garlic, thyme, and apple cider vinegar. Cover with 2.4 litres water and bring to a boil. Skim any scum that floats on the top. Let simmer for 24 hours. Add water as needed.

Let the broth cool and then strain it, making sure all of the marrow is released from the center of the bones and into the broth. Add sea salt.

> Store in an airtight container in the refrigerator for up to 5 days or in the freezer for up to 5 months.

CHICKEN BROTH

Makes 2.4 litres

1.4kg chicken bones: necks and backs or carcass
1 onion, quartered
3 carrots, sliced
3 celery stalks, sliced
1 small leek, chopped
1 medium parsnip, sliced
1 head garlic, halved
1 small piece ginger, chopped
1 bunch thyme
5 whole black peppercorns
1 bay leaf
Sea salt to taste

Place the chicken bones in a large pot. Add the onion, carrots, celery, leek, parsnip, garlic, ginger, thyme, peppercorns, and bay leaf. Cover with 2.4 litres water and bring to a boil. Reduce to a simmer and skim any scum off of the top. Let simmer for 24 hours. Let cool then strain. Add sea salt.

> Store in an airtight container in the refrigerator for up to 5 days or in the freezer for up to 5 months.

BROTH SHOPPING LIST

Dry Goods
apple cider vinegar

Meat and Poultry
1.8kg beef knuckle bones
1.4kg chicken bones: necks and backs or carcass

Vegetables
6 carrots
1 head celery
1 head garlic
1 ginger root
1 small leek
1 medium parsnip
3 onions

Herbs
2 bay leaves
2 bunches thyme

ASPARAGUS SOUP

Makes 4 servings

450g asparagus, trimmed

2 tablespoons avocado oil

1 teaspoon minced garlic

45g sliced leeks

960ml chicken or vegetable broth

30g baby spinach

1 teaspoon lemon juice

Sea salt and pepper to taste

Chop the asparagus into thirds and set aside. Heat the avocado oil in a large pot over medium heat. Add the garlic and leeks and cook until the leeks are translucent. Add the broth and bring to a boil. Add the asparagus and cook until tender, about 5 minutes. Remove from heat.

Blend the cooked vegetables, baby spinach, and lemon juice in a blender until smooth. Season with sea salt and pepper. The soup can be served hot or chilled.

> Store ¼ of the soup in an airtight container in the refrigerator for lunch.

> Store the remaining ½ of the soup in an airtight container in the freezer for Day 13 Maintenance dinner and Day 14 Maintenance lunch.

———— Days 9 and 10 Revitalize; Days 13 and 14 Maintenance

CARROT GINGER SOUP

Makes 4 servings

2 tablespoons avocado oil

1 teaspoon minced garlic

1 teaspoon minced ginger

40g chopped white onion

450g peeled sliced carrots, sliced 2.5cm thick

720ml chicken or vegetable broth

1 teaspoon turmeric

½ teaspoon ground cumin

Sea salt to taste

1 teaspoon lemon juice

Heat the avocado oil in a medium pot over medium heat. Add garlic, ginger, and onions and cook until the onions are translucent. Add the carrots, broth, turmeric, cumin, and sea salt. Continue cooking until the carrots are soft to touch, about 12 minutes. Remove from heat and let cool.

Blend with the lemon juice and purée until smooth and creamy. The soup can be served hot or chilled.

> Store ¼ of the soup in an airtight container in the refrigerator for lunch.

> Store the remaining ½ of the soup in an airtight container in the freezer for Day 16 Maintenance dinner and Day 17 Maintenance lunch.

—— Days 7 and 8 Revitalize; Days 16 and 17 Maintenance

CAULIFLOWER SOUP

Makes 4 servings

975g cauliflower
480ml chicken or vegetable broth
1 tablespoon grass-fed butter
1 teaspoon lemon juice
Sea salt and pepper to taste

Boil the cauliflower and broth in a medium saucepan over high heat for 5 minutes. Remove from heat.

Blend with the butter and lemon juice in a blender or food processor until smooth and creamy. Season with salt and pepper. Soup can be served hot or chilled.

> Store ¼ of the soup in an airtight container in the refrigerator for lunch.

> Store the remaining ½ soup in an airtight container in the freezer for Day 9 Maintenance dinner and Day 10 Maintenance lunch.

> It will last for up to 5 days in the fridge or up to 5 months in the freezer.

◆——— Days 2 and 3 Revitalize; Days 9 and 10 Maintenance

GET YOUR GREENS ON SOUP

Makes 4 servings

350g broccoli florets
480ml chicken or vegetable broth
60g spinach
50g cashews
Sea salt and pepper to taste

Boil the broccoli and broth in a medium saucepan over high heat. Remove from heat.

Blend with the spinach and cashews until smooth and creamy. Season with salt and pepper. Soup can be served hot or chilled.

> Store ¼ of the soup in an airtight container in the refrigerator for lunch.

> Store the remaining ½ soup in an airtight container in the freezer for Day 20 Maintenance dinner and Day 21 Maintenance lunch.

> It will last for up to 5 days in the fridge or up to 5 months in the freezer.

◆——— Days 13 and 14 Revitalize; Days 20 and 21 Maintenance

DRESSINGS

These four core dressings should be made in the Revitalize phase and will be used throughout the Revitalize and Maintenance programs.

LEMON VINAIGRETTE

Yields 600ml

480ml extra virgin olive oil
8 tablespoons lemon juice
1 shallot, chopped
2 teaspoons Dijon mustard
1 tablespoon chopped chives
Sea salt and pepper to taste

Whisk together olive oil, lemon juice, shallot, mustard, and chives in a medium bowl. Season with sea salt and pepper.

> Store in an airtight container in the refrigerator for up to 2 weeks.

APPLE CIDER VINAIGRETTE

Yields 600ml

180ml apple cider vinegar

360ml extra virgin olive oil

2 small shallots, chopped

2 teaspoons Dijon mustard

Sea salt and pepper to taste

Whisk together apple cider vinegar, olive oil, shallots, and mustard in a medium bowl. Season with sea salt and pepper.

> Store in an airtight container in the refrigerator for up to 2 weeks.

TAHINI DRESSING

Yields 480ml

135ml tahini

120ml extra virgin olive oil

5 tablespoons freshly squeezed lemon juice

120ml water

3 teaspoons chopped coriander

Sea salt and pepper to taste

Blend tahini, olive oil, lemon juice, water, and coriander in a blender until smooth and creamy. Season with sea salt and pepper.

> Store in an airtight container in the refrigerator for up to 2 weeks.

ASIAN VINAIGRETTE

Yields 600ml

180ml apple cider vinegar

3 tablespoons wheat-free tamari

2 limes, juiced

3 teaspoons grated ginger

1½ teaspoons minced garlic

3 teaspoons Dijon mustard

3 tablespoons chopped coriander

360ml toasted sesame oil

Blend apple cider vinegar, tamari, lime juice, ginger, garlic, mustard, coriander, and sesame oil in a blender until smooth.

Store in an airtight container in the refrigerator for up to 2 weeks.

YOUR LIFELONG MAINTENANCE PROGRAM:

MOVING FORWARD

by Kerry Bajaj, Health Coach

You did it! You completed your 2-Week Revitalize Program, and now you're looking younger and slimmer, zipping around with lots of energy. So what's your next step?

You might be tempted to jump right back into the sugary, starchy foods you used to love . . . but take a moment. Think about what that way of eating brought you—and what your 2-Week Revitalize Program did for you. Let your body's responses to food be your new guide to choosing what to eat. Meanwhile, your lifelong Maintenance Program allows for some more flexibility.

You'll notice that in the Maintenance Program you'll begin to reintroduce foods that we kept out of the Revitalize Program. You might be able to enjoy all of these foods—or you might have a reaction to some or all. Symptoms might include nausea, indigestion, aching joints, headache, acne or skin problems, fatigue, depression, or anxiety. You'll likely respond within the next two or three hours, but it might take two or three days. After your time away, you're likely to be even more sensitive to any problem food.

We tell patients to monitor their reactions carefully so they can determine which foods they need to avoid. If you have a negative reaction to a food, cut it out for another three months. Then reintroduce it, ideally eating a large amount and then noticing your reactions for the next few hours . . . and the next few days. If you tolerate it well, terrific! If you have a negative reaction again, wait another three months or even longer. The healthier your gut and your overall body become, the more foods you can tolerate. But you may discover that you simply don't react well to some foods and you will want to continue to avoid them. Here is where you become your own physician and your own nutritionist, empowered to choose the foods your body loves while avoiding those it cannot tolerate well.

Meanwhile, if a food makes you feel nauseous or achy, take two tablets of Alka-Seltzer Gold or a tablespoon of buffered vitamin C powder in water. And for more information on how and when to reintroduce foods, see www.bewell.com/blog/feel-great-after-cleanse.

Maintenance: The Overview

Foods to Embrace:

- Nonstarchy vegetables, including the nightshades (aubergine, peppers of all types, and tomatoes)
- Organic or free-range chicken, turkey, lamb, duck, wild game, and grass-fed beef and pork
- Organic pastured eggs
- Wild-caught fish and seafood/shellfish
- Small fish, such as black cod, herring, sardines, and trout
- Fermented soy (natto, tempeh, miso)
- Raw almonds, cashews, walnuts, hazelnuts, Brazil nuts, sesame seeds, pumpkin seeds
- Unsweetened almond, rice, hemp, and coconut milk
- Raw milk cheese, sheep and goat's milk products, grass-fed butter, ghee
- Noncaffeinated green or herbal teas, spring or sparkling water, fresh vegetable juices
- Coconut, avocado, sesame, flaxseed, MCT, and extra virgin olive oil
- Vinegar (apple cider, white wine, red wine, balsamic, and rice)
- Herbs and spices
- Cacao nibs, unsweetened cocoa powder, 100 percent raw cacao

Foods to Enjoy in Moderation*:

- 1 to 2 servings of low-sugar fruits daily: green apples, berries of all types, and citrus fruits

---

* Your consumption should depend on your ability to tolerate these foods, which will vary from person to person, and which may vary in you over time.

- 2 to 3 servings of moderately high-sugar fruits weekly: red apples, cantaloupe, guavas, melons, papayas, peaches, and plums.

- 1 serving of starchy vegetables daily

- 1 to 2 servings of beans and pulses daily depending on your carb tolerance

- 2 to 3 servings of gluten-free grains weekly (quinoa, brown or wild rice, buckwheat, teff, millet, amaranth, gluten-free pasta, and oats) depending on your carb tolerance

- Plain organic, grass-fed cow's milk whole yogurt—no low-fat or partial-fat products

- Small amounts of dark chocolate—no more than a couple of squares a day

Foods to Avoid

- Factory-farmed meats

- Farmed fish and high-mercury fish (tuna, swordfish)

- Processed foods

- Dried fruits

- Salted and roasted nuts and all peanut products

- Added sugars and natural sweeteners, including agave, honey, and maple syrup

- Artificial sweeteners

- Fruit juices and energy drinks

- Processed seed and vegetable oils such as canola, sunflower, safflower, corn, soy, margarine, and shortening

- Commercial salad dressings, ketchup, relish, barbecue sauce, mayonnaise

- Candy, energy bars, and protein bars

If you would like to use a sweetener, you can enjoy small amounts of stevia, lakanto, monk fruit, or xylitol, as well as small amounts of raw honey.

Customizing the Maintenance Program

We're all different. Some of us can follow a 90–10 plan, eating "right" 90 percent of the time and "splurging" the other 10 percent. People like this can have a dinner out with pasta and wine, and then they're easily able to get back on track the next day. I fall into this camp when it comes to sweets. I eat tons of veggies and green smoothies, I have a daily meditation practice, and I exercise five times a week. My foundation is strong and I feel great. However, I do enjoy the occasional dessert. Then I drink a bunch of water and get right back on track.

However, I've noticed that some people do best sticking to the plan all the time. My fellow health coach Megan has an autoimmune disease, so she never strays from her diet. Any deviation is likely to cause her symptoms to flare up, and it's just not worth it. Another health coach, Laura, has celiac disease, so she might deviate from the plan with a glass of wine or a scoop of ice cream, but she doesn't touch even a speck of gluten under any circumstances. I'm the same way about alcohol: I never drink any, because even a few sips makes me feel terrible.

What's the moral of the story? Sometimes we need moderation, sometimes we need "100 percent," and sometimes we can switch back and forth. When you get to know your own body, you'll figure out which approach is right for you and whether you need to vary it depending on circumstances.

What about Snacks During Maintenance?

Over the years, we've noticed that some of our clients love snacking between meals while others are happier sticking with three meals a day. The choice is yours, which is why we haven't built snacks into your Maintenance meal plans. Instead, we've included a list of healthy snacks on page 305, and you'll find recipes for those snacks in the Recipes section. Include snacks as the spirit moves you—and remember: fermented foods and bone broth both make healthy, gut-healing snacks as well.

The Maintenance Program: Gut Healing

- Include fermented foods in your diet several times a week. Good choices include 40g of unpasteurized sauerkraut or kimchi, or 230ml of kefir (fermented milk).

- Continue to enjoy bone broth, especially during times when you are feeling run down or feel a cold coming on. Add it to any meal or use it as a snack. Feel free to sub it in for any of the soups in the Maintenance meal plans.

- Start taking the probiotics that Dr. Lipman recommends on page 163.

The Maintenance Program: Supplements

- Start taking a multivitamin
- Start taking a fish oil
- Start taking vitamin D
- Start taking a probiotic

Bonus Healthy Eating Tips

Chew your food well. Digestion begins in the mouth with the manual breakdown of food, and salivary amylase starts to break down carbohydrates. We teach our kids to chew, but sometimes we forget to chew our food—it's important!

Get help. If you're a klutz in the kitchen, this might be a good time to phone a friend. Get some support so you'll be set up to succeed over the next two weeks. You may just need a pep talk, or you may even have a friend who would join you for grocery shopping and meal preparation.

Make eating a mindful experience. Give thanks for your food, and remember to set down your fork, breathe, and enjoy the company of others between bites.

Eat when you're hungry and stop when you are 80 percent full. Overeating creates a burden for your whole digestive system to manage.

Try fasting overnight to rest your digestive system for at least ten hours at night. For example, if you eat breakfast at 7:00 A.M., try not to eat anything after 9:00 P.M. This means your body won't have to do the hard work of digestion, and will have time for rest and repair.

Eat your probiotics. Have some unpasteurized sauerkraut or kimchi before a meal—about 40g will be plenty to stimulate your body's digestive juices and aid digestion.

Make mealtime special. Tonight when you're having dinner, create some ambience. Light a candle, use cloth napkins, and play some music. See how much more enjoyable the meal is when you set a relaxing mood.

Sit down and relax while you eat. Eating in a rush and under stress is not healthy and may lead to digestive problems. I recently saw a woman walking down the street in New York City eating a bag of microwave popcorn as she walked—I would bet you that she has digestive problems!

Practice reading food labels. Spend a few minutes checking out some nutrition labels on various food items. The two most important things that I tell people to look for are: 1) The number of ingredients in the food. If the list is a mile long, stay away! 2) The grams of sugar per serving. Remember that 4 grams of sugar is the equivalent of a teaspoon! Simply looking for those two pieces of information when you check out food labels will empower you to make much better choices.

Snack on Brazil nuts. Brazil nuts are high on selenium, which can support your thyroid health, but a little bit goes a long way. Incorporate two Brazil nuts as part of a snack today—your thyroid will thank you.

Try a new vegetable you've never had before. This is one of my favorite things to do when I'm grocery shopping: I look for a veggie I've never tried before, like an unusual variety of squash, and find a way to incorporate it into the next meal. If you can't find a veggie you've *never* tried, then find one you haven't had in a long time, like leeks or Brussels sprouts.

Eat greens at breakfast. Whenever my diet is subpar for a few days, I challenge myself to eat greens with breakfast, lunch, and dinner until I get back on track. For breakfast, I add powdered greens to a shake, have spinach with eggs, or add kale to a smoothie.

Clean out the cupboards. Now that you're reaching or have reached the end of your Revitalize Program, you have likely realized that some of the foods you used to eat all the time were not serving you well at all. Do some "spring cleaning" in your kitchen and toss or donate the foods you no longer want to eat.

The Maintenance Program: Stress Relief

Keep going with at least 10 minutes a day . . . and if you're really enjoying your meditation practice, consider extending your practice to 20 or 30 minutes.

I personally love meditation, but every so often, my practice can get stale. When it does, I read a book or two about meditation to reinvigorate my practice. I also like to go on a meditation retreat once a year. If these ideas intrigue you, check out our recommendations in the Resources section.

As with your 2-Week Revitalize Program, you can always substitute the yoga poses on page 329 for meditation and/or breathing practice.

Bonus Stress Reduction Tips

Drop your shoulders. So many of us carry stress in the shoulders. Today, make it a point to pay attention to hunched shoulders. When you notice that your shoulders are traveling up to your ears, drop them down and take a deep breath. You may have to do this many times throughout the day.

Just say no. Find at least one task, obligation, or activity that doesn't inspire you and say no to it. Running around from one commitment to the next is not very relaxing, and you may be happier doing less. Saying yes to one less event will create more time and freedom in your day.

Turn up the radio. Find a time to incorporate music into your day—it could be while you're commuting to work, cooking dinner, or winding down before bed. Let yourself notice how quickly music can shift your mood.

Work your gratitude muscle. Take a pen and blank sheet of paper and set the clock for ten minutes. Make a list of things you are grateful for, and don't stop until the time runs out.

Take an "electronic Sabbath." Choose one day a week with no e-mail, text, phone, or TV. If a whole day is impossible, then set aside half of a day to completely unplug.

Laugh out loud. Today your goal is to infuse an extra dose of laughter into your day. You can be creative with how you do this: spend a few minutes joking around with friends, find humor in an ordinary situation, or watch a funny TV show or movie. Laughter is the best antidote to stress.

Let go. So often we want things to be different than they are, and we can get quite riled up when things don't go our way. During a moment when you feel agitated or frustrated, practice letting go. Take a deep breath, give up the struggle, and simply allow things to be as they are.

Get a massage. There are so many ways to incorporate massage into your life, even without spending $100 at the spa. Some of my patients swear by stopping at a salon for a 15-minute chair massage once a week. You can also massage your feet using a tennis ball, or lie on the floor and place a tennis ball under your shoulders, take a deep breath, and feel the tension dissolve.

Lend a hand. Nothing feels better than helping another person in need. Do something kind for someone today. It could be as simple as smiling at a stranger, holding the door open, or making a phone call to check on a loved one.

The Maintenance Program: Exercise

I hope by now you've seen how great exercise can make you feel, and how helpful it is for feeling young and slim. You can use the Maintenance routine on pages 317–326, or you can explore some of the other forms of movement discussed in Chapter 5. Or perhaps you'd like to find your own personal blend of both. Your goal is to keep moving at least 30 minutes a day, five days a week, focusing on core support, strength, flexibility, fascia release, and cardio stimulation. Experiment with various activities until you find the ones you love and look forward to, celebrating the movement that is your birthright.

Bonus Exercise Tips

Don't compare. There's always going to be someone in better shape than you—but so what? Keep your focus on your own body, your own sense of well-being, and your own pleasure.

Plan ahead. I tell clients to take a few moments on Sunday night or Monday morning to visualize the week ahead. Figure out where, when, and how you'll get your weekly exercise. If you leave it to chance, something more important always seems to come along. If you plan it, you are far more likely to do it.

Get creative. If your schedule changes, if you travel, or if something else keeps you from your usual routine, find a creative alternative. Maybe you can take a brisk walk through the corridors of your hotel, find a local fitness center, or go dancing at a local club. Don't get hung up on duplicating your normal routine or even your normal 30 minutes—just find some ways to let your body move.

The Maintenance Program: Sleep

It's so easy to skimp on sleep, but folks, please treat sleep like the sacred healing activity that it is. Maybe your bedtime can go a little bit later, but make sure to keep up with your wind-down routine and keep your bedroom electronics free.

Bonus Sleep Tips

Bask in the sun. Try to get some exposure to bright, natural light during the day in order to support your circadian rhythms and promote deep, restful sleep.

Fight the slump. If you're struggling with the 3 P.M. slump, drink a big glass of water or go for a brisk five-minute walk instead of reaching for caffeine. If you work in an office, a brisk walk around the hallways might be all you need.

Don't panic. If you can't fall asleep within 45 minutes, try one of the breathing activities on pages 327–328 to help calm your body and mind so you can achieve a healthy sleep.

Deprive your senses. To sleep better, you'll need a quiet, dark room. Blackout curtains, an old-fashioned sleep mask, earplugs, plus a white noise machine (optional) will help block out common sleep disrupters like street noise, streetlights, and snoring partners.

Rest your belly. To rest easier, eat light at night, at least three hours before bed. This will help ensure that the digestive process is well under way and nearing completion before you hit the hay. Eating close to bedtime forces your body to work well into the wee hours, digesting when it should be resting.

Cool down. Lower the temperature in your bedroom to 68 degrees or even cooler. We sleep best in a warm bed within a cold room.

Pay attention. Listen to your body as you improve your sleep habits. How many hours of sleep feel best? How much time do you need to wind down at night? Keep track of what's working.

Young and Slim for Life

Okay, so there's no such thing as the fountain of youth. But I promise you: this program is the next best thing! If you give your body what it needs to support optimal function, you will enjoy a healthy weight, a sense of well-being, and a deep wellspring of vitality. You'll look good, feel good, and live well. Enjoy!

MAINTENANCE: WEEK ONE

DAY 1
Breakfast: Raspberry Tahini Smoothie (page 273)
Lunch: Scallop Rocket Salad (pages 216–217)
Dinner: Grass-Fed Beef (or Turkey) Chili (pages 288–289)
Beverages: 1.8 litres filtered water
Supplements: 1 good-quality multivitamin; 2,000–5,000 units vitamin D; 1–2 grams fish oil; 1 probiotic
Exercise: Routine B (pages 317–326) at any time of your choosing
De-stress: 4–7–8 Breathing + Meditation Practice, in the morning or evening, or, alternatively, a restorative yoga pose in the morning and/or evening
Sleep: 9 P.M.–10 P.M.: Electronic sundown, wind-down, and lights out

DAY 2
Breakfast: 1.8 litres sheep's or goat's milk yogurt + berries + nuts
Lunch: Grass-Fed Beef (or Turkey) Chili (pages 288–289)
Dinner: Tomato Soup (page 299) + side salad
Beverages: 1.8 litres filtered water
Supplements: 1 good-quality multivitamin; 2,000–5,000 units vitamin D; 1–2 grams fish oil; 1 probiotic
Exercise: Routine B (pages 317–326) at any time of your choosing
De-stress: 4–7–8 Breathing + Meditation Practice, in the morning or evening, or, alternatively, a restorative yoga pose in the morning and/or evening
Sleep: 9 P.M.–10 P.M.: Electronic sundown, wind-down, and lights out
DAY 3
Breakfast: Apple Pie Smoothie (page 271)
Lunch: Tomato Soup (page 299) + side salad
Dinner: Seared Cod with Lemon Asparagus and Tahini (page 280)
Beverages: 1.8 litres filtered water
Supplements: 1 good-quality multivitamin; 2,000–5,000 units vitamin D; 1–2 grams fish oil; 1 probiotic
Exercise: Routine B (pages 317–326) at any time of your choosing
De-stress: 4–7–8 Breathing + Meditation Practice, in the morning or evening, or, alternatively, a restorative yoga pose in the morning and/or evening
Sleep: 9 P.M.–10 P.M.: Electronic sundown, wind-down, and lights out

DAY 4
Breakfast: Banana Almond-Butter Pancakes (pages 274–275) + berries
Lunch: Cod Tacos with Fermented Slaw (pages 280–281)
Dinner: Cauliflower Mock and Cheese (pages 294–295)
Beverages: 1.8 litres filtered water
Supplements: 1 good-quality multivitamin; 2,000–5,000 units vitamin D; 1–2 grams fish oil; 1 probiotic
Exercise: Routine B (pages 317–326) at any time of your choosing
De-stress: 4–7–8 Breathing + Meditation Practice, in the morning or evening, or, alternatively, a restorative yoga pose in the morning and/or evening
Sleep: 9 P.M. –10 P.M.: Electronic sundown, wind-down, and lights out
DAY 5
Breakfast: Chocolate Almond-Buttercup Smoothie (page 272)
Lunch: Cauliflower Mock and Cheese (pages 294–295)
Dinner: Peruvian Chicken and Sautéed Leafy Greens (page 293)
Beverages: 1.8 litres filtered water
Supplements: 1 good-quality multivitamin; 2,000–5,000 units vitamin D; 1–2 grams fish oil; 1 probiotic
Exercise: Routine B (pages 317–326) at any time of your choosing
De-stress: 4–7–8 Breathing + Meditation Practice, in the morning or evening, or, alternatively, a restorative yoga pose in the morning and/or evening
Sleep: 9 P.M.–10 P.M.: Electronic sundown, wind-down, and lights out

DAY 6
Breakfast: Banana Almond-Butter Pancakes (pages 274–275) + berries
Lunch: Peruvian Chicken Salad with Beetroot, Goat Cheese, and Pumpkin Seeds (pages 293–294)
Dinner: Cheesy Broccoli Soup (page 298) + side salad
Beverages: 1.8 litres filtered water
Supplements: 1 good-quality multivitamin; 2,000–5,000 units vitamin D; 1–2 grams fish oil; 1 probiotic
Exercise: Routine B (pages 317–326) at any time of your choosing
De-stress: 4–7–8 Breathing + Meditation Practice, in the morning or evening, or, alternatively, a restorative yoga pose in the morning and/or evening
Sleep: 9 P.M. –10 P.M.: Electronic sundown, wind-down, and lights out
DAY 7
Breakfast: 1 Grain-Free Muffin (page 275) + 230ml kefir
Lunch: Cheesy Broccoli Soup (page 298) + side salad
Dinner: Olive-Roasted Halibut Filet with Melted Leeks and Grape Tomatoes (page 278)
Beverages: 1.8 litres filtered water
Supplements: 1 good-quality multivitamin; 2,000–5,000 units vitamin D; 1–2 grams fish oil; 1 probiotic
Exercise: Routine B (pages 317–326) at any time of your choosing
De-stress: 4–7–8 Breathing + Meditation Practice, in the morning or evening, or, alternatively, a restorative yoga pose in the morning and/or evening
Sleep: 9 P.M. –10 P.M.: Electronic sundown, wind-down, and lights out

MAINTENANCE
WEEK ONE
SHOPPING LIST

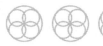

Dairy

    450g grass-fed butter

    60g soft goat cheese

    200g goat Gouda or favorite goat cheese

    230ml kefir

    200g manchego cheese

    1 jar sauerkraut or favorite fermented vegetable

    tahini

    170g sheep or goat yogurt, plain

Dry Goods

    1 jar raw almond butter

    almond meal

    1 box almond milk, unsweetened

    1 jar applesauce, unsweetened

    apple cider vinegar

    arrowroot powder

    avocado oil

    bicarbonate of soda

    1 box beef broth

    chilli pepper

    2 boxes chicken or vegetable broth

    chipotle chile powder

    chocolate protein powder

    ground cinnamon

    1 box coconut milk

    1 bottle coconut water

    ground coriander

    ground cumin

liquid stevia
maple syrup
nutmeg, ground
1 jar olive tapenade
115g raw pumpkin seeds
protein powder
1 box quinoa
sea salt
tomato paste
One 400g box chopped tomatoes
turmeric
1 small bottle vanilla extract

Meat, Poultry, and Seafood
2 boneless skinless chicken breasts
Two 170g cod filets
1 dozen eggs
450g ground grass-fed beef
Two 170g halibut filets

Produce
Fruit:
1 avocado
1 bag mixed berries (blueberry, raspberry, or strawberry)
5 bananas
3 lemons
1 bag frozen raspberries
½ pint raspberries or blueberries
1 pint strawberries

Greens:
1 bunch rocket
450g baby spinach
1 bunch kale
mesclun salad
450g mixed greens

Vegetables:
1 bunch asparagus
100g peeled beetroot
1 large head broccoli
1 head butter lettuce

900g butternut squash, peeled and cubed

2 carrots

1 large head cauliflower or 2.2kg of florets

1 bunch celery

2 heads garlic

1 pint grape tomatoes

2 jalapeño peppers

1 large leek

2 onions

1 red pepper

1 red onion

1 yellow pepper

Herbs:

1 bunch coriander

1 bunch oregano

1 bunch parsley

1 bunch thyme

Storage Tips

Keep herbs in a jar with an inch of water in the bottom.

MAINTENANCE: WEEK TWO

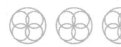

DAY 8
Breakfast: Green Smoothie (pages 272–273)
Lunch: Olive-Roasted Halibut Filet with Quinoa Tabouleh (pages 278–279)
Dinner: Lamb and Root Vegetable Curry (pages 285–286)
Beverages: 1.8 litres filtered water
Supplements: 1 good-quality multivitamin; 2,000–5,000 units vitamin D; 1–2 grams fish oil; 1 probiotic
Exercise: Routine B (pages 317–326) at any time of your choosing
De-stress: 4–7–8 Breathing + Meditation Practice, in the morning or evening, or, alternatively, a restorative yoga pose in the morning and/or evening
Sleep: 9 P.M.–10 P.M.: Electronic sundown, wind-down, and lights out

DAY 9
Breakfast: Hard-Boiled Eggs with Kimchi (page 274)
Lunch: Roast Rack of Lamb with Rocket, Fennel, Pomegranate, and Tahini Dressing (pages 285–286)
Dinner: Cauliflower Soup (page 230) + side salad
Beverages: 1.8 litres filtered water
Supplements: 1 good-quality multivitamin; 2,000–5,000 units vitamin D; 1–2 grams fish oil; 1 probiotic
Exercise: Routine B (pages 317–326) at any time of your choosing
De-stress: 4–7–8 Breathing + Meditation Practice, in the morning or evening, or, alternatively, a restorative yoga pose in the morning and/or evening
Sleep: 9 P.M.–10 P.M.: Electronic sundown, wind-down, and lights out
DAY 10
Breakfast: Carrot Cake Smoothie (page 272)
Lunch: Cauliflower Soup (page 230) + side salad
Dinner: Wild Salmon Collard Rolls (page 276)
Beverages: 1.8 litres filtered water
Supplements: 1 good-quality multivitamin; 2,000–5,000 units vitamin D; 1–2 grams fish oil; 1 probiotic
Exercise: Routine B (pages 317–326) at any time of your choosing
De-stress: 4–7–8 Breathing + Meditation Practice, in the morning or evening, or, alternatively, a restorative yoga pose in the morning and/or evening
Sleep: 9 P.M.–10 P.M.: Electronic sundown, wind-down, and lights out

DAY 11
Breakfast: 170g sheep's or goat's milk yogurt + berries + nuts
Lunch: Wild Salmon Collard Rolls (page 276)
Dinner: Coconut Oil Vegetable Stir-Fry and Quinoa Bowl (pages 296–297)
Beverages: 1.8 litres filtered water
Supplements: 1 good-quality multivitamin; 2,000–5,000 units vitamin D; 1–2 grams fish oil; 1 probiotic
Exercise: Routine B (pages 317–326) at any time of your choosing
De-stress: 4–7–8 Breathing + Meditation Practice, in the morning or evening, or, alternatively, a restorative yoga pose in the morning and/or evening
Sleep: 9 P.M.–10 P.M.: Electronic sundown, wind-down, and lights out
DAY 12
Breakfast: Hard-Boiled Eggs with Kimchi (page 274)
Lunch: Coconut Oil Vegetable Stir-Fry and Quinoa Bowl (pages 296–297)
Dinner: Chicken Parmesan with Garlicky Broccoli (pages 290–291)
Beverages: 1.8 litres filtered water
Supplements: 1 good-quality multivitamin; 2,000–5,000 units vitamin D; 1–2 grams fish oil; 1 probiotic
Exercise: Routine B (pages 317–326) at any time of your choosing
De-stress: 4–7–8 Breathing + Meditation Practice, in the morning or evening, or, alternatively, a restorative yoga pose in the morning and/or evening
Sleep: 9 P.M.–10 P.M.: Electronic sundown, wind-down, and lights out

DAY 13
Breakfast: Raspberry Tahini Smoothie (page 273)
Lunch: Chicken Parmesan and Rocket Salad (pages 290–291)
Dinner: Asparagus Soup (page 228) + side salad
Beverages: 1.8 litres filtered water
Supplements: 1 good-quality multivitamin; 2,000–5,000 units vitamin D; 1–2 grams fish oil; 1 probiotic
Exercise: Routine B (pages 317–326) at any time of your choosing
De-stress: 4–7–8 Breathing + Meditation Practice, in the morning or evening, or, alternatively, a restorative yoga pose in the morning and/or evening
Sleep: 9 P.M.–10 P.M.: Electronic sundown, wind-down, and lights out
DAY 14
Breakfast: 1 Grain-Free Muffin (page 275) + 230ml kefir
Lunch: Asparagus Soup (page 228) + side salad
Dinner: Vegetable Shrimp Pad Thai (page 279)
Beverages: 1.8 litres filtered water
Supplements: 1 good-quality multivitamin; 2,000–5,000 units vitamin D; 1–2 grams fish oil; 1 probiotic
Exercise: Routine B (pages 317–326) at any time of your choosing
De-stress: 4–7–8 Breathing + Meditation Practice, in the morning or evening, or, alternatively, a restorative yoga pose in the morning and/or evening
Sleep: 9 P.M.–10 P.M.: Electronic sundown, wind-down, and lights out

MAINTENANCE
WEEK TWO
SHOPPING LIST

Dairy/Miscellaneous
    230ml kefir
    1 jar kimchi
    1 small bottle maple syrup
    Two 170g containers goat or sheep milk yogurt, plain

Dry Goods
    1 bag almond meal
    1 bag arrowroot powder
    1 box bicarbonate of soda
    450g raw cashews
    ground cinnamon
    1 box coconut milk
    curry powder
    liquid stevia
    nutmeg
    protein powder
    sea salt
    tahini
    1 jar tomato sauce, unsweetened

Meat, Poultry, and Seafood
    2 boneless skinless chicken breasts
    1 grass-fed rack of lamb, about 680g
    340g wild salmon
    450g medium wild shrimp

Produce
    Fruit:
    1 avocado
    1 bag frozen blueberries

1 pack pomegranate seeds
½ pint raspberries or blueberries
1 bag frozen raspberries

Greens:
150g rocket
450g baby spinach
1 bunch collard greens
225g mixed greens

Vegetables:
4 bulbs baby bok choy
1 head broccoli
150g butternut squash, diced and peeled
4 large carrots
1 fennel bulb
1 garlic bulb
1 ginger root
1 garlic bulb
1 onion
1 large parsnip
1 red onion
1 red pepper
1 medium spaghetti squash
1 yellow pepper

Herbs:
1 bunch basil
bay leaves
1 bunch coriander

Storage Tips
Keep herbs in a jar with an inch of water in the bottom.

MAINTENANCE: WEEK THREE

DAY 15
Breakfast: Apple Pie Smoothie (page 271)
Lunch: Vegetable Shrimp Pad Thai (page 279)
Dinner: Grass-Fed Beef (or Turkey) Chili (pages 288–289)
Beverages: 1.8 litres filtered water
Supplements: 1 good-quality multivitamin; 2,000–5,000 units vitamin D; 1–2 grams fish oil; 1 probiotic
Exercise: Routine B (pages 317–326) at any time of your choosing
De-stress: 4–7–8 Breathing + Meditation Practice, in the morning or evening, or, alternatively, a restorative yoga pose in the morning and/or evening
Sleep: 9 P.M.–10 P.M.: Electronic sundown, wind-down, and lights out

DAY 16
Breakfast: Poached Eggs and Greens (page 273)
Lunch: Grass-Fed Beef (or Turkey) Chili (pages 288–289)
Dinner: Carrot Ginger Soup (page 229) + side salad
Beverages: 1.8 litres filtered water
Supplements: 1 good-quality multivitamin; 2,000–5,000 units vitamin D; 1–2 grams fish oil; 1 probiotic
Exercise: Routine B (pages 317–326) at any time of your choosing
De-stress: 4–7–8 Breathing + Meditation Practice, in the morning or evening, or, alternatively, a restorative yoga pose in the morning and/or evening
Sleep: 9 P.M.–10 P.M.: Electronic sundown, wind-down, and lights out
DAY 17
Breakfast: Chocolate Almond-Buttercup Smoothie (page 272)
Lunch: Carrot Ginger Soup (page 229) + side salad
Dinner: Ginger Miso Salmon Stir-Fry (pages 281–282)
Beverages: 1.8 litres filtered water
Supplements: 1 good-quality multivitamin; 2,000–5,000 units vitamin D; 1–2 grams fish oil; 1 probiotic
Exercise: Routine B (pages 317–326) at any time of your choosing
De-stress: 4–7–8 Breathing + Meditation Practice, in the morning or evening, or, alternatively, a restorative yoga pose in the morning and/or evening
Sleep: 9 P.M.–10 P.M.: Electronic sundown, wind-down, and lights out

DAY 18
Breakfast: 1 Grain-Free Muffin (page 275) + 230ml kefir
Lunch: Ginger Miso Salmon Filet with Mixed Greens (pages 281–282)
Dinner: Cauliflower Mock and Cheese (pages 294–295) + side salad
Beverages: 1.8 litres filtered water
Supplements: 1 good-quality multivitamin; 2,000–5,000 units vitamin D; 1–2 grams fish oil; 1 probiotic
Exercise: Routine B (pages 317–326) at any time of your choosing
De-stress: 4–7–8 Breathing + Meditation Practice, in the morning or evening, or, alternatively, a restorative yoga pose in the morning and/or evening
Sleep: 9 P.M.–10 P.M.: Electronic sundown, wind-down, and lights out
DAY 19
Breakfast: Green Smoothie (pages 272–273)
Lunch: Cauliflower Mock and Cheese (pages 294–295) + side salad
Dinner: Apple-Glazed Turkey Meatloaf with Sweet Potato Fries (page 287)
Beverages: 1.8 litres filtered water
Supplements: 1 good-quality multivitamin; 2,000–5,000 units vitamin D; 1–2 grams fish oil; 1 probiotic
Exercise: Routine B (pages 317–326) at any time of your choosing
De-stress: 4–7–8 Breathing + Meditation Practice, in the morning or evening, or, alternatively, a restorative yoga pose in the morning and/or evening
Sleep: 9 P.M.–10 P.M.: Electronic sundown, wind-down, and lights out

DAY 20
Breakfast: Poached Eggs and Greens (page 273)
Lunch: Apple-Glazed Turkey Meatloaf with Garden Salad and Lemon Vinaigrette (pages 287–288)
Dinner: Get Your Greens On Soup (pages 230–231) + side salad
Beverages: 1.8 litres filtered water
Supplements: 1 good-quality multivitamin; 2,000–5,000 units vitamin D; 1–2 grams fish oil; 1 probiotic
Exercise: Routine B (pages 317–326) at any time of your choosing
De-stress: 4–7–8 Breathing + Meditation Practice, in the morning or evening, or, alternatively, a restorative yoga pose in the morning and/or evening
Sleep: 9 P.M.–10 P.M.: Electronic sundown, wind-down, and lights out
DAY 21
Breakfast: Vanilla Chia Pudding (pages 276–277)
Lunch: Get Your Greens On Soup (pages 230–231) + side salad
Dinner: Cheesy Spaghetti Squash Egg Cups (pages 297–298) + side salad
Beverages: 1.8 litres filtered water
Supplements: 1 good-quality multivitamin; 2,000–5,000 units vitamin D; 1–2 grams fish oil; 1 probiotic
Exercise: Routine B (pages 317–326) at any time of your choosing
De-stress: 4–7–8 Breathing + Meditation Practice, in the morning or evening, or, alternatively, a restorative yoga pose in the morning and/or evening
Sleep: 9 P.M.–10 P.M.: Electronic sundown, wind-down, and lights out

MAINTENANCE WEEK THREE SHOPPING LIST

Dairy
    1 bottle kefir
    115g manchego cheese

Dry Goods
    almond butter
    1 box almond milk, unsweetened
    1 bag raw almonds
    1 bottle apple cider vinegar
    1 jar applesauce, unsweetened
    avocado oil
    1 bag cacao nibs
    1 bag chia seeds
    1 box chicken or vegetable broth
    chocolate protein powder
    ground cinnamon
    1 bag coconut flour
    1 box coconut milk
    coconut oil
    1 box coconut water
    extra virgin olive oil
    ground cumin
    liquid stevia
    nutmeg
    protein powder
    sea salt
    sesame seeds
    tamari, wheat-free
    tomato paste
    750g carton chopped tomatoes

turmeric
vanilla extract
white miso

Meat, Poultry, and Seafood
1 dozen eggs
450g ground turkey, dark or white meat
Two 200g salmon filets

Produce
Fruit:
1 avocado
2 limes
½ pint raspberries or blueberries

Greens:
450g baby spinach
1 bunch kale
mesclun salad
450g mixed greens

Vegetables:
3 bulbs baby bok choy
1 small head broccoli
2 carrots
1 bulb garlic
2 onions
2 red onions
1 red pepper
1 sweet potato
1 yellow pepper

Herbs:
1 bunch coriander
1 ginger root
1 bunch Italian parsley

Storage Tips
Keep herbs in a jar with an inch of water in the bottom.

MAINTENANCE: WEEK FOUR

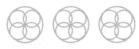

DAY 22
Breakfast: Carrot Cake Smoothie (page 272)
Lunch: Cheesy Spaghetti Squash Egg Cups (pages 297–298) + side salad
Dinner: Grass-Fed Beef Burger with Quick Probiotic Pickle and Sweet Potato Wedges (pages 284–285)
Beverages: 1.8 litres filtered water
Supplements: 1 good-quality multivitamin; 2,000–5,000 units vitamin D; 1–2 grams fish oil; 1 probiotic
Exercise: Routine B (pages 317–326) at any time of your choosing
De-stress: 4–7–8 Breathing + Meditation Practice, in the morning or evening, or, alternatively, a restorative yoga pose in the morning and/or evening
Sleep: 9 P.M.–10 P.M.: Electronic sundown, wind-down, and lights out

DAY 23
Breakfast: Vanilla Chia Pudding (pages 276–277)
Lunch: Grass-Fed Beef Burger and Mixed Greens Salad (pages 284–285)
Dinner: Tomato Soup (page 299) + side salad
Beverages: 1.8 litres filtered water
Supplements: 1 good-quality multivitamin; 2,000–5,000 units vitamin D; 1–2 grams fish oil; 1 probiotic
Exercise: Routine B (pages 317–326) at any time of your choosing
De-stress: 4–7–8 Breathing + Meditation Practice, in the morning or evening, or, alternatively, a restorative yoga pose in the morning and/or evening
Sleep: 9 P.M.–10 P.M.: Electronic sundown, wind-down, and lights out
DAY 24
Breakfast: Raspberry Tahini Smoothie (page 273)
Lunch: Tomato Soup (page 299) + side salad
Dinner: Asian Chicken Stir-Fry (pages 291–292)
Beverages: 1.8 litres filtered water
Supplements: 1 good-quality multivitamin; 2,000–5,000 units vitamin D; 1–2 grams fish oil; 1 probiotic
Exercise: Routine B (pages 317–326) at any time of your choosing
De-stress: 4–7–8 Breathing + Meditation Practice, in the morning or evening, or, alternatively, a restorative yoga pose in the morning and/or evening
Sleep: 9 P.M.–10 P.M.: Electronic sundown, wind-down, and lights out

DAY 25
Breakfast: 1 Grain-Free Muffin (page 275) + 230ml kefir
Lunch: Asian Shaker Salad (pages 291–292)
Dinner: Warm Lentil Salad, Roasted Courgette, and Goat Cheese (pages 295–296)
Beverages: 1.8 litres filtered water
Supplements: 1 good-quality multivitamin; 2,000–5,000 units vitamin D; 1–2 grams fish oil; 1 probiotic
Exercise: Routine B (pages 317–326) at any time of your choosing
De-stress: 4–7–8 Breathing + Meditation Practice, in the morning or evening, or, alternatively, a restorative yoga pose in the morning and/or evening
Sleep: 9 P.M.–10 P.M.: electronic sundown, wind-down, and lights out
DAY 26
Breakfast: Apple Pie Smoothie (page 271)
Lunch: Beet Lentil Salad with Rocket and Goat Cheese (pages 295–296)
Dinner: Seared Salmon Filet with Lemon Asparagus and Tahini (pages 282–283)
Beverages: 1.8 litres filtered water
Supplements: 1 good-quality multivitamin; 2,000–5,000 units vitamin D; 1–2 grams fish oil; 1 probiotic
Exercise: Routine B (pages 317–326) at any time of your choosing
De-stress: 4–7–8 Breathing + Meditation Practice, in the morning or evening, or, alternatively, a restorative yoga pose in the morning and/or evening
Sleep: 9 P.M.–10 P.M.: Electronic sundown, wind-down, and lights out

DAY 27
Breakfast: Poached Eggs and Greens (page 273)
Lunch: Salmon Tacos with Fermented Slaw (pages 282–283)
Dinner: Cheesy Broccoli Soup (page 298) + side salad
Beverages: 1.8 litres filtered water
Supplements: 1 good-quality multivitamin; 2,000–5,000 units vitamin D; 1–2 grams fish oil; 1 probiotic
Exercise: Routine B (pages 317–326) at any time of your choosing
De-stress: 4–7–8 Breathing + Meditation Practice, in the morning or evening, or, alternatively, a restorative yoga pose in the morning and/or evening
Sleep: 9 P.M.–10 P.M.: Electronic sundown, wind-down, and lights out
DAY 28
Breakfast: 170g sheep's or goat's milk yogurt + berries + nuts
Lunch: Cheesy Broccoli Soup (page 298) + side salad
Dinner: Turkey Shepherd's Pie (page 221)
Beverages: 1.8 litres ounces filtered water
Supplements: 1 good-quality multivitamin; 2,000–5,000 units vitamin D; 1–2 grams fish oil; 1 probiotic
Exercise: Routine B (pages 317–326) at any time of your choosing
De-stress: 4–7–8 Breathing + Meditation Practice, in the morning or evening, or, alternatively, a restorative yoga pose in the morning and/or evening
Sleep: 9 p.m.–10 p.m.: electronic sundown, wind-down, and lights out

MAINTENANCE
WEEK FOUR
SHOPPING LIST

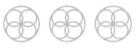

Dairy

    1 jar kefir

    1 jar sauerkraut or favorite fermented vegetable

    170g sheep or goat yogurt

Dry Goods

    1 box almond milk

    1 jar apple cider vinegar

    1 jar applesauce, unsweetened

    1 jar avocado oil

    chia seeds

    ground cinnamon

    1 box coconut milk

    1 box coconut water

    Dijon mustard

    1 bag lentils

    liquid stevia

    nutmeg

    protein powder

    sea salt

    tahini

    vanilla extract

Meat, Poultry, and Seafood

    2 boneless skinless chicken breasts

    1 dozen eggs

    340g ground grass-fed beef

    Four 200g wild salmon filets

Produce

Fruit:

2 avocados

4 lemons

1 lime

½ pint raspberries

1 bag frozen raspberries

Greens:

1 head butter lettuce

225g mixed greens

Vegetables:

2 bunches asparagus

150g peeled cooked beetroot

3 large carrots

1 bunch celery

2 English cucumbers

1 bulb garlic

1 ginger root

2 jalapeño peppers

1 small head red cabbage

2 red onions

1 bunch baby spinach

1 sweet potato

1 tomato

1 pint grape tomatoes

1 small head green cabbage

1 medium courgette

Herbs:

1 bunch coriander

Storage Tips

Keep herbs in a jar with an inch of water in the bottom.

MAINTENANCE RECIPES

by Chef Tricia Williams

The following smoothies can be made with Be Well Vanilla Whey Protein Powder, Be Well Chocolate Whey Protein Powder, and Be Well Sustain Vegetarian Protein Powder, or you may also use your favorite brand. Look for either a whey protein powder from grass-fed cows with less than 4 grams of sugar per serving, or a non-GMO pea protein powder.

APPLE PIE SMOOTHIE

Makes 1 serving

200g unsweetened apple sauce
150g ice
½ teaspoon cinnamon
Pinch nutmeg
½ teaspoon vanilla extract
1 scoop protein powder
240ml coconut water or filtered water

Blend all ingredients on high speed until smooth and creamy.

CARROT CAKE SMOOTHIE

Makes 1 serving

150g chopped carrots, cooked
120ml coconut milk
150g ice
1 scoop protein powder
½ teaspoon cinnamon
Pinch nutmeg
Pinch sea salt
Liquid stevia, to taste (optional)

Blend all ingredients with 120ml water on high speed until smooth and creamy.

CHOCOLATE ALMOND-BUTTERCUP SMOOTHIE

Makes 1 serving

2 tablespoons almond butter
150g ice
240ml coconut milk
1 scoop chocolate protein powder
Liquid stevia, to taste (optional)

Blend all ingredients on high speed until smooth and creamy.

GREEN SMOOTHIE

Makes 1 serving

240ml almond milk or coconut milk
150g ice
15g baby spinach
50g kale, stems removed
¼ avocado
1 scoop protein powder
Liquid stevia, to taste (optional)

Blend all ingredients on high speed until smooth and creamy.

RASPBERRY TAHINI SMOOTHIE

Makes 1 serving

2 tablespoons tahini
125g frozen raspberries
150g ice
240ml almond milk
1 scoop protein powder
Liquid stevia, to taste (optional)

Blend all ingredients on high speed until smooth and creamy.

POACHED EGGS AND GREENS

Makes 1 serving

1 tablespoon avocado oil
60g baby spinach or your favorite greens
Sea salt to taste
1 teaspoon apple cider vinegar
2 eggs

Heat the avocado oil in a cast iron frying pan over medium heat. Add the baby spinach. Season with sea salt and cook for 2 minutes. Remove from heat.

Add about 1½ inches of water to a medium frying pan. Place over medium-high heat. Add the apple cider vinegar. Once the water comes to a boil, reduce the heat to a simmer and crack in the eggs. Poach for about for 4 minutes. Remove the poached eggs from the water with a slotted spoon and place over the greens.

HARD-BOILED EGGS WITH KIMCHI

Makes 2 servings

4 eggs
Pinch sea salt
2 teaspoons apple cider vinegar
One 450ml jar kimchi

Place the eggs in a small pot. Cover with 720ml water. Add the salt and apple cider vinegar. Cook over medium heat, bringing to a rolling boil. Remove from heat and cover the pan. Let the eggs stand for 13 minutes.

Drain the eggs and run them under cold water to cool them. Peel the eggs and cut them in half. Set aside.

Remove the kimchi from the jar and roughly chop it. Divide it into two even portions and top each with 2 hard-boiled eggs.

> Store half in an airtight container in the refrigerator for Day 12 Maintenance breakfast.

> It will last in the refrigerator for up to 3 days.

—◆—— Days 9 and 12 Maintenance

BANANA ALMOND-BUTTER PANCAKES

Makes 2 servings

2 eggs
2 bananas, mashed
2 tablespoons almond butter
1 tablespoon coconut flour
½ teaspoon cinnamon
Pinch sea salt
1 teaspoon grass-fed butter

Mix the eggs, bananas, almond butter, coconut flour, cinnamon, and salt in a medium bowl until thoroughly combined.

Melt grass-fed butter in a cast iron frying pan over medium heat. Spoon a tablespoon of batter in to make each pancake. Cook for 2 minutes on each side or until golden brown.

> Divide pancake recipe in half. Store 1 serving of pancakes in the fridge. They can be warmed in a toaster for Day 6 Maintenance breakfast.

◆───── Days 4 and 6 Maintenance

GRAIN-FREE MUFFINS

Yields 8 muffins

4 tablespoons butter, room temperature
3 tablespoons maple syrup
4 eggs
1 teaspoon apple cider vinegar
100g almond meal
100g arrowroot powder
½ teaspoon bicarbonate of soda
Pinch sea salt
1 teaspoon cinnamon
Pinch nutmeg
190g mixed berries (blueberry, raspberry, or strawberry)

Preheat the oven to 350 degrees Fahrenheit.

Mix together the butter and maple syrup in a large bowl. Add in the eggs one at a time, mixing well. Add the apple cider vinegar, almond meal, arrowroot powder, bicarbonate of soda, sea salt, cinnamon, and nutmeg. Mix until thoroughly combined. Carefully fold in the berries.

Spoon the batter into nonstick muffin pans. Bake for 12 to 15 minutes.

> Store the remaining 7 muffins in an airtight container in the freezer. Defrost the muffins and reheat in a toaster oven.

◆───── Days 7, 14, 18, and 25 Maintenance

WILD SALMON COLLARD ROLLS

Makes 2 servings

340g wild salmon
Sea salt
4 large collard green leaves
2 tablespoons Tahini Dressing (page 232)
300g grated carrots
25g sliced red onion
½ avocado, sliced

Preheat the oven to 375 degrees Fahrenheit.

Pat the salmon dry with a paper towel and season with sea salt. Place on a roasting tray and cook for 15 to 18 minutes. Let cool. Flake the salmon into small pieces and set aside.

Remove the hard stems from the collard leaves. Lay them out on a cutting board. Spoon ½ tablespoon of Tahini Dressing across the bottom of each leaf. Add the salmon, carrots, onion, and avocado to each leaf, being sure to distribute evenly. Tightly roll collards into wraps.

> Store half in an airtight container in the refrigerator for lunch.

◆——— Days 10 and 11 Maintenance

VANILLA CHIA PUDDING

Makes 4 servings

480ml coconut milk
Liquid stevia, to taste
½ teaspoon vanilla extract
Pinch sea salt
100g chia seeds
45g berries (optional)
15g Cinnamon Cacao Granola (optional) (page 277)

Whisk together the coconut milk, liquid stevia, vanilla extract, and sea salt in a large mixing bowl. Gradually whisk in the chia seeds, making sure no clumps have formed. Cover the mixture with plastic wrap and refrigerate for 2 hours. Top it with berries and Cinnamon Cacao Granola, if using.

———— Days 21 and 23 Maintenance

CINNAMON CACAO GRANOLA

Yields approximately 2 cups

75g raw cashews

40g raw sliced almonds

65g raw pumpkin seeds

3 tablespoons cacao nibs

1 tablespoon sesame seeds

1 teaspoon cinnamon

¼ teaspoon sea salt

Liquid stevia, to taste

1 tablespoon olive oil

Preheat the oven to 175 degrees Fahrenheit.

Mix together the cashews, almonds, pumpkin seeds, cacao nibs, and sesame seeds in a medium bowl. Add the cinnamon, sea salt, stevia, and olive oil. Mix until the nuts-seeds mixture is well coated. Spread the mixture evenly onto a roasting tray. Bake for 45 minutes or until the mixture is dry. Let it cool.

Store in an airtight container for up to 2 months.

OLIVE-ROASTED HALIBUT FILETS

Makes 2 servings

2 tablespoons olive tapenade
Two 200g halibut filets

Preheat the oven to 375 degrees Fahrenheit.

Spread the olive tapenade evenly on the tops of the halibut filets. Place on a roasting tray and cook for approximately 12 minutes.

> Store 1 halibut filet in an airtight container in the refrigerator for lunch.

Dinner:
OLIVE-ROASTED HALIBUT FILET WITH MELTED LEEKS AND GRAPE TOMATOES

1 tablespoon grass-fed butter
135g thinly sliced leeks
Sea salt and pepper to taste
8 grape tomatoes
1 Olive-Roasted Halibut Filet

Heat the butter in a cast iron frying pan over medium-low heat. Stir in the leeks, making sure they are evenly coated with butter. Season with the sea salt and pepper. Cook for 20 minutes or until soft. Remove from heat.

While the leeks are cooking, slice the grape tomatoes in half. Plate the leeks with grape tomatoes and top with the Olive-Roasted Halibut Filet.

Lunch:
OLIVE-ROASTED HALIBUT FILET WITH QUINOA TABOULEH

90g quinoa, cooked
25g chopped red onion
5g chopped parsley
6 grape tomatoes, halved
2 tablespoons Lemon Vinaigrette (page 231)
Sea salt to taste
1 Olive-Roasted Halibut Filet

Mix together the quinoa, red onion, parsley, grape tomatoes, Lemon Vinaigrette, and sea salt. Mix until thoroughly combined. Plate and top with the Olive-Roasted Halibut Filet.

◆───── Days 7 and 8 Maintenance

VEGETABLE SHRIMP PAD THAI

Makes 2 servings

2 tablespoons avocado oil

35g sliced onions

90g sliced red peppers

90g sliced yellow peppers

450g Spaghetti Squash, cooked (page 225)

2 to 3 tablespoons Asian Vinaigrette (page 233)

450g medium shrimp, cleaned

Sea salt to taste

2 teaspoons coriander leaves

50g raw cashews

Heat 1 tablespoon of the avocado oil in a cast iron frying pan over medium heat. Add the onions and peppers and cook until the onions are translucent. Add in the cooked Spaghetti Squash and continue to heat until the Spaghetti Squash is warmed. Remove from heat and place in a large bowl. Toss with Asian Vinaigrette.

Wipe the cast iron pan clean.

Pat the shrimp dry with paper towels. Season with sea salt. Heat the remaining tablespoon of avocado oil in the cast iron frying pan over high heat. Add the shrimp and sear for 2 minutes on each side or until slightly golden. Top the spaghetti squash mix with the shrimp, coriander leaves, and raw cashews. This dish can be served hot or cold.

> Store half in an airtight container in the refrigerator for lunch.

◆───── Days 14 and 15 Maintenance

SEARED COD FILETS

Makes 2 servings

Two 200g cod filets

Sea salt and pepper to taste

1 tablespoon avocado oil

Season the cod filet with sea salt and pepper. Heat the avocado oil in a cast iron frying pan over high heat. When the pan is hot, sear the cod until golden brown, about 3 minutes on each side. Remove from heat and allow to cool.

> Store 1 Seared Cod Filet in an airtight container in the refrigerator for lunch.

DINNER:
SEARED COD WITH LEMON ASPARAGUS AND TAHINI

12 spears or more medium asparagus

1 tablespoon avocado oil

Sea salt to taste

1 teaspoon lemon zest

1 Seared Cod Filet

1 tablespoon Tahini Dressing (page 232)

Preheat the oven to 375 degrees Fahrenheit.

Place the asparagus on a roasting tray and coat with avocado oil. Season with sea salt and roast for 8 to 12 minutes. Remove from heat and plate. Sprinkle the lemon zest on the asparagus. Top with the Seared Cod Filet. Spoon Tahini Dressing on top of the cod fish. Serve.

LUNCH: COD TACOS WITH FERMENTED SLAW

½ avocado, pitted

1 teaspoon finely chopped jalapeño

1 teaspoon lime juice

½ teaspoon chopped coriander

Sea salt

1 Seared Cod Filet

5 large butter lettuce leaves

75g sauerkraut or favorite fermented vegetable

Mash the avocado in a small bowl using the back of a fork. Add the jalapeño, lime juice, coriander, and sea salt. Mix well. Set aside.

Place the Seared Cod Filet in a small bowl, flaking the fish into small pieces with a fork.

Spread out the lettuce cups and start building tacos. Divide the Seared Cod Filet flakes into lettuce cups. Top each one with the sauerkraut and avocado mixture.

⋙——— Days 3 and 4 Maintenance

GINGER MISO SALMON FILETS

Makes 2 servings

2 tablespoons white miso

Juice of 1 lime

½ teaspoon grated ginger

1 teaspoon wheat-free tamari

1 teaspoon chopped coriander

Sea salt to taste

Two 200g salmon filets

Preheat the oven to 375 degrees Fahrenheit.

Mix together the miso, lime juice, ginger, tamari, coriander, and sea salt in a bowl. Set aside.

Place the salmon filets in a baking pan and bake for 12 to 14 minutes depending on the thickness of the fish. Remove from the oven and spread the miso mixture evenly over the filets.

> Store 1 Ginger Miso Salmon Filet in an airtight container in the refrigerator for lunch.

DINNER: GINGER MISO SALMON STIR-FRY

1½ tablespoons coconut oil

130g small broccoli florets

55g sliced baby bok choy

Sea salt to taste

1 Ginger Miso Salmon Filet

Heat the coconut oil in a cast iron frying pan over medium heat. Add the broccoli, bok choy, and sea salt to the frying pan. Sauté for 10 minutes or until the vegetables are soft. Plate the vegetables and top with the Ginger Miso Salmon Filet.

LUNCH: GINGER MISO SALMON WITH MIXED GREENS

200g mixed greens

15g sliced red onion

1 tablespoon Asian Vinaigrette (page 233)

1 Ginger Miso Salmon Filet

Place the mixed greens and red onion in a bowl and toss with Asian Vinaigrette. Serve with the cold Ginger Miso Salmon Filet.

—◆—— Days 17 and 18 Maintenance

SEARED SALMON FILETS

Makes 2 servings

Two 200g salmon filets

Sea salt and pepper to taste

1 tablespoon avocado oil

Season the salmon filet with sea salt and pepper. Heat the avocado oil in a cast iron frying pan over high heat. When the pan is hot, sear the salmon until golden brown, about 3 minutes on each side. Remove from heat and allow to cool.

> Store 1 Seared Salmon Filet in an airtight container in the refrigerator for lunch.

DINNER: SEARED SALMON FILET WITH LEMON ASPARAGUS AND TAHINI

12 spears or more medium asparagus

1 tablespoon avocado oil

Sea salt to taste

1 teaspoon lemon zest

1 Seared Salmon Filet

1 tablespoon Tahini Dressing (page 232)

Preheat the oven to 375 degrees Fahrenheit.

Place the asparagus on a roasting tray coat with the avocado oil. Season with the sea salt and roast for 8 to 12 minutes. Remove from heat and plate. Sprinkle the lemon zest on the asparagus. Top with the Seared Salmon Filet. Spoon the Tahini Dressing on top of the salmon. Serve.

LUNCH: SALMON TACOS WITH FERMENTED SLAW

½ avocado, pitted

1 teaspoon finely chopped jalapeño

1 teaspoon lime juice

½ teaspoon chopped coriander

Sea salt

1 Seared Salmon Filet

5 large butter lettuce leaves

75g sauerkraut or favorite fermented vegetable

Mash the avocado in a small bowl using the back of a fork. Add the jalapeño, lime juice, coriander, and sea salt. Mix well. Set aside.

Place the Seared Salmon Filet in a small bowl, flaking the fish into small pieces with a fork.

Spread out the lettuce cups and build tacos. Divide the Seared Salmon Filet flakes into lettuce cups. Top each one with sauerkraut and the avocado mixture.

————— Days 26 and 27 Maintenance

GRASS-FED BEEF BURGER

Makes 2 servings

340g ground grass-fed beef
Sea salt and pepper
1 tablespoon avocado oil

Preheat the oven to 375 degrees Fahrenheit.

Form 2 even patties out of ground grass-fed beef. Season with salt and pepper. Heat the avocado oil in a cast iron frying pan on high heat. Sear the patties in the frying pan for about 2 minutes on each side. Place the frying pan in the oven and continue cooking for approximately 8 minutes for medium, or longer if you prefer a more well-done burger.

> Store 1 burger in an airtight container in the refrigerator for lunch.

 DINNER:
GRASS-FED BEEF BURGER WITH QUICK PROBIOTIC PICKLE AND SWEET POTATO WEDGES

150g English cucumber, thinly sliced
240ml apple cider vinegar
2 teaspoons sea salt
1 sweet potato, sliced lengthwise into wedges
2 teaspoons avocado oil
Sea salt to taste
1 Grass-Fed Beef Burger
1 tomato, sliced
1 red onion, sliced
100g mixed greens
2 teaspoons extra virgin olive oil

Preheat the oven to 375 degrees Fahrenheit.

To pickle the cucumber, toss the cucumber slices with apple cider vinegar and sea salt in a medium bowl. Let the mixture stand for 20 minutes, tossing it every 5 minutes. Drain the mixture.

While cucumbers are pickling, place the sweet potato wedges on a roasting tray, coat with avocado oil, and season with sea salt. Bake for 20 minutes or until tender.

Top the Grass-Fed Beef Burger with tomato, red onion, and pickled cucumbers. Serve with the mixed greens topped with olive oil.

LUNCH:
GRASS-FED BEEF BURGER AND MIXED GREENS SALAD

200g mixed greens

1 slice red onion

150g cucumbers, sliced

6 grape tomatoes

1 tablespoon Apple Cider Vinaigrette (page 232)

1 Grass-Fed Beef Burger

Toss the mixed greens, red onion, cucumber, and grape tomatoes in a medium bowl. Add the Apple Cider Vinaigrette and mix well. Serve with the Grass-Fed Beef Burger on the side.

———— Days 22 and 23 Maintenance

ROAST RACK OF LAMB

Makes 2 servings

1 grass-fed rack of lamb

Sea salt and pepper to taste

1 tablespoon avocado oil

Preheat the oven to 375 degrees Fahrenheit.

Season the lamb with sea salt and pepper. Heat the avocado oil in a cast iron frying pan. Once the pan is hot, sear the lamb approximately 2 minutes on each side. Roast the lamb for 15 minutes. Remove from heat and allow to cool for 10 minutes.

Slice the rack into chops.

> Store half in an airtight container in the refrigerator for lunch.

DINNER:
LAMB AND ROOT VEGETABLE CURRY

150g chopped butternut squash
130g chopped parsnips
2 tablespoons avocado oil
Sea salt and pepper
2 teaspoons mild curry
½ recipe Roast Rack of Lamb
1 teaspoon chopped coriander
2 teaspoons sheep's yogurt (optional)

Toss the butternut squash, parsnips, avocado oil, sea salt, pepper, and curry in a medium bowl. Mix until the vegetables are evenly coated. Spread the mixture evenly on a roasting tray.

Roast for 20 minutes at 375 degrees Fahrenheit, until soft and slightly caramelized. Plate and top with ½ Roast Rack of Lamb. Sprinkle the coriander on top and drizzle with the yogurt, if using.

LUNCH:
ROAST RACK OF LAMB WITH ROCKET, FENNEL, POMEGRANATE, AND TAHINI DRESSING

50g rocket
30g sliced fennel
1 tablespoon Tahini Dressing (page 232)
90g pomegranate seeds
½ recipe Roast Rack of Lamb

Toss the rocket and fennel in a bowl with the Tahini Dressing. Mix until the greens are evenly coated. Sprinkle the pomegranate seeds on top. Top with the Roast Rack of Lamb.

Days 8 and 9 Maintenance

APPLE-GLAZED TURKEY MEATLOAF

Makes 2 servings

2 tablespoons avocado oil

90g chopped red pepper

90g chopped yellow pepper

50g chopped onion

2 tablespoons chopped parsley

450g ground turkey

Sea salt and pepper

2 tablespoons unsweetened apple sauce

Preheat the oven to 325 degrees Fahrenheit.

Heat the avocado oil in a cast iron frying pan. Once the pan is hot, add the peppers and onion. Cook until the onions are translucent. Remove from heat and allow to cool.

Combine the pepper-onion mixture, parsley, and ground turkey in a large bowl. Mix well and season with salt and pepper. Divide the ground turkey mixture into two parts. Form two even loaves and place them on a roasting tray. Coat the tops of the loaves with applesauce.

Bake for 25 minutes. Remove from heat and allow to cool.

> Store 1 Apple-Glazed Turkey Meatloaf in an airtight container in the refrigerator for lunch.

DINNER:
APPLE-GLAZED TURKEY MEATLOAF WITH SWEET POTATO FRIES

1 sweet potato, sliced lengthwise

2 tablespoons avocado oil

Sea salt

1 teaspoon minced garlic

60g baby spinach

1 Apple-Glazed Turkey Meatloaf

Preheat the oven to 375 degrees Fahrenheit.

Place the sweet potatoes on a roasting tray and coat with 1 tablespoon of avocado oil. Season with sea salt. Bake for 18 to 20 minutes or until soft.

Heat the remaining tablespoon of avocado oil in a cast iron frying pan. Add the garlic and spinach and sauté for 2 minutes. Plate the spinach and sweet potato fries with Apple-Glazed Turkey Meatloaf.

✦ LUNCH:
APPLE-GLAZED TURKEY MEATLOAF WITH GARDEN SALAD AND LEMON VINAIGRETTE

200g mesclun salad

1 cup broccoli florets

20g thinly sliced carrots

1½ tablespoons Lemon Vinaigrette (page 231)

1 Apple-Glazed Turkey Meatloaf, sliced

Mix together the mesclun salad, broccoli, carrots, and Lemon Vinaigrette in a medium bowl. Top with slices of Apple-Glazed Turkey Meatloaf.

◆——— Days 19 and 20 Maintenance

GRASS-FED BEEF (OR TURKEY) CHILI

Makes 4 servings

2 tablespoons avocado oil

450g grass-fed ground beef or ground turkey

Sea salt and pepper to taste

½ medium onion, diced

1 red pepper, diced

1 yellow pepper, diced

1 jalapeño pepper, seeded and diced

2 stalks celery, diced

1 medium carrot, peeled and diced

5 garlic cloves, crushed

1 teaspoon ground cumin

1 teaspoon ground coriander

1 teaspoon chipotle chile powder

1 teaspoon turmeric

2 teaspoons tomato paste

240ml beef broth

400g strained chopped tomatoes

¼ avocado, sliced (optional)

2 teaspoons sheep's milk yogurt (optional)

Heat 1 tablespoon of avocado oil in a large pot over medium-high heat. Add the meat and season with sea salt and pepper. Break up the meat using a wooden spoon, stirring as the meat browns. Once the beef is browned, remove the meat from the pot and set aside.

Add the remaining tablespoon of avocado oil to the pot and cook over medium-high heat. Add the onions, peppers, jalapeño, celery, carrot, and garlic. Stir occasionally and cook for about 6 minutes or until the vegetables are soft.

Add in the meat, cumin, coriander, chipotle, turmeric, and tomato paste, stirring until the ingredients are well combined. Add the beef broth and strained tomatoes. Cook over medium-low heat for 40 minutes. Garnish with the avocado slices or yogurt, if using.

> Store ¼ of the chili in an airtight container in the refrigerator for lunch.

> Store the remaining ½ chili in an airtight container in the freezer for Day 15 Maintenance dinner and Day 16 Maintenance lunch.

Days 1, 2, 15, and 16 Maintenance

CHICKEN PARMESAN

Makes 2 servings

2 boneless skinless chicken breasts

2 teaspoons avocado oil

Sea salt to taste

4 tablespoon of Green Goodness (see recipe below)

100g tomato sauce

Preheat the oven to 375 degrees Fahrenheit.

Rub the chicken breasts with avocado oil and season with sea salt. Place on a roasting tray and cook in the oven for 20 minutes. Remove from heat and spread Green Goodness on top. Spoon the tomato sauce on top of the Green Goodness. Return to the oven and continue to cook for 6 minutes.

> Store 1 Chicken Parmesan breast in an airtight container in the refrigerator for lunch.

GREEN GOODNESS

Yields 600ml

300ml raw cashews

Sea salt

15g basil, blanched and shocked

Blend the cashews and 160ml water in a blender; let stand for 15 minutes. Add the sea salt and basil. Purée on high speed until smooth and creamy.

> Leftovers can be used as a snack. It will last in an airtight container in the refrigerator for up to 1 week.

DINNER:
CHICKEN PARMESAN WITH GARLICKY BROCCOLI

2 tablespoons avocado oil
350g broccoli florets
2 teaspoons minced garlic
Sea salt to taste
1 Chicken Parmesan breast

Heat the avocado oil in a cast iron frying pan over medium heat. Add the broccoli and garlic, making sure the broccoli is well coated. Add 120ml water and the sea salt. Cover and cook for 6 to 8 minutes.

Remove from heat and serve with Chicken Parmesan breast.

LUNCH:
CHICKEN PARMESAN AND ROCKET SALAD

50g rocket or mixed greens
25g sliced onion
1 tablespoon Lemon Vinaigrette (page 231)
1 Chicken Parmesan breast, sliced into strips

Toss the rocket, onion, and Lemon Vinaigrette together in a medium bowl. Mix well until the greens are evenly coated. Top with the Chicken Parmesan strips.

◆——— Days 12 and 13 Maintenance

ASIAN CHICKEN

2 boneless skinless chicken breasts
1 tablespoon avocado oil
Sea salt

Preheat the oven to 375 degrees Fahrenheit.

Coat the chicken with the avocado oil and season with sea salt. Place on a roasting tray and cook in the oven for 25 minutes. Let cool and slice into cubes.

> Store 1 Asian Chicken breast in an airtight container in the refrigerator for lunch.

DINNER:
ASIAN CHICKEN STIR-FRY

1 tablespoon coconut oil

1 teaspoon grated ginger

1 teaspoon minced garlic

25g sliced onions

50g white cabbage, chopped into 2.5cm squares

50g red cabbage, chopped into 2.5cm squares

25g carrot rounds, sliced 1cm thick

1 Asian Chicken breast

1 tablespoon Asian Vinaigrette (page 233)

1 teaspoon chopped coriander (optional)

Heat the coconut oil in a cast iron frying pan. Add the ginger, garlic, and onions. Cook for 2 minutes. Add the white cabbage, red cabbage, and carrots. Cook for 6 to 8 minutes. Remove from heat. Add the Asian Chicken breast, Asian Vinaigrette, and coriander, if using. Toss together and plate.

LUNCH:
ASIAN SHAKER SALAD

75g thinly sliced red cabbage

75g thinly sliced white cabbage

50g sliced red onion

1 Asian Chicken breast, chopped

1 teaspoon sesame seeds

1 teaspoon chopped parsley

2 tablespoons Asian Vinaigrette (page 233)

In a large 450g jar, layer the red cabbage, white cabbage, onion, Asian Chicken breast, sesame seeds, and parsley. Pour in the Asian Vinaigrette and seal the jar tightly. Shake jar until salad is well coated with dressing.

———— Days 24 and 25 Maintenance

PERUVIAN CHICKEN

Makes 2 servings

1 tablespoon minced garlic
240ml apple cider vinegar
1½ teaspoons sea salt
2 chicken breasts
4 sprigs oregano

Preheat the oven to 375 degrees Fahrenheit.

Place the garlic, apple cider vinegar, and sea salt in a medium bowl; mix together. Place the chicken breasts in the vinegar mixture, making sure they are well coated. Top the chicken with 2 oregano sprigs, cover, and refrigerate for 15 to 20 minutes for a quick marinade.

Place the remaining 2 oregano sprigs on a roasting tray. Place the marinated chicken breasts on top of the oregano. Bake for 26 minutes.

> Store 1 Peruvian Chicken breast in an airtight container in the refrigerator for lunch.

DINNER:
PERUVIAN CHICKEN AND SAUTÉED LEAFY GREENS

1 tablespoon coconut oil
1 teaspoon minced garlic
150g kale, stems removed
45g baby spinach
Sea salt and pepper to taste
1 Peruvian Chicken breast

Heat the coconut oil in a cast iron frying pan. Add the garlic and kale. Sauté for 2 minutes, and then add the baby spinach, sea salt, and pepper. Continue cooking for 1 minute. Remove from heat. Serve with Peruvian Chicken.

Lunch:

PERUVIAN CHICKEN SALAD WITH BEETROOT, GOAT CHEESE, AND PUMPKIN SEEDS

200g mesclun salad

1 tablespoon Apple Cider Vinaigrette (page 232)

75g peeled, sliced beetroot

1 tablespoon pumpkin seeds

2 tablespoons crumbled goat cheese

1 Peruvian Chicken breast, sliced

Toss the mesclun salad in a medium bowl with the Apple Cider Vinaigrette. Top it with beet slices. Sprinkle the pumpkin seeds and goat cheese on top. Fan the Peruvian Chicken slices over the salad.

———— Days 5 and 6 Maintenance

CAULIFLOWER MOCK AND CHEESE

Makes 4 servings

2 tablespoons avocado oil

50g diced red onion

1 teaspoon minced garlic

1 teaspoon grass-fed butter

1 teaspoon chopped thyme

1 teaspoon turmeric

2.2kg small cauliflower florets

Sea salt to taste

60g grated manchego cheese

75g grated goat Gouda

Preheat the oven to 350 degrees Fahrenheit.

Heat the avocado oil in a medium pan and add onion and garlic. Cook until the onions are translucent. Remove from heat. Add the butter, thyme, and turmeric. Stir until the butter is melted.

Combine the cauliflower and the onion mixture in a large mixing bowl. Add the sea salt and mix until evenly coated. Transfer to a 2-quart baking dish. Cover evenly with manchego and goat Gouda. Bake for 25 minutes. If you would like more color to the cheese, place under the grill for 3 to 4 minutes.

> Store ¼ recipe Cauliflower Mock and Cheese in an airtight container in the refrigerator for lunch.

> Store the other ½ recipe in an airtight container in the freezer for Day 18 Maintenance dinner and Day 19 Maintenance lunch.

—— Days 4, 5, 18, and 19 Maintenance

LENTIL SALAD

Makes 2 servings

75g cooked lentils
35g chopped red onion
50g diced celery
10g chopped parsley
1 teaspoon Dijon mustard
2 tablespoons Apple Cider Vinaigrette (page 232)
Sea salt and pepper to taste

Mix together the lentils, red onion, celery, parsley, Dijon mustard, and Apple Cider Vinaigrette in a medium bowl. Season with sea salt and pepper.

> Store half in an airtight container in the refrigerator for lunch.

DINNER:
WARM LENTIL SALAD, ROASTED COURGETTE, AND GOAT CHEESE

1 tablespoon avocado oil

150g courgette rounds, sliced 0.5cm thick

Sea salt and pepper to taste

½ recipe Lentil Salad

1 tablespoon soft goat cheese

Heat the avocado oil in a sauté pan on high heat. Cook the courgette and season it with sea salt and pepper. Cook for 2 minutes on each side until slightly golden. Remove from heat and transfer courgette to a plate. Reduce to medium heat and add the Lentil Salad to the pan to warm. Sprinkle the warmed Lentil Salad on top of the courgette. Crumble the goat cheese on top.

LUNCH:
BEET LENTIL SALAD WITH ROCKET AND GOAT CHEESE

200g rocket or mixed greens

½ recipe Lentil Salad

115g peeled, sliced beetroot

1 tablespoon soft goat cheese

Place the rocket and Lentil Salad in a bowl and mix well. Top with beet slices and crumbled goat cheese.

Days 25 and 26 Maintenance

COCONUT OIL VEGETABLE STIR-FRY AND QUINOA BOWL

Makes 2 servings

2 tablespoons coconut oil

1 teaspoon minced garlic

1 teaspoon grated ginger

35g sliced red onion

75g sliced baby bok choy

60g sliced red pepper

60g sliced yellow pepper

90g broccoli florets

Sea salt and pepper to taste

1 teaspoon wheat-free tamari

1 teaspoon chopped coriander

175g cooked quinoa

Heat the coconut oil in a cast iron frying pan over medium heat. Add the garlic, ginger, red onion, baby bok choy, peppers, and broccoli. Sauté until the broccoli is soft, about 8 minutes. Season with sea salt and pepper. Remove from heat and toss with the tamari and coriander. Let cool. Top the cooked quinoa with stir-fried vegetables.

> Store half in an airtight container in the refrigerator for lunch.

—— Days 11 and 12 Maintenance

CHEESY SPAGHETTI SQUASH EGG CUPS

Makes 4 servings

2 teaspoons avocado oil

50g diced onion

30g baby spinach

600g cooked Spaghetti Squash (page 225)

1 tablespoon coconut flour

Sea salt and pepper to taste

3 eggs

60g grated manchego cheese or your favorite goat or sheep cheese

Preheat the oven to 350 degrees Fahrenheit.

Heat the avocado oil in a cast iron frying pan over medium heat. Add the onions and cook until translucent. Add the spinach and cook for 1 minute. Remove from heat and transfer to a large bowl. Add the cooked Spaghetti Squash, coconut flour, sea salt, and pepper. Spoon into nonstick muffin cups. Sprinkle with the manchego or other cheese. Bake for 25 minutes. Serve 2 Cheesy Spaghetti Squash Egg Cups.

> Store 2 Cheesy Spaghetti Squash Egg Cups in an airtight container in the refrigerator for lunch.

> Store the remaining 6 Cheesy Spaghetti Squash Egg Cups in an airtight container for snacks. They will last for up to 3 days in the refrigerator or up to 5 months in the freezer.

—◆—— Days 21 and 22 Maintenance

CHEESY BROCCOLI SOUP

Makes 4 servings

2 tablespoons avocado oil

50g diced onion

25g diced carrots

50g diced celery

350g broccoli, florets and stems

720ml chicken or vegetable broth

Pinch chilli

Sea salt to taste

1 teaspoon lemon juice

85g grated manchego cheese

85g grated goat Gouda

90g cooked quinoa (optional)

Heat the avocado oil in a medium pot over medium heat. Add the onion, carrots, and celery. Cook until the onions are translucent. Add the broccoli, broth, chilli, and sea salt. Cook until the broccoli is tender, approximately 8 minutes. Remove from heat and let cool. Place in a blender and add the lemon juice, manchego, Gouda, and quinoa, if using. Purée until smooth and creamy.

> Store ¼ recipe in an airtight container in the refrigerator for lunch.

> Store the remaining ½ in an airtight container in the freezer for Day 27 Maintenance dinner and Day 28 Maintenance lunch.

—◆—— Days 6, 7, 27, and 28 Maintenance

TOMATO SOUP

Makes 4 servings

3 tablespoons avocado oil

1 teaspoon minced garlic

50g diced celery

25g diced carrots

50g diced onion

One 750g carton chopped tomatoes

240ml chicken or vegetable broth

1 teaspoon thyme

1 bay leaf

1 tablespoon grass-fed butter

Sea salt and pepper to taste

Heat the avocado oil in a medium pot over medium heat. Add the garlic, celery, carrots, and onion. Cook until the onion is translucent. Add the chopped tomatoes, broth, thyme, and bay leaf. Cook for 20 minutes. Remove from heat and place in a blender with the grass-fed butter. Season with sea salt and pepper. Purée at high speed until mixture is smooth and creamy.

> Store ¼ recipe in an airtight container in the refrigerator for lunch.

> Store the remaining ½ recipe in an airtight container in the freezer for Day 23 Maintenance dinner and Day 24 Maintenance lunch.

◆—— Days 2, 3, 23, and 24 Maintenance

GRAIN-FREE BREAD

Yields 1 loaf

2 tablespoons grass-fed butter, room temperature
4 eggs
1 teaspoon apple cider vinegar
175g almond meal
175g arrowroot powder
½ teaspoon bicarbonate of soda
1 teaspoon sea salt

Preheat the oven to 325 degrees Fahrenheit.

Mix together the butter, eggs, and apple cider vinegar in a large bowl until thoroughly combined. Add the almond meal, arrowroot powder, bicarbonate of soda, and sea salt, mixing well.

Transfer to a 20cm x 10cm loaf pan. Bake for 30 minutes. Remove from oven and let cool.

> Store in an airtight container in the refrigerator for 3 days or in the freezer for up to 5 months.

ADDITIONAL VEGETARIAN RECIPES

Use these recipes as an alternative to meat dishes in both the 2-Week Revitalize and 6-Week Maintenance programs.

LENTIL WALNUT SALAD

Makes 2 servings

150g cooked lentils
35g diced celery
20g chopped carrots
35g diced red onion
45g roughly chopped walnuts
1 tablespoon roughly chopped parsley
Sea salt and pepper to taste
4 tablespoons Apple Cider Vinaigrette (page 232)

Toss together the lentils, celery, carrots, red onion, walnuts, and parsley in a medium bowl. Season with sea salt and pepper. Toss in the Apple Cider Vinaigrette until thoroughly combined.

> Store half in an airtight container in the refrigerator for lunch.

DINNER:
WARM LENTIL WALNUT SALAD OVER ROCKET

½ recipe Lentil Walnut Salad
50g rocket

Warm the Lentil Walnut Salad in a cast iron frying pan over low heat for 4 minutes, stirring occasionally. Serve over rocket.

LUNCH:
LENTIL WALNUT SALAD WITH BABY SPINACH

100g Lentil Walnut Salad
60g baby spinach

Toss together Lentil Walnut Salad and spinach in a medium bowl.

Shopping List for this recipe:

ground black pepper
1 bunch rocket
1 bunch baby spinach
1 carrot ·
1 stalk celery
lentils
1 bunch parsley
1 red onion
sea salt
walnuts

ROASTED ROOT VEGETABLES AND LENTILS

Makes 2 servings

260g chopped parsnip, 1cm

300g cubed butternut squash

2 tablespoons avocado oil

Sea salt to taste

4 thyme sprigs

115g lentils, cooked

2 tablespoons chopped parsley

3 tablespoons Apple Cider Vinaigrette (page 232)

Preheat the oven to 375 degrees Fahrenheit.

Place the parsnip, butternut squash, and avocado oil in a medium bowl. Toss until the vegetables are well coated. Season with the sea salt. Place on a roasting tray and cover with the thyme sprigs. Roast for 20 minutes or until golden. Remove from the oven and discard the thyme sprigs.

Place the roasted vegetables, lentils, parsley, and Apple Cider Vinaigrette in a bowl. Toss until the vegetables and lentils are thoroughly coated. Season with sea salt.

> Store half in an airtight container in the refrigerator for lunch.

DINNER:
ROASTED ROOT VEGETABLES AND LENTILS WITH SAUTÉED GREENS

1 tablespoon avocado oil

1 teaspoon minced garlic

200g of Swiss chard, spinach, or favorite greens

Sea salt to taste

½ recipe Roasted Root Vegetables and Lentils

Heat the avocado oil in a cast iron frying pan over medium-low heat. Add the garlic and Swiss chard and sauté for 2 minutes. Season with the sea salt. Serve with the Roasted Root Vegetables and Lentils.

LUNCH:
ROASTED ROOT VEGETABLES, LENTILS, AND GARDEN SALAD

½ recipe Roasted Root Vegetables and Lentils

200g mesclun salad

In a medium bowl toss Roasted Root Vegetables and Lentils with mesclun salad.

Shopping List for this recipe:

1 small butternut squash
lentils
1 bunch mesclun
2 parsnips

1 bunch parsley
1 bunch Swiss chard, spinach, or favorite greens
1 bunch thyme

LENTIL STEW*
Makes 4 servings

2 tablespoons avocado oil
25g diced carrots
50g diced celery
50g diced onions
1 teaspoon minced garlic
280g lentils, rinsed
800g tomato sauce
½ teaspoon ground cumin
1 bay leaf
Sea salt to taste
50g baby spinach (optional)

Heat the avocado oil in a large pan. Add the carrots, celery, onions, and garlic. Cook until the onions are translucent. Add the lentils, tomato sauce, 750ml water, cumin, and bay leaf. Cook for 35 minutes. Remove and discard the bay leaf. Season with sea salt. Remove from heat and stir in the baby spinach, if using.

> Store ¾ of the Lentil Stew recipe in an airtight container in the refrigerator.

> It will last for up to 3 days in the fridge or up to 5 months in the freezer.

Shopping List for this recipe:

2 bunches baby spinach
bay leaf
1 carrot
2 stalks celery
ground cumin
1 garlic clove
lentils
1 onion
One 900g can tomato sauce

---

*   Lentil Stew is to be eaten during the Maintenance Program only.

MAINTENANCE SNACK RECOMMENDATIONS

Here are some snacks you can enjoy on your Maintenance Program. However, we ask you to be mindful of the reason you are having a snack. Rather than mindlessly grazing out of boredom, we ask that you only have a snack if you are hungry. The time of day when most people choose to have a snack is either mid-morning or mid-afternoon. We don't encourage you to snack after 8 P.M. You'll see that these snacks are nutrient dense, and most include healthy fats and protein, which are great for supporting your energy on a busy day.

¼ Cinnamon Cacao Granola recipe (page 277)
1 tablespoon almond butter + 1 small apple
50g Vanilla Chia Pudding (pages 276–277) + 125g berries
55g goat's or sheep's milk cheese
1 slice Grain-Free Bread (page 300)
125g berries
1 green juice (no added fruit)
2 tablespoons Green Goodness (page 290) + 1 cucumber
2 tablespoons Tahini Dressing (page 232) + 1 carrot
½ grapefruit
1 Grain-Free Muffin (page 275)
1 Cheesy Spaghetti Squash Egg Cup (pages 297–298)
2 gluten-free buckwheat crackers + ¼ avocado
1 hardboiled egg
1 pear
Handful raw nuts
1 stalk celery + 1 tablespoon almond butter

EXERCISES

by Jim Clarry, Personal Trainer and Dr. Keren Day, Active Release Technique Provider

I'm very excited to share with you two workout routines: a gentle but effective workout for the 2-Week Revitalize period, which will get you started, and a more vigorous workout for your lifelong Maintenance Program.

Feeling old and getting fat seems like the inevitable destiny of everyone over 40 in our youth-oriented culture—but I'm here to tell you that it doesn't have to be that way. If you're feeling old and fat, there is no better antidote than to get your body moving.

Our culture of convenience has allowed our bodies to deteriorate. We've become immobile, weak, and misshapen creatures that hardly resemble our vigorous, vital ancestors. Luckily, there is a solution: to integrate, slowly but surely, some of those ancestors' basic daily habits. This workout approach is *progressive:* once you're in the Maintenance phase, you'll keep finding new ways to add intensity and challenge to your workout so you continue to build strength, stamina, and flexibility. It's also *formal*—it relies on my knowledge of basic physiology and the many ways you can address your body's needs and stimulate your DNA's true potential.

I know you're busy, so I've kept it short and sweet—and effective. All you need to commit is a grand total of 30 minutes a day, five days a week. That includes your warm-up, cooldown, and everything in between—which is all you need to meet our five key goals:

1. Core support

2. Strength

3. Flexibility

4. Fascia release

5. Cardio stimulation

In either phase, if you want you can substitute one or two days each week with vigorous activities such as dancing, hiking, bicycling, or anything that you perceive to be challenging. The variety, mental challenges, and fun of varying your workouts offer tremendous value.

I know that for many people, making all the dietary changes that Dr. Lipman recommends can create some challenges. If you're used to eating sweet foods or drinking large amounts of caffeine, you might have some difficult days before your body readjusts. With precisely that in mind, I've designed a gentle, supportive exercise program for your first two weeks. You will embark on a transformative process that begins with small steps.*

After your first two weeks on the Revitalize Program, you should be feeling great! Your new healthy diet and lifestyle will give you lots of energy, and you will have primed the body's systems for more vigorous work. I'm happy to support your new level of health with this second workout.

If you move through the Maintenance workout as quickly as possible, without stopping to rest between sets, you'll get a real cardio workout by sufficiently stressing your cardiovascular system and provoking central adaptations in the heart and lungs. This is actually a better workout than a more obvious cardio activity, such as jogging, because your peripheral muscles—the ones in your arms, shoulders, hips, and legs—are getting more work, with many more muscles included.

Once you've mastered this second workout, what's next? No worries—you can keep progressing and improving without adding any time. I've included instructions for how to add intensity to your Maintenance workout so you can keep it at just the right level of challenge for wherever you happen to be.

Ready? Then let's get started.

Equipment You Will Need

Don't worry: you only need a few things, and they're all cheap, light, and easy to store—or to take with you if you happen to be traveling. A foam roller is just a long cylinder made out of foam rubber. You're going to love the way it helps you release your fascia and opens you up. And the mini band—which looks like a large rubber band—is a great way to work your muscles without using weights.

I also suggest you have a timer so you can count off the seconds as you hold and release. You can look at the second hand or digital timer on your watch, or you can use your smart

---

*   If you're already exercising regularly, feel free to stick with your own, more vigorous workout.

phone. You can even buy an app for interval training or one that works as a metronome, ticking off the seconds.

- Foam roller

- Timer

- Mini band (for the Maintenance Phase only)

Your Revitalize Workout: Routine A

Warm-up: Shoulder Stretch and Box Breathing

- Lie down on your back on a hard, flat surface with both arms extended over your head, as far away from your feet as possible.

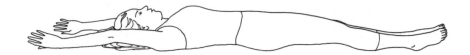

- Inhale slowly through your nose for a count of four, breathing deep into your belly. Put one hand on your lower abdomen. It should rise as you inhale.

- Hold for a count of four.

- Exhale slowly through your nose for a count of four.

- Hold the exhale for a count of four.

- Repeat for two minutes. If you have a little extra time and find this type of breathing relaxing or energizing, feel free to repeat as often as you like.

Ankle Mobility 1

- Stand facing a wall.

- Lean back slightly as you place the ball of one foot at the base of the wall.

- While keeping that knee straight, lean your body toward the wall. Hold for ten seconds.

- Lean away from the wall. Relax for five seconds.

- Repeat for a total of eight times. Then switch feet and repeat for a total of eight times.

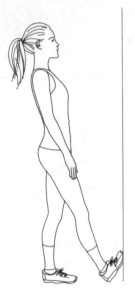 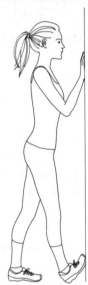

Ankle Mobility 2

- Sit on a chair, toward the edge.

- Turn the top of your foot downward, stretching the top of your foot and the front of your shin.

- Hold the stretch ten seconds. Relax for five seconds.

- Repeat the stretch-relax sequence eight times. Then switch feet and repeat nine times.

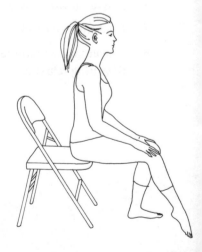

Dynamic Hamstring Stretch

- Stand facing a chair or bench.

- Put your hands on the bench or chair and bend your knees slightly.

- Flatten your back while maintaining a neutral head position (see below). Keep your core tight (see below). Gradually straighten your knees, extending your hamstrings.

- Hold the stretch for ten seconds.

- Relax for five seconds.

- Repeat the stretch ten–relax five cycle eight times.

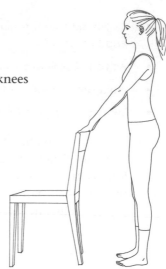

Couch Stretch

- Kneel on your sofa with your left knee, your left leg bent underneath you with the top of your foot pressed against the couch cushion.

- Put your right foot on the floor.

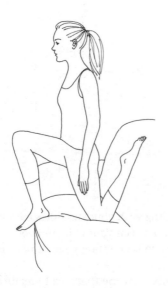
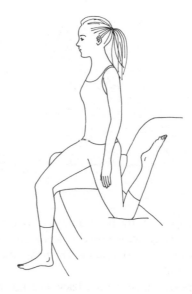

- Slowly raise your torso to a neutral-spine* position so you are standing straight and tall.

- As you raise your torso, squeeze your butt and abs (see note below).

- Hold the position for two minutes.

- Switch and repeat for two minutes on the other leg.

  Note: If you find this position challenging and want to make it a bit easier on yourself, move your right knee away from the sofa. The farther away your knee is, the less severe the stretch. Never overdo. Find a position that is just a little bit challenging . . . and then work up gradually, at your own pace, until you are doing the full stretch.

V-Sit

- Sit on the floor with your legs slightly bent as you extend them in front of you while keeping your back straight.
- Slowly work your legs apart as far as they will go and then slowly straighten them out.

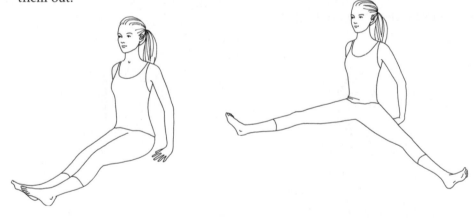

---

*   "Neutral spine" is the position you have while standing with your shoulders back and your chin level, pointing neither up nor down. Tuck your fist between your chin and your collarbone to get the feel of where it should be. The temptation will be to keep lifting your chin, so make sure to keep it at neutral.

In this position, your lower back muscles are activated, causing that area to retain its natural arch. Keep your abdomen tense. If you are having trouble connecting to your lower back or *lumbar* muscles, lie facedown on the floor with your arms stretched overhead. Then lift your arms and legs away from the floor. The arch you feel in your lower back is where your lumbar area is—that's the area you want to tighten up for this exercise.

- Remain in this straight-legged position—back straight—for ten seconds.

- Then relax by slightly bending your knees for five seconds.

- Next, as you exhale, bend forward at your hips until you feel more resistance. Be sure to keep your chest up and maintain a "lumbar lordosis": normal inward curvature of the lower back.

- Keep leaning forward for ten seconds.

- Then slowly straighten up and relax for five seconds.

Wall Sits

- Stand with your back against a smooth wall.

- Walk your feet out about one foot away from the wall.

- Slide your back down along the wall to the point where you can manage to hold the position for 30 seconds. You might need to experiment to find this point—and, as you get stronger, you might be able to go lower. Use your own judgment about how much you can do and do not overdo.

- When you have found your "sweet spot," hold the position for 30 seconds. Stand up, shake out, and relax for 5 seconds.

- Repeat the hold + relax sequence two more times.

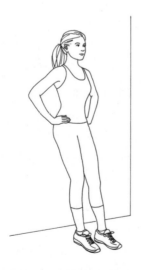
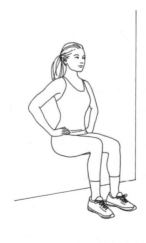

Plank

- Get down on your hands and knees.

- Place your forearms on the floor with your hands flat, palms down, and your forearms parallel to each other. Keep your elbows directly below your shoulders.

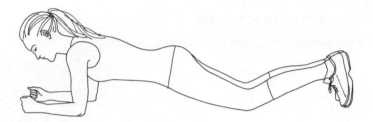

- Lift your knees from the floor, letting your only points of contact with the floor be your toes, elbows, and forearms. Keep your head, shoulders, hips, and knees in one straight line, like a plank. If this is too difficult, put a pillow below your knees and perform it on your hands and knees. Your goal is to hold the position for 30 seconds. You might need to experiment to find this point—and, as you get stronger, you might be able to go lower. Use your own judgment about how much you can do and don't overdo.

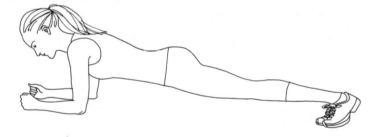

- When you have held the position for 30 seconds, relax for 5 seconds. Repeat for a total of three sequences of hold + relax.

Cooldown: Fascia Release

Please perform all three exercises.

IT Band Foam Rolling

- Lie on your side and place the foam roller just below the greater trochanter: that big bony structure on your hip. Try to keep your arms straight; for modification, bend the arms.

- Slowly roll the foam down the side of your leg, stopping just above your knee joint. Be careful not to cross the knee joint or press on that bony area above, as that can cause pain and irritation to those sensitive areas.

- Take the movement slowly—it should take eight to ten seconds in each direction.

- Repeat three or four times on each side. You'll get best results if you do this every other day.

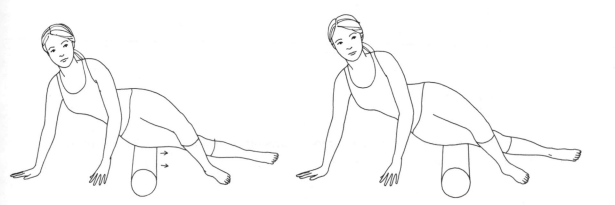

Quadratus Lumborum Foam Rolling with Counterstretch

- Lie on your side and put the foam roller above the iliac crest: the bone on your hip that you would normally rest your hands on.

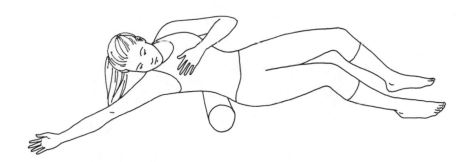

- Slowly move the roller up toward your ribs.

- Once you get halfway between your ribs and your hips, reach the opposite arm slowly up over your head, reaching back slightly. At the end of the movement, slowly lower the arm back down. Take eight to ten seconds to complete the movement.

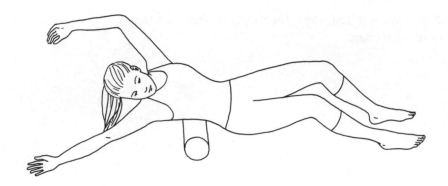

- Repeat this movement three or four times on each side. You'll get best results if you do this every other day.

Pec Stretch with Counter Rhomboid/Midback Stretch

- Place the foam roller vertically and lie on it so that the base of your occiput (your head) and sacrum (bottom of your spine) sit comfortably on the roller.
- Stretch both arms out so your body forms a T. If you need more balance, keep your knees bent (about your hips' width apart).

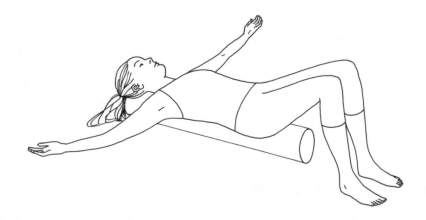

- Slowly lift your right arm up toward the ceiling and then slightly over to the opposite shoulder. The movement should take eight to ten seconds.

- Repeat five times with each arm.

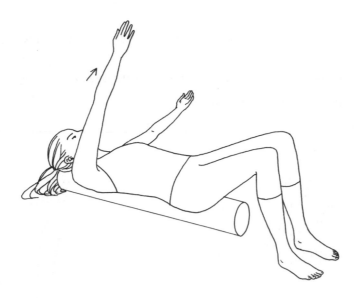

Your Maintenance Workout: Routine B

Warm-up: Shoulder Stretch and Box Breathing

- Lie down on your back on a hard, flat surface with both arms extended over your head, as far away from your feet as possible.

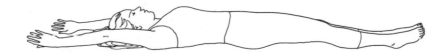

- Inhale slowly through your nose for a count of four, breathing deep into your belly. Put one hand on your lower abdomen. It should rise as you inhale.

- Hold for a count of four.

- Exhale slowly through your nose for a count of four.

- Hold the exhale for a count of four.

- Keep repeating the sequence until two minutes have passed.

Couch Stretch

- Kneel on your sofa with your left knee, your left leg bent underneath you with the top of your foot pressed against the couch cushion.

- Put your right foot on the floor.

- Slowly raise your torso to a neutral-spine position so you are standing straight and tall.

- As you raise your torso, squeeze your butt and abs (see note on page 312).

- Hold the position for two minutes.

- Switch and repeat on the other leg for two minutes.

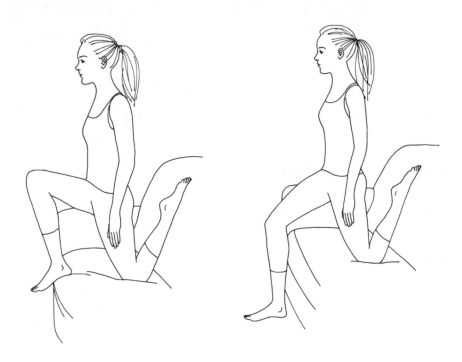

Glute Bridge

One missing link for most people is the ability to connect to their glutes—that is, their butt muscles. The glutes are the most powerful muscles in your body. This exercise will help create a mind-body connection that carries over to everyday movements such as squatting, lifting heavy objects, walking, and keeping an erect posture.

- Lie down on your back on a hard, flat surface. Your feet should be on the floor and your knees bent at a 90-degree angle.

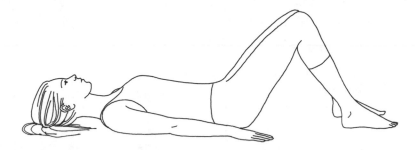

- Press through the feet and lift your hips until your butt is as far away from the floor as possible while you squeeze your butt cheeks—your glutes—together.

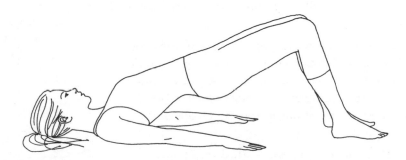

- Hold for ten seconds.
- Lower your hips to the floor and rest for five seconds.
- Repeat for a total of eight times.

After you've mastered this, try taking one foot off the floor and extending your leg while you lift and squeeze. Try to keep the knee straight and leg parallel to the floor.

Dynamic Hamstring Stretch

- Stand facing a chair or bench.

- Put your hands on the bench or chair and bend your knees slightly.

- Flatten your back while maintaining a neutral head position (see note on page 312). Keep your core tight (see below). Gradually straighten your knees, extending your hamstrings.

- Hold the stretch for ten seconds.

- Relax for five seconds.

- Repeat the stretch ten–relax five cycle for a total of eight times.

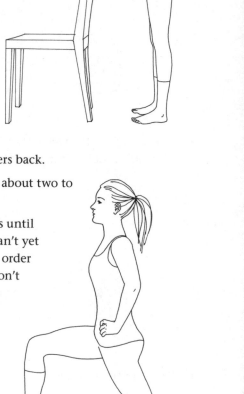

Isometric Lunge

- Stand with your feet shoulder width apart, your spine long and straight, and your shoulders back.

- Step forward with one foot into a wide stance, about two to two and a half feet apart.

- While keeping a vertical spine, lower your hips until both knees are bent about 90 degrees. If you can't yet manage this, just go down as far as you can in order to successfully complete the whole exercise. Don't overdo. As you get stronger, you can challenge yourself more.

- Hold the lunge for 10 seconds, then stand up and relax for 5 seconds.

- Repeat the lunge + relax sequence a total of eight times.

Inverted Row

Much of what we do has us slumped over, eventually causing a posture that is unappealing and dysfunctional. This will help you open your chest and pull your shoulders back. Think of it as an upside down push-up.

- Place two kitchen chairs with their backs facing each other about two feet apart.

- Put a broomstick or similar sturdy pole on top of the chairs through their backs.

- Lie down faceup between the chairs with the pole over your chest. Place your feet flat on the floor, knees bent.

- With an underhand grip—your palms facing your head—take hold of the pole and pull your chest as close to it as you can. Work on squeezing your shoulder blades together while keeping your hips in line with your chest.

- See how long you can hold without losing form. Gradually work up to holding for 30 seconds.

- When you can hold for 30 seconds, try this exercise with your legs completely straight, keeping only your heels in contact with the floor.

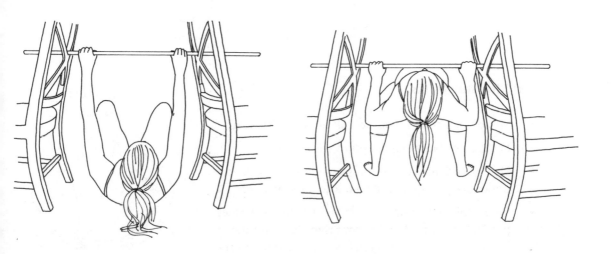

Push-ups

The part of the push-up that is easiest is the time when your elbows are straight. The hard part comes when your elbows are bent. Likewise, push-ups are easiest when you are balancing on your knees and harder when you're balancing on your toes—and hardest of all when your feet are elevated. So start your push-ups from the easiest position, with your knees on the ground and your elbows almost straight.

Work up to 30 seconds of holding that position without moving. Move on to that position with elbows bent . . . then with your toes on the floor . . . then with your feet elevated. Take your time progressing—it's better to have a steady, confident hold than to move on to the next pose while you're still wobbly in the one before.

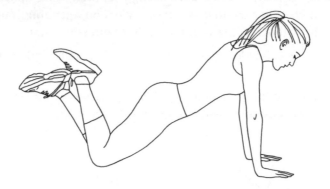

Lateral Monster Walks

- Stand upright with your feet shoulder width apart.

- Place a resistance band around your ankles.

- Hold your hands on your hips while keeping your upper body straight and your knees slightly bent.

- While looking straight ahead and keeping your feet parallel to each other, lift your right foot and step to the side. You will experience the resistance of the band, which is what you want.

- Place your right foot down, still parallel with your left, but in a wider stance.

- Lift your left foot and move it toward your right without losing tension on the band.

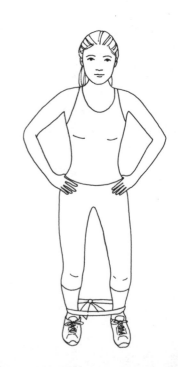

- Place your left foot down while still parallel to the right.

- Repeat three more times going in the same direction.

- Then switch directions, taking four sets of steps to the left.

- Repeat—for a total of five sets (a set = four steps to the right + four steps to the left).

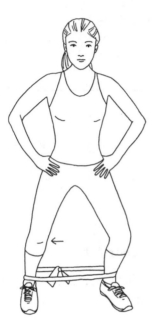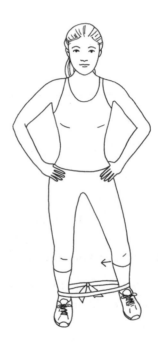

Foam Rolling

IT Band Foam Rolling

- Lie on your side and place the foam roller just below the greater trochanter: that big bony structure on your hip.

- Slowly roll the foam down the side of your leg, stopping just above your knee joint. Be careful not to cross the knee joint or press on that bony area above, as that can cause pain and irritation to those sensitive areas.

- Take the movement slowly—it should take eight to ten seconds in each direction.

- Repeat three or four times on each side. You'll get best results if you do this every other day.

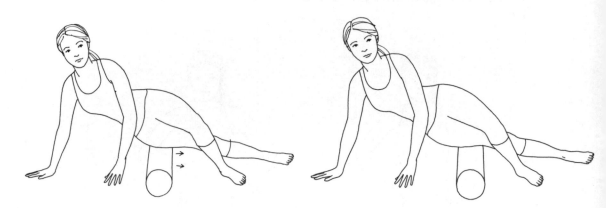

Quadratus Lumborum Foam Rolling with Counterstretch

- Lie on your side and put the foam roller above the iliac crest: the bone on your hip that you would normally rest your hands on.

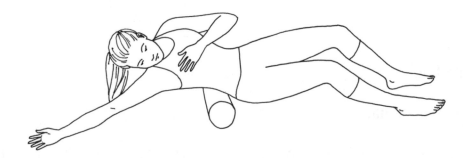

- Slowly move the roller up toward your ribs.

- Once you get halfway between your ribs and your hips, reach the opposite arm slowly up over your head, reaching back slightly. At the end of the movement, slowly lower the arm back down. Take eight to ten seconds to complete the movement.

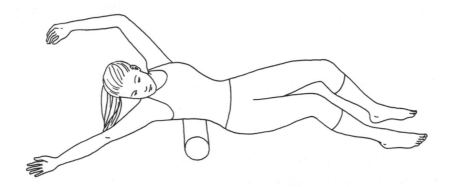

- Repeat that movement three or four times. You'll get best results if you do this every other day.

Pec Stretch with Counter Rhomboid/Midback Stretch

- Place the foam roller vertically and lie on it so that the base of your occiput (your head) and sacrum (bottom of your spine) sit comfortably on the roller.

- Stretch both arms out so your body forms a T. If you need more balance, keep your knees bent and move them farther apart.

- Slowly lift your right arm up toward the ceiling and then slightly over to the opposite shoulder. The movement should take eight to ten seconds.

- Repeat five times with each arm.

Cooldown: Shoulder Stretch and Box Breathing

- Lie down on your back on a hard, flat surface with both arms extended over your head, as far away from your feet as possible.

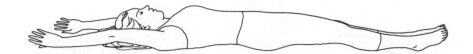

- Inhale slowly through your nose for a count of four, breathing deep into your belly. Put one hand on your lower abdomen. It should rise as you inhale.

- Hold for a count of four.

- Exhale slowly through your nose for a count of four.

- Hold the exhale for a count of four.

- Repeat for five minutes. If you have a little extra time and find this type of breathing relaxing or energizing, feel free to repeat as often as you like.

STRESS REDUCTION
PRACTICES:

MINDFUL BREATHING
AND MEDITATION

4–7–8 Breathing Practice

Time: Approximately one minute

- Place the tip of your tongue so that it's touching the place where the backs of your top front teeth meet the roof of your mouth.

- Exhale completely, making a whooshing or sighing sound.

- Close your mouth and inhale through your nose for four counts.

- Hold your breath for seven counts.

- Exhale through your mouth for eight counts.

- Repeat the cycle four times.

Mindful Breathing Practice

Time: Ten minutes

- Choose a quiet and comfortable spot that is free of distractions.

- Set a timer for ten minutes.

- Take a comfortable seated position. You can sit cross-legged on the floor, or you can sit in a chair. If you are sitting on the floor, you may want to use a cushion so your hips are raised. Keep your spine erect.

- Now begin paying attention to your breath as you inhale and exhale. The purpose of this practice is not to control the breath or slow it down but simply to bring your awareness to your breathing. You can feel the sensation of the breath around your nostrils.

- During your practice, your attention will wander away from the breath. This is not a problem—it doesn't mean you're doing anything wrong. Simply note that the attention has wandered, and bring your focus back to your breath as you inhale and as you exhale.

Meditation Practice

Time: Ten minutes

- Choose a quiet and comfortable spot that is free of distractions.

- Set a timer for ten minutes.

- Take a comfortable seated position. You can sit cross-legged on the floor, or you can sit in a chair. If you are sitting on the floor, you may want to use a cushion so your hips are raised. Keep your spine erect.

- Choose an object to concentrate on. It could be a mantra such as *Om* or an uplifting image such as a full moon or a rose.

- Begin meditating on that mantra or image. During your practice, your attention will wander away from the object of concentration. Simply note that the attention has wandered, and bring your focus back to your object of concentration.

A RESTORATIVE YOGA SEQUENCE

by Bobby Clennell

Practice these three restorative poses to give yourself a lift when you are physically fatigued.

Reclining Bound Angle Pose

Time: One to ten minutes
Benefits: Loosens your hips and relaxes your lower back. Dissipates abdominal tension. Regulates blood pressure. Alleviates menstrual pain. Reduces fatigue.

- Sit on a yoga mat with your legs straight out in front of you and a bolster or a stack of blankets folded into a rectangle to support your spine behind you. Place a blanket at the far end to support your head. Have a looped yoga belt close at hand.

- Cup your hands and press your fingers and thumbs into the floor. Pull your spine in and up and sit up straight so that your pubic bone (in front) and sacrum (at the back) are parallel to each other. Press your shoulder blades against your back and lengthen your front torso through the top of your sternum bone.

- Bend your knees and bring the soles of your feet together, and then drop your knees out to the sides. Slip the looped yoga belt over your head and shoulders

329

and around your lower hips. Hook it around your feet and ankles. Slide your feet toward you and tighten the belt.

- Place your hands behind you and, leaning back, lower your spine down along the bolster, first leaning on your hands and then your elbows.

- Check that your head is not tipping back or falling to one side. Make sure that you are not sinking on one side—distribute the weight of the left and right sides of your torso evenly along the bolster or blanket stack.

- Turn your arms out at the shoulder sockets and roll your shoulders away from your neck so your palms face up. Allow your inner thighs to extend out to the sides.

- Relax your facial muscles, your eyes, and your tongue. Settle your groin deep into your pelvis. As your groin drops toward the floor, so will your knees.

- To start, remain in this pose for one minute. Gradually extend your stay anywhere from five to ten minutes. To come out of the pose, use your hands to press your thighs together, and slip your feet out of the strap. Roll over onto one side. Wait for a few moments. Push yourself away from the floor, head trailing the torso.

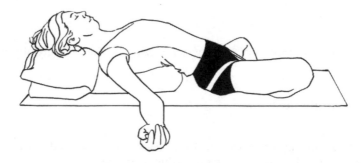

Practice notes: If you don't have a strap, set yourself up in the same way but sit close to and facing a wall. Turn your toes out (with the soles of the feet still together) and brace them against the wall. This will prevent your feet from sliding away from you.

If you experience a painful stretch in the inner thighs, support them with additional rolled blankets.

Inverted Relaxation Pose

Time: Five to ten minutes
Benefits: Regulates blood pressure. Relieves swollen ankles and varicose veins. Restores tired feet and legs. Relieves mild backache and respiratory ailments. Calms anxiety. Relieves symptoms of mild depression and insomnia.

- Place a yoga mat with the narrow end against the wall. Place a bolster or a stack of folded blankets across the mat a few inches from the wall.

- Kneel to the side of the mat, facing into the room.

- Lean sideways over the bolster, and pivoting on your hips, swing your legs up the wall so your pelvis rests on the bolster and your heels and sitting bones are supported against the wall.

- Rest your head and the top of your shoulders on the mat and spread your arms out to your sides, relaxing your hands and wrists. Keep your legs held vertically in place.

- Release the weight of your belly toward the back of your pelvis.

- Soften your eyes and turn them down toward your heart.

- Remain in this pose for five to fifteen minutes. To come out, slide back off the support. Cross your legs and rest them on the support. Reverse your crossed legs. Roll to your side. Wait for a few moments before pushing yourself away from the floor, head trailing the torso.

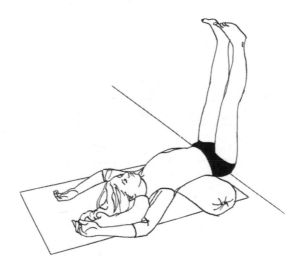

Supported Relaxation

Time: Five to ten minutes
Benefits: Opens the chest. Reduces nasal congestion. Improves breath awareness and pattern. Relaxes the nerves, mind, and body.

- Sit on a yoga mat with your legs bent in front of you and a bolster or a stack of rectangularly folded blankets behind you to support the length of your spine. Place a folded blanket at the far end to support your head.

- Lean back onto your elbows. Recline back, placing your spine evenly along the bolster.

- Straighten your legs. Carefully place them, one at a time, on the floor to rest on the center of the backs of the thighs and calves. Let your feet fall out to the sides.

- Elongate the back of your neck and rest your head on the center of the back of your skull. Spread your arms out to the sides, turned outward at a 45-degree angle, with your palms facing up. Roll your shoulders away from your ears.

- Consciously relax your muscles and joints. Draw the senses in; relax the skin on your face. Soften your eyes, tongue, and throat. Let go completely. Allow your breath to become soft and quiet.

- Remain in this pose for five to ten minutes. To come up, bend your knees and roll off the bolster onto your right side. Wait for a few moments before pushing yourself away from the floor, head trailing the torso.

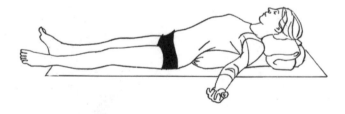

APPENDIX A:

YOGA FOR STRENGTH

by Bobby Clennell

Bobby Clennell has provided you with some restorative yoga poses to use as part of your daily stress relief. If you'd like to practice yoga for strengthening, here is a sequence to get you started.

Standing Forward Bend Pose

Benefits: Warms you up for the strengthening poses. Brings flexibility through the pelvis and spine. Relieves mental strain and physical tiredness.

- Stand up straight and tall on your yoga mat with your feet hip width apart.

- Holding your legs firm, raise your arms above your head, palms facing forward. Exhale and, sweeping your arms forward and down, bend forward from the hips.

- Reach down and press your fingers and thumbs onto the floor beside your feet and look up. Take one or two breaths.

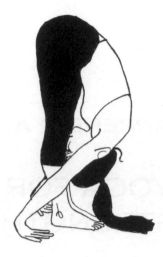

- On an exhalation, extend your torso down and release your head toward the floor. To bend farther forward, lift your inner thighs up into your pelvis and lift your sit bones. If possible, press your palms back and down. Allow your breath to become quiet and even. Hold this pose for 20 to 30 seconds.

Practice note: If your hands do not reach the floor without bending your legs, hold your shins or place your hands on blocks. Those with herniated discs: do not practice the final pose where the head is down.

Triangle Pose

Benefits: Develops strength and flexibility through the legs, arms, spine, and chest.

- Stand up straight and tall on your yoga mat.

- With an inhalation, jump your feet three and a half to four feet apart and swing your arms out to the sides. Fully stretch your arms and legs and raise your chest.

- Turn your left foot in and your right foot out. Take a few breaths.

- Exhale and bend sideways over your right leg.

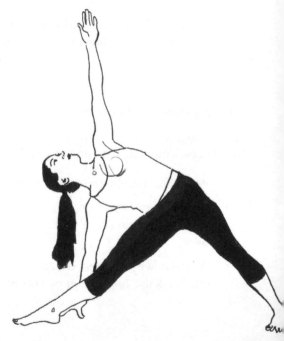

- Take hold of your right shin. As your hand grips your shin, firm both legs by pulling up your kneecaps.

- Press your pelvis forward and roll your left hip, torso, and left shoulder back. Breathing normally, raise your left arm and look up.

- Try touching your right hand to the floor, keeping your pelvis pressed forward, aligned over your right foot as you do so. Hold the pose for 20 to 30 seconds. Repeat on the other side.

Practice note: For a less strenuous way of practicing, do this pose with your shoulders and buttocks against the wall and your hand on a block to help keep your shoulders, hips, and feet in alignment.

Extended Side Angle Pose

Benefits: Develops strength and flexibility through the legs, arms, spine, and chest. Tones the waist and stomach muscles.

- Stand up straight and tall on your yoga mat.

- With an inhalation, jump your feet four to four and a half feet apart and swing your arms out to the sides. Fully stretch your arms and legs and raise your chest. Take a couple of breaths.

- Turn your left foot in and your right foot out. Holding your legs firm, exhale and bend your right knee to form a square, so your shin is upright and your thigh is parallel to the floor. Place your right hand on the floor to the outside of your right foot.

- Extend your left arm up. Tuck your tailbone in. Press your right knee and thigh back to align it above your right ankle.

- Anchor your left foot firmly to the floor. Turning your right arm in, extend it over your ear and look up.

- Breathe evenly and hold the pose steadily for 20 to 30 seconds. Repeat on the other side.

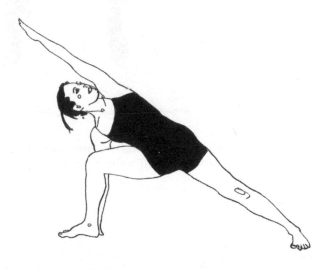

Practice note: If you cannot easily reach the floor with your hand, place it on a block.

Half Moon Pose

Benefits: Strengthens the legs. Helps develop poise and balance.

- Stand up straight and tall on your yoga mat. With an inhalation, jump your feet three and a half to four feet apart and swing your arms out to your sides. Fully stretch your arms and legs. Turn your left foot in and your right foot out.

- Exhaling, extend your torso sideways to the right.

- Hold your right shin bone and come into Triangle Pose (see page 334). Take a couple of normal breaths.

- Bend your right knee, slide your left foot in toward the right, and reach out to place your right hand on the floor about one foot ahead of your right foot.

- On an exhalation, straighten your right leg and simultaneously raise your left leg to the level of your left hip. Keep both legs firm and straight. Raise your left arm. Look up. Breathe evenly and hold the pose for 20 to 30 seconds. Repeat on the other side.

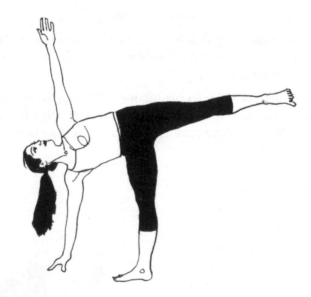

Practice note: If your hand does not reach the floor without your knee bending, place it on a block. You can also practice this pose with your back against the wall while you are learning to balance.

Post-Workout Relaxation

Benefits: Recovers you at the end of your practice. Enables the absorption of the benefits of your practice.

- Sit upright on your yoga mat with your legs outstretched in front of you.

- Bend your knees. Lean back onto your elbows.

- Lie down evenly along your spine.

- Straighten your legs one at a time and rest them on the floor at the center of the back of your thighs and calves. Then let your feet fall out to the sides.

- With your hands, elongate the back of your neck and position your head at the center of the back of your skull. Turn your upper arms outward and rest them at your sides with the palms facing up. Roll your shoulders away from your ears.

- Consciously relax your muscles and joints. Relax the skin on your face. Relax your eyes, tongue, and throat. Let go completely. Allow the breath to become soft and quiet.

- Remain in this pose for five minutes. To come up, bend your knees, roll over onto one side, and push yourself away from the floor, head trailing the torso.

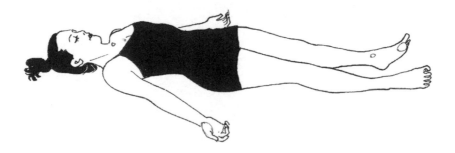

APPENDIX B:

ADRENAL SUPPORT

My go-to supplements for adrenal support are a group of unique herbal ingredients known as *adaptogens*. They got this name from their ability to adapt to the body's needs, so if you are feeling exhausted and depleted, they can boost your energy, while if you are feeling wired and agitated, they can help calm you down. If you feel both tired *and* wired, adaptogens can help you feel both more energized and calmer.

Generally, adaptogens help strengthen your body's response to stress and enhance its ability to cope with anxiety and fight fatigue—slowly and gently, without jolts or crashes. Though their effects may initially be subtle and take time to make themselves felt, I assure you that their benefits are real and undeniable. Indeed, they have been used in Chinese medicine and Indian Ayurvedic medicine for centuries to boost energy and resilience in the face of stress.

Consult Your Doctor
Before Taking Adaptogens

Please don't make the mistake of thinking that just because adaptogens are herbs and "all natural" you can take them carelessly. They are very powerful medicine, and while they are right for many people, they are not right for everyone. Be sure to consult your physician before taking any of the herbs I discuss in this book and, ideally, take them only under the care of someone who is experienced in herbal medicine. Take special care to follow the cautions noted for each of the herbs that follow.

Which Adaptogens Should You Use?

I prefer combination adaptogenic herb formulas. The ones I consider most important include Asian ginseng, eleuthero, ashwagandha, and *Rhodiola rosea*. You can take them individually or in a combination formula (see Resources). When you are buying a formula, look for one that has at least three of the above adaptogens, and make sure it has some *Rhodiola*.

Asian Ginseng

For thousands of years, Asian ginseng has been one of the most valued—and expensive—medicinal plants in the world. It's believed to affect the body by influencing metabolism within individual cells, and it has been studied extensively for its ability to help the body withstand stress. Western herbalists say that it restores and strengthens the body's immune response, promotes longevity, and enhances the growth of normal cells. Research indicates that it promotes a sense of well-being and may protect against some kinds of cancer.

Dose: 100 to 200 milligrams per day of a standardized extract. Most standardized ginseng extracts supply approximately 4 to 7 percent ginsenosides. Or take 1 to 2 grams per day of the dried, powdered root, usually found in gelatin capsules.

Caution: At the recommended dose, ginseng is generally safe, but occasionally it might cause agitation, palpitations, or insomnia. Consuming large amounts of caffeine with large amounts of ginseng might increase the risk of overstimulation and gastrointestinal upset. If you have high blood pressure, make sure to monitor your blood pressure while taking it. Ginseng is not recommended for pregnant or breastfeeding women.

Eleuthero

Eleuthero is used in traditional Chinese medicine for muscle spasms, joint pain, insomnia, and fatigue. In Germany, its use is approved for chronic fatigue syndrome, impaired concentration, and convalescing after illness. Western herbalists note that it improves memory, induces feelings of well-being, and can lift mild depression.

Dose: 2 to 3 grams per day of the dried root

Caution: As with Asian ginseng, eleuthero is generally safe. But occasionally it has been associated with agitation, palpitations, or insomnia in patients with cardiovascular disorders. If you have high blood pressure, monitor your blood pressure while taking it. I generally don't recommend it for pregnant or breastfeeding women, even though limited research has not turned up evidence of harmful effects in the fetus.

Ashwagandha

Ashwagandha has been used for thousands of years in Ayurvedic medicine. Like Asian ginseng, ashwagandha is used to help increase vitality, energy, endurance, and stamina; promote longevity; and strengthen the immune system. Today, herbalists often recommend it for people with high blood pressure, insomnia, chronic fatigue syndrome, and impotence associated with anxiety or exhaustion. It enhances endocrine function, especially of the thyroid and adrenals. Ayurvedic healers have long prescribed the herb to treat exhaustion brought on by both physical and mental strain.

Dose: 3 to 6 grams per day of the dried root

Caution: Avoid during pregnancy, if you are taking sedatives, or if you have severe gastric irritation or ulcers. People who are sensitive to the nightshade group of plants—peppers, tomatoes, aubergine, and potatoes—should also be careful with ashwagandha, as it is a nightshade.

Rhodiola Rosea

Rhodiola rosea acts like a hormone thermostat, especially as it pertains to the stress hormone cortisol, which is almost always out of whack during times of stress or exhaustion. Getting your cortisol back in rhythm is crucial—and *Rhodiola* helps to do just that, raising or lowering your cortisol response as needed. Rhodiola has also demonstrated a remarkable ability to support cellular energy metabolism. And it positively affects brain function, depression, and heart health. In my experience, most patients who take *Rhodiola* start feeling better within a few weeks to a month.

Dose: 200 to 600 milligrams per day of a *Rhodiola rosea* extract standardized to contain 2 to 3 percent rosavins and 0.8 to 1 percent salidroside. Or 2 to 3 grams per day of the nonstandardized root.

Caution: Avoid if you have manic depression or are bipolar. *Rhodiola* is not recommended for pregnant or breastfeeding women. Although it's unusual, at high doses *Rhodiola* can cause insomnia.

APPENDIX C:

SUPPORT FOR MENOPAUSE

My patients struggling with menopause find that a number of herbal supplements can bring relief. Ideally, you would work with a functional medicine practitioner to develop the herbal regimen that's right for you. However, you might consider experimenting with some or all of the following supplements, following the doses recommended on the bottle.

Black Cohosh

This is one of the most well-studied supplements for menopause. Several researchers have found that it helps with symptoms, especially with hot flashes.

Dose: 40 to 80 milligrams twice a day of a standardized extract

Caution: Don't take black cohosh if you have liver problems.

Wild Yam

Many of my patients use wild yam pills or creams as an alternative to hormone therapy. Some of the natural compounds in these yams appear similar to estrogen and progesterone. So far, clinical studies have not found that they ease menopause symptoms but I have seen them help some of my patients, and they might be helpful to you too.

Dose for cream: Depending on the concentration of the product, the recommended dose is usually 1 teaspoon of the cream applied daily to any of the following places: inner wrists, breasts, abdomen, or inner thighs.

Dose for powder: 250 milligrams, one to three times a day

Adaptogens

See Appendix B for adaptogens that might be helpful with menopausal symptoms. This class of herb—especially ginseng—seems to help many women with menopause symptoms, in particular with boosting mood and helping hot flashes.

Caution: Note the caution on page 339 so you use adaptogens safely.

DHEA

Dehydroepiandrosterone—better known as DHEA—is a naturally energizing hormone found in the human body, where it is produced by the adrenals as part of the stress response. Natural levels of DHEA hormone drop in our bodies after age 30, and there is some evidence—rather mixed—that supplements can help combat some symptoms of aging. Indeed, I have observed that DHEA supplements do indeed help some menopause symptoms: in particular, low libido and hot flashes.

If you are considering DHEA, I recommend getting your blood levels checked, and supplement only if your reading is low. The beauty of DHEA supplementation is that you can always check your levels to see whether you actually need it or if your supplements are causing your levels to rise too high.

Dose: Start at a small dose, such as 10 milligrams a day, and see whether it helps.

Flaxseed and Flaxseed Oil

These healthy fats might help some women with mild menopause symptoms. They are a good source of lignans, which tend to balance female hormones. However, not all studies of these supplements have shown benefits in relieving hot flashes.

Dose: 1 to 2 tablespoons of ground flaxseed or flaxseed oil a day

Red Clover

Many of my patients have used red clover to ease their menopause symptoms. Thanks to red clover's natural plant estrogens, they have met with some success. So far, though, the research results have been mixed.

Dose: 40 milligrams a day, in tincture or capsule form

APPENDIX D:

SLEEP SUPPORT

Instead of taking a sleeping pill, there are many natural sleep aids that can help you fall asleep and stay asleep—without the side effects of prescription drugs. You can take these nutrients separately, or find a formula that contains some or all of the following nutrients:

Amino Acids

- **GABA (gamma-aminobutyric acid)** promotes relaxation by quelling overstimulated nerve cells. (Dose: 200 to 500 milligrams)

- **L-theanine** helps form GABA. It is the main amino acid found in green tea, but you can take it separately. It is known for its ability to calm without compromising mental clarity. (Dose: 100 to 300 milligrams)

- **5-HTP (5-hydroxytryptophan)** is a building block of melatonin, a key hormone that regulates our sleep-wake cycles. It converts to serotonin, the "feel good" natural antidepressant that is also involved in deep, restful sleep. (Dose: 50 to 100 milligrams)

Herbs

- Valerian root
- Passionflower

- Lemon balm
- Chamomile

You can buy these as teas or as herbal supplements. Follow the dosage on the bottle.

Hormones

- **Melatonin** is a naturally occurring hormone that is released in cycles throughout the day to synchronize your circadian rhythm so you are alert during the day and at rest during the night. (Dose: 0.5 to 1 milligram)

Minerals

- Magnesium is a wonderful calming mineral that can help induce sleep. (Dose: 300 to 600 mg)

The Be Well Sleep Formula (see Resources) contains most of these nutrients, all in one pill.

APPENDIX E:

OPTIMIZING YOUR VITAMIN D LEVELS

To get the most accurate determination of how much vitamin D you need, ask your physician to test the levels in your blood (the 25-OH vit D level). This is one of the most important blood tests to get done as most people have low vitamin D levels. Optimal levels are 50 to 80 nanograms/milliliter (ng/ml). Since most physicians don't recommend high enough amounts, here are my guidelines:

If your blood level is above 45 ng/ml and for maintenance, I recommend 2,000 to 4,000 IU daily depending on age, weight, season, how much time you spend outdoors, where you live, skin color, and, obviously, blood levels. In other words, if you are older, larger, living in the northern latitudes during the winter, are not getting sun, and have dark skin, I recommend the higher maintenance dose.

If your blood level is 35 to 45 ng/ml, I recommend you correct it with 5,000 IU of vitamin D3 a day for three months under a doctor's supervision and then recheck your blood levels.

If your blood level is less than 35 ng/ml, I recommend you correct it with 10,000 IU of vitamin D3 a day under a doctor's supervision and then recheck your blood levels after three months. It usually takes a good six months to optimize your vitamin D levels if you're deficient. Once you're at the optimal level, drop down to the maintenance dose of 2,000 to 4,000 IU a day.

RESOURCES

Frank Lipman, M.D.

32 West 22nd Street, 5th Floor
New York, NY 10010
Telephone: (212) 255-1800
Fax: (212) 255-0714
www.bewell.com/drfranklipman

The author of this book, Dr. Lipman is available for appointments in his New York office. His website and blog also include a great deal of useful information.

Be Well by Dr. Frank Lipman

www.bewell.com/book

This is the line of leading-edge supplements that Dr. Lipman uses to treat thousands of patients in his practice.

Telephone: (888) 434-9483
Customer Support: booksupport@bewell.com

Be Well Health Coaching

Dr. Lipman has personally trained a team of health coaches who are available for one-on-one appointments to help you create a tailored plan and support you every step of the way to reach your health goals.

www.bewell.com/health-coach

More Be Well Resources

Blog: www.bewell.com/blog
Facebook: www.facebook.com/drfranklipman,
www.facebook.com/bewellbydrfranklipman
Pinterest: www.pinterest.com/drfranklipman
Twitter: @drfranklipman, @bewellteam
Instagram: @bewellbydrfranklipman
YouTube:www.youtube.com/user/
drfranklipman

Chef Tricia Williams

Telephone (212) 227-8610
www.FoodmattersNYC.com

BOOKS

Anatomy of an Epidemic by Robert Whitaker
The Autoimmune Solution by Amy Myers, M.D.
Best Green Drinks Ever by Katrine van Wyk
Best Green Eats Ever by Katrine van Wyk
The Big Fat Surprise by Nina Teicholz
The Blue Zones by Dan Buettner
Brain Maker by David Perlmutter, M.D.
The Disease Delusion by Dr. Jeffrey S. Bland
Drug Muggers by Suzy Cohen, R.Ph.
Full Catastrophe Living by Jon Kabat-Zinn
Goddesses Never Age by Christiane Northrup, M.D.

Grain Brain by David Perlmutter, M.D.
  Mindfulness: A Practical Guide to Awakening by
  Joseph Goldstein
  Minding My Mitochondria, 2nd Edition, by Terry
  L. Wahls, M.D.
  The New Health Rules by Frank Lipman, M.D.
  The Paleo Cure by Chris Kresser
  Revive by Frank Lipman, M.D.
  Thrive by Arianna Huffington
  Total Renewal by Frank Lipman, M.D.
  Wheat Belly by William Davis, M.D.
  Why Meditate? by Matthieu Ricard
  Why We Get Fat by Gary Taubes

ENVIRONMENTAL SUPPORT AND INFORMATION
Air Filters

AllerAir
www.allerair.com

IQAir
www.iqair.com

Moso Natural
www.mosonatural.com

Cleaning Products

EWG'S Guide to Healthy Cleaning
www.ewg.org/guides/cleaners

Gimme the Good Stuff
http://gimmethegoodstuff.org/safe-product-guides

Home Products

Allergy Buyers Club
www.allergybuyersclub.com

Baby Earth
www.babyearth.com

EcoChoices Natural Living Store
www.ecochoices.com

Gaiam
www.gaiam.com

Green Home
www.greenhome.com

Lifekind
www.lifekind.com

Nonprofits

Center for Children's Health and the Environment
www.childenvironment.org

Environmental Working Group
www.ewg.org

Healthy Child Healthy World
www.healthychild.org

Institute for Responsible Technology
www.responsibletechnology.org

Just Label It
www.justlabelit.org

Non-GMO Project
www.nongmoproject.org

Ubuntu Education Fund
www.ubuntufund.org

Water Filters

Aquasana
www.aquasana.com

Berkey Filters
www.berkeyfilters.com

PUR
www.pur.com

FOOD

All-Natural Condiments

Tessemae's All Natural
www.tessemaes.com

Coconut Products

Coconut Aminos (soy sauce alternative)
https://www.coconutsecret.com/aminos2.html

Edward & Sons
http://www.edwardandsons.com/native_shop_coconut.itml

This online grocer carries Native Forest brand coconut milks: BPA-free cans of organic, non-GMO coconut milk.

Virgin coconut oil, coconut flour
www.tropicaltraditions.com

Fermented Foods

Immunitrition
www.immunitrition.com

Wise Choice Market
www.wisechoicemarket.com/organic-raw-fermented-vegetables/

Food Organizations/Nonprofits

Center for Food Safety
www.centerforfoodsafety.org

Community Supported Agriculture (CSA)
www.localharvest.org/csa/

Eat Well Guide
www.eatwellguide.org

Environmental Working Group
www.ewg.org

This site features a great downloadable guide to the fruits and vegetables with the most and least pesticides so you'll know which ones you must buy organic and which conventionally grown produce is okay when organic isn't available.

Farmers' Markets
www.ams.usda.gov/farmersmarkets

This is a national listing of farmers' markets.

Local Harvest
www.localharvest.org

Use this website to find farmers' markets, family farms, and other sources of sustainably grown food in your area.

Non-GMO Shopping Guide
www.nongmoshoppingguide.com

Organic Consumers Association
www.organicconsumers.org

Seafood Watch
www.seafoodwatch.org

Weston A. Price Foundation
www.westonaprice.org

Gluten-Free Food Sources and Information

Bob's Red Mill
www.bobsredmill.com

Cappello's Pasta
https://cappellosglutenfree.com

Glutenfree.com
www.glutenfree.com

Nuts.com
https://nuts.com/cookingbaking/gluten-free-flour/
Gluten-free flours

On the Go Paleo
http://www.onthegopaleo.net

Top Six Gluten-Free Pastas
http://www.bewell.com/blog/top-6-gluten-free-pastas/

Grass-Fed Meats and Poultry

Eat Wild
www.eatwild.com

Grassland Beef
www.grasslandbeef.com

Vital Choice
www.vitalchoice.com

Wise Choice Market
www.wisechoicemarket.com/bone-broth

You can buy bone broth here if you don't want to make your own.

Online Grocery Stores

Green Pasture
www.greenpasture.org

Mountain Rose Herbs
www.mountainroseherbs.com

Radiant Life Company
www.radiantlifecatalog.com

Thrive Market
www.thrivemarket.com

Wild Mountain Paleo Market
https://www.wildmountainpaleo.com

Organic and Raw Chocolate

eatingEVOLVED
http://eatingevolved.com

Fine & Raw Chocolate
http://fineandraw.com

Lily's Sweets
htpp://lilyssweets.com

Wei of Chocolate
http://weiofchocolate.com

Teas and Coffee Alternatives

Breakaway Matcha
www.breakawaymatcha.com

Dandy Blend
http://www.dandyblend.com/

DoMatcha Green Tea
http://www.domatcha.com

Green Tea
http://www.traditionalmedicinals.com/
product_categories/green-teas/

Guyaki Yerba Mate
http://guayaki.com/product/47/Traditional-
Yerba-Mate-Tea-Bags.html

Teechino
http://teeccino.com/

Wild and Organic Fish

Vital Choice
www.vitalchoice.com

Wild Planet
www.wildplanetfoods.com

FUNCTIONAL MEDICINE

Institute for Functional Medicine
Telephone: (800) 228-0622
www.functionalmedicine.org
    You can find a list of functional medicine practitioners at this site.

KITCHEN TOOLS

Ceramcor
www.ceramcor.com

Le Creuset
www.lecreuset.com

Paderno World Cuisine Spiralizers
http://www.padernousa.com/4-blade-spiralizer/

Vitamix
www.vitamix.com

MEDITATION

Buddhify
www.Buddhify.com

Calm
www.calm.com

Headspace
www.headspace.com

Mindapps
www.mindapps.se

YogaGlo
https://www.yogaglo.com/

RECIPES

Against All Grain
www.againstallgrain.com

Balanced Bites and Diane Sanfilippo
www.balancedbites.com

Candice Kumai
www.candicekumai.comt

Deliciously Organic
www.deliciouslyorganic.net

Dr. Frank Lipman on Pinterest
www.pinterest.com/drfranklipman

Elana's Pantry
www.elanaspantry.com

Guilty Kitchen
www.guiltykitchen.com

The Healthy Apple
www.thehealthyapple.com

Hemsley + Hemsley
www.hemsleyandhemsley.com

My New Roots
http://www.mynewroots.org/site/

Nourished Kitchen
http://nourishedkitchen.com

Rubies & Radishes
www.rubiesandradishes.com

The Spunky Coconut
www.thespunkycoconut.com

SKIN CARE

Annmarie Gianni
http://www.annmariegianni.com/

Beauty Counter
http://www.beautycounter.com/

CV Skinlabs
http://cvskinlabs.com

Joanna Vargas Skincare
www.joannavargas.com

Naturopathica
www.naturopathica.com

Pratima Skin Care
http://www.pratimaskincare.com/

Ren Skincare
http://renskincare.com/usa/

S.W. Basics
http://swbasicsofbk.com/

Tata Harper
http://www.tataharperskincare.com

SLEEP RESOURCES

Fisher Wallace Stimulator
http://www.fisherwallace.com
      Brain stimulation for depression, insomnia, and anxiety.

f.lux
www.justgetflux.com

YOGA SUPPLIES AND CLASSES

Manduka
www.manduka.com

My YogaWorks Online Yoga Classes
www.MyYogaworks.com

YogaGlo
www.yogaglo.com

ENDNOTES

Introduction

1. Danielle Simmons, Ph.D., "Epigenetic Influences and Disease." *Nature Education* 1, no. 1 (2008): 6; Anne Brunet and Shelley L. Berger, "Epigenetics of Aging and Aging-related Disease," *The Journals of Gerontology Series A: Biological Sciences and Medical Sciences* 69, Supplement 1 (2014): S17–S20; Duke Medicine News and Communications, "'Epigenetics' Means What We Eat, How We Live and Love, Alters How Our Genes Behave," (October 25, 2005): http://corporate.dukemedicine.org/news_and _publications/news_office/news/9322.

Chapter 1

1. Qing Yang, "Gain Weight by 'Going Diet?' Artificial Sweeteners and the Neurobiology of Sugar Cravings," *Yale Journal of Biology and Medicine* 83, no. 2 (June 2010): 101–8: http://www.ncbi.nlm.nih.gov /pmc/articles/PMC2892765/; David S. Ludwig, M.D., Ph.D., "Artificially Sweetened Beverages Cause for Concern," *JAMA* 302, no. 22 (December 2009): 2477–78; Lisa Conti, "Artificial Sweeteners Confound the Brain; May Lead to Diet Disaster," *Scientific American* (May 2008): http://www .scientificamerican.com/article/artificial-sweeteners-confound-the-brain/.

2. Magalie Lenoir et al, "Intense Sweetness Surpasses Cocaine Reward," *PLOS One* (August 1, 2007): http://journals.plos.org/plosone/article?id=10.1371/journal.pone.0000698.

3. The Scripps Research Institute, "Scripps Research Study Shows Compulsive Eating Shares Same Addictive Biochemical Mechanism with Cocaine, Heroin Abuse" (March 23, 2010): http://www.scripps .edu/news/press/2010/2010329.html.

4. Yang, "Gain Weight by 'Going Diet?'"; Alison Abbot, "Sugar Substitutes Linked to Obesity," *Nature,* 513, no. 7518: 279–454: http://www.nature.com/news/sugar-substitutes-linked-to-obesity-1.15938; Fernando de Matos Feijó et al. "Saccharin and aspartame, compared with sucrose, induce greater weight gain in adult Wistar rats, at similar total caloric intake levels," *Appetite,* 60, no.1 (January 2013): 203–7: http://www.sciencedirect.com/science/article/pii/S0195666312004138; Jotham Suez et al.,

"Artificial sweeteners induce glucose intolerance by altering the gut microbiota," *Nature* 514 (October 9, 2014): 181–86: http://www.nature.com/nature/journal/v514/n7521/full/nature13793.html.

5. Harvard T. H. Chan School of Public Health, "Omega-3 Fatty Acids: An Essential Contribution," *The Nutrition Source,* http://www.hsph.harvard.edu/nutritionsource/omega-3-fats/; Jump, Donald B., Ph.D., "What's Good About Dietary Fat?," *Research Newsletter,* Linus Pauling Institute, Oregon State University, Spring/Summer 2008: http://lpi.oregonstate.edu/files/pdf/newsletters/ss08.pdf#page=8.

Chapter 2

1. Lydia A. Bazzano, M.D., Ph.D., M.P.H. et al, "Effects of Low-Carbohydrate and Low-Fat Diets: A Randomized Trial," *Annals of Internal Medicine* 161, no. 5 (September 2, 2014): http://annals.org/article.aspx?articleid=1900694; Jeff S. Volek et al, "Carbohydrate Restriction has a More Favorable Impact on the Metabolic Syndrome than a Low Fat Diet," *Lipids* 44, no. 4 (April 2009): 297–309: http://link.springer.com/article/10.1007%2Fs11745-008-3274-2.

2. Kristine Yaffe, M.D. et al, "The Metabolic Syndrome, Inflammation, and Risk of Cognitive Decline," *JAMA* 292, no. 18 (2004):2237–42: http://jama.jamanetwork.com/article.aspx?articleid=199762; S. Bhashyam et al, "Aging is associated with myocardial insulin resistance and mitochondrial dysfunction," *American Journal of Physiology. Heart and Circulatory Physiology* 293, no. 5 (November 2007): H3063–71: http://www.unboundmedicine.com/harrietlane/ub/citation/17873028/Aging_is_associated_with_myocardial_insulin_resistance_and_mitochondrial_dysfunction_.

3. A. S. Ryan, "Insulin resistance with aging: effects of diet and exercise," *Sports Medicine* 30, no. 5 (November 2000):327–46: http://www.ncbi.nlm.nih.gov/pubmed/11103847.

Chapter 3

1. Joe Alcock et al, "Is eating behavior manipulated by the gastrointestinal microbiota? Evolutionary pressures and potential mechanisms," *BioEssays* (2014): http://onlinelibrary.wiley.com/doi/10.1002/bies.201400071/abstract;jsessionid=F6B7EFFC0AAABB48927933F7877B1332.f02t03; Jeffrey Norris, "Do Gut Bacteria Rule Our Minds? In an Ecosystem Within Us, Microbes Evolved to Sway Choices," UCSF News Center, University of California San Francisco (August 15, 2014): https://www.ucsf.edu/news/2014/08/116526/do-gut-bacteria-rule-our-minds.

2. GM Watch, "GM soy linked to health damage in pigs—a Danish Dossier": http://gmwatch.eu/gm-reality/13882-gm-soy-linked-to-health-damage-in-pigs-a-danish-dossier.

3. Institute of Science in Society, "A Roundup of Roundup® Reveals Converging Pattern of Toxicity from Farm to Clinic to Laboratory Studies," ISIS Report (January 19, 2015): http://www.i-sis.org.uk/Roundup_of_Roundup.php; Tom Laskawy, "Gut punch: Monsanto could be destroying your microbiome" (May 23, 2013): www.grist.org; http://grist.org/food/gut-punch-monsanto-could-be-destroying-your-microbiome/; Tom Philpott, "USDA Scientist: Monsanto's Roundup Herbicide Damages Soil," *Mother Jones* (August19, 2011): http://www.motherjones.com/tom-philpott/2011/08/monsantos-roundup-herbicide-soil-damage; Jack Kaskey, "Monsanto Weedkiller is 'Probably Carcinogenic,' WHO Says," *Bloomberg Business* (March 20, 2015): http://www.bloomberg.com/news/articles/2015-03-20/who-classifies-monsanto-s-glyphosate-as-probably-carcinogenic-; Elizabeth Grossman, "Study Links Widely Used Pesticides to Antibiotic Resistance," civileats.com (March 24, 2015): http://civileats.com/2015/03/24/study-links-widely-used-pesticides-to-antibiotic-resistance/;

William Abraham. Glyphosate formulations and their use for the inhibition of 5-enolpyruvylshiki-mate-3-phosphate synthase. US Patent 7,771,736 B2, filed August 29, 2003, and issued August 10, 2010.

4. Suez, et al, "Artificial sweeteners induce glucose intolerance by altering the gut microbiota."

5. Anna Sapone et al, "Spectrum of gluten-related disorders: consensus on new nomenclature and classification,"*BMC Medicine* 10: http://www.biomedcentral.com/1741-7015/10/13; Ari LeVaux, "Meet the Controversial MIT Scientist Who Claims She Discovered a Cause of Gluten Intolerance," AlterNet.org (February 27, 2014): http://www.alternet.org/food/meet-controversial-mit-scientist-who -claims-have-discovered-cause-gluten-sensitivty.

6. Brad Plumer, "How GMO crops conquered the United States," Vox.com (August 12, 2014): http:// www.vox.com/2014/8/12/5995087/genetically-modified-crops-rise-charts; Institute for Responsible Technology, "GMOs in Food, A summary of crops, foods and food ingredients have been genetically modified as of May, 2010": http://www.responsibletechnology.org/gmo-basics/gmos-in-food.

Chapter 5

1. Saurabh S. Thosar et al, "Taking Short Walking Breaks Found to Reverse Negative Effects of Prolonged Sitting," *Medicine & Science in Sports & Exercise* (2014): http://www.sciencedaily.com /releases/2014/09/140908083748.htm

2. Gabrielle Roth, *Maps to Ecstasy: The Healing Power of Movement* (Novato, CA: New World Library, 1998).

3. Jay Williams, "How much sex is considered exercise?" upwave.com: http://www.cnn.com/2013/09/17 /health/sex-calorie-burn-upwave/.

4. Eric Dash, "Ideas and Trends; Sex May Be Happiness but Wealth Isn't Sexiness," *New York Times* (July 11, 2004): http://www.nytimes.com/2004/07/11/weekinreview/ideas-trends-sex-may-be -happiness-but-wealth-isn-t-sexiness.html.

5. Katherine Chatfield, "10 Health Rules for Women," bodyandsoul.com.au: http://www.bodyandsoul .com.au/health/health+advice/10+health+rules+for+women,8017.

Chapter 6

1. K. A. Scott et al, "Effects of Chronic Social Stress on Obesity," *Current Obesity Reports* 1, no. 1 (March 2012): 16–25, www.ncbi.nlm.nih.gov/pubmed/22943039; S. J. Melhorn et al, "Meal Patterns and Hypothalamic NPY Expression During Chronic Social Stress and Recovery," *American Journal of Physiology: Regulatory, Integrative, and Comparative Physiology,* 299, no. 3 (September 2010): R813–R833: www .ncbi.nlm.nih.gov/pmc/articles/PMC2944420/; Lydia E. Kuo et al, "Neuropeptide Y acts directly in the periphery on fat tissue and mediates stress-induced obesity and metabolic syndrome,"*Nature Medicine* 13 (2007): 803–11; Published online: July 1, 2007, Corrected online: July 24, 2007. http:// www.nature.com/nm/journal/v13/n7/full/nm1611.html.

2. Sally S. Dickerson et al, "When the Social Self Is Threatened: Shame, Physiology, and Health," *Journal of Personality,* 72, no. 6 (December 2004): 1191–1216: http://onlinelibrary.wiley.com/doi/10.111 1/j.1467-6494.2004.00295.x/abstract.

3. Suzanne B. Hanser, "Music Therapy and Stress Reduction Research," *Journal of Music Therapy* 22, no. 4 (1985): 193–206: http://jmt.oxfordjournals.org/content/22/4/193.abstract; Amy Novotney, "Music as Medicine," American Psychological Association, 44, no. 10 (November 2013): http://www.apa.org /monitor/2013/11/music.aspx.

4. Clara Strauss et al, "Mindfulness-Based Interventions for People Diagnosed with a Current Episode of an Anxiety or Depressive Disorder: A Meta-Analysis of Randomised Controlled Trials," *PLOS One* (April 24, 2014): http://www.plosone.org/article/info:doi%2F10.1371%2Fjournal.pone.0096110; T. L. Jacobs et al, "Self-reported mindfulness and cortisol during a Shamatha meditation retreat,"*Health Psychology* 32, no. 10 (March 25, 2013): 1104–9: http://www.ncbi.nlm.nih.gov/pubmed/23527522; Lee S. Berk et al, "Cortisol and Catecholamine stress hormone decrease is associated with the behavior of perceptual anticipation of mirthful laughter," *The FASEB Journal,* 22 (2008): http://www.fasebj .org/cgi/content/meeting_abstract/22/1_MeetingAbstracts/946.11.

Chapter 7

1. Jonnelle Marte, "10 Things the Sleep-Aid Industry Won't Tell You," Marketwatch.com (May 23, 2013): http://www.marketwatch.com/story/10-things-the-sleep-aid-industry-wont-tell-you-2013-05-22; Maureen Mackey, "Sleepless in America: A $32.4 Billion Business," *The Fiscal Times* (July 23, 2012): http://www.thefiscaltimes.com/Articles/2012/07/23/Sleepless-in-America-A-32-4-Billion-Business.

2. Cleveland Clinic, "Sleep Disorders in the Older Child and Teen," https://my.clevelandclinic.org/ccf /media/files/Sleep_Disorders_Center/09_Adolescent_factsheet.pdf.

3. R. Morgan Griffin, "9 Surprising Reasons to Get More Sleep," WebMd: http://www.webmd.com /sleep-disorders/features/9-reasons-to-sleep-more.

4. Claire E. Sexton et al, "Poor sleep quality is associated with increased cortical atrophy in community-dwelling adults," (September 3, 2014): http://www.neurology.org/content/early/2014/09/03 /WNL.0000000000000774.

5. "Losing 30 minutes of sleep per day may promote weight gain and adversely affect blood sugar control," presented March 5, at ENDO 2015, the annual meeting of the Endocrine Society in San Diego; http://www.sciencedaily.com/releases/2015/03/150306082541.htm.

6. "Scientists find mechanism to reset body clock," *University of Manchester News* (March 21, 2014): http:// www.manchester.ac.uk/discover/news/article/?id=11803; "Body clock link could aid obesity treatments," *University of Manchester News* (September 4, 2014): http://www.manchester.ac.uk/discover /news/article/?id=12689.

7. Jane Kay, "Loss of night: Artificial light disrupts sex hormones of birds," *Environmental Health News* (Sept. 4, 2014): http://www.environmentalhealthnews.org/ehs/news/2014/aug/wingedwarnings6lossofnight.

8. Deborah Weinstein, "Merck looks to wake up sleep aids category with suvorexant," Medical, Marketing, and Media Online (February 8, 2012): mmm-online.com; http://www.mmm-online.com /merck-looks-to-wake-up-sleep-aids-category-with-suvorexant/article/226461/.

9. Sophie Billioti de Gage et al, "Benzodiazepine use and risk of Alzheimer's disease: case-control study," *BMJ* (September 9, 2014): http://www.bmj.com/content/349/bmj.g5205.

10. T. B. Huedo-Medina et al, "Effectiveness of non-benzodiazepine hypnotics in treatment of adult insomnia: meta-analysis of data submitted to the Food and Drug Administration," *BMJ* (December 17, 2012): http://www.ncbi.nlm.nih.gov/pubmed/23248080.

Chapter 8

1. "Last Week Tonight with John Oliver: Marketing to Doctors (HBO)," https://www.youtube.com/watch?v=YQZ2UeOTO3I; Alix Spiegel, "How to Win Doctors and Influence Prescriptions," NPR (October 21, 2010): http://www.npr.org/templates/story/story.php?storyId=130730104; Adriane Fugh-Berman and Shahram Ahari, "Following the Script: How Drug Reps Make Friends and Influence Doctors," *PLOS Medicine* 4, no. 4 (April 2007): http://www.ncbi.nlm.nih.gov/pmc/articles/PMC1876413/; J. P. Orlowski and L. Wateska, "The effects of pharmaceutical firm enticements on physician prescribing patterns. There's no such thing as a free lunch," *Chest,* 102, no. 1 (1992): 270–73: http://journal.publications.chestnet.org/article.aspx?articleid=1065179.

2. "Dangerous Drugs," Drugwatch.com, http://www.drugwatch.com/dangerous-drugs.php; "Prescription Drug Side Effects," Prescription Drug Side Effects, Drugwatch.com, http://www.drugwatch.com/side-effects/; "Adverse Drug Reactions," worstpills.org, https://www.worstpills.org/public/page.cfm?op_id=4; Michael B. Kelley, "Prescription Drugs Now Kill More People In The US Than Heroin And Cocaine Combined," *Business Insider* (September 26, 2012): http://www.businessinsider.com/painkillers-kill-more-americans-than-heroin-and-cocaine-2012-9.

3. Ian Forgacs and Aathavan Loganayagam, "Overprescribing proton pump inhibitors," *BMJ* 333, no. 7634 (January 5, 2008): http://www.ncbi.nlm.nih.gov/pmc/articles/PMC2174763/; Sheila Wilhelm et al, "Perils and Pitfalls of Long-term Effects of Proton Pump Inhibitors," *Expert Review of Clinical Pharmacology* 6, no. 4 (2013): 443-451: http://www.medscape.com/viewarticle/809193_3; "Overuse of Proton Pump Inhibitors is Expensive & Dangerous," *Physician's Weekly Newsletter* (June 26, 2012): http://www.physiciansweekly.com/proton-pump-inhibitors-overuse/.

4. Hershel Jick, M.D., et al, "Antidepressants and the Risk of Suicidal Behaviors," *JAMA* 292, no. 3 (2004): http://jama.jamanetwork.com/article.aspx?articleid=199120; "Suicide & Antidepressants," Drugwatch.com, http://www.drugwatch.com/ssri/suicide/.

5. Carol Coupland et al, "Antidepressant use and risk of adverse outcomes in older people: population based cohort study," *BMJ* 343 (August 2, 2011): http://www.bmj.com/content/343/bmj.d4551; Jennifer Anderson, "Some Antidepressants Dramatically Increase Risk of Falls in Older People," *AARP Bulletin* (August 23, 2011): http://www.aarp.org/health/drugs-supplements/info-08-2011/some-antidepressants-increase-senior-fall-risk.html.

6. Larry Husten, "One Quarter of US Adults 45 and Over Taking Statins," CardioBrief (February 17, 2011): http://cardiobrief.org/2011/02/17/one-quarter-of-us-adults-45-and-over-taking-statins/; Kristina Fiore, "One U.S. Patient in Four Takes Statins," *MedPage Today* (February 16, 2011): http://www.medpagetoday.com/PublicHealthPolicy/PublicHealth/24913.

7. "Strong statin-diabetes link seen in large study of Tricare patients," *MedicalXpress* (May 7, 2015): http://medicalxpress.com/news/2015-05-strong-statin-diabetes-link-large-tricare.html.

8. Brady Dennis and Lenny Bernstein, "New guidelines could have far more Americans taking statin drugs for cholesterol," *Washington Post* (November 12, 2013): http://www.washingtonpost.com/national/health-science/new-guidelines-could-have-far-more-americans-taking-statin-drugs-for-cholesterol/2013/11/12/7f249318-4be4-11e3-be6b-d3d28122e6d4_story.html.

9. Jeanne Garbarino, "Cholesterol and Controversy: Past, Present and Future,"*Scientific American* (November 15, 2011): http://blogs.scientificamerican.com/guest-blog/2011/11/15/cholesterol-confusion-and-why-we-should-rethink-our-approach-to-statin-therapy/; John G. Canto et al, "Number of Coronary

Heart Disease Risk Factors and Mortality in Patients With First Myocardial Infarction," *JAMA* 306, no. 19 (2011): 2120–27: http://jama.jamanetwork.com/article.aspx?articleid=1104631; Richard A. Kronmal et al, "Total Serum Cholesterol Levels and Mortality Risk as a Function of Age, A Report Based on the Framingham Data," *Archives of Internal Medicine* 153, no. 9 (1993): 1065–73: http://archinte.jamanetwork.com/article.aspx?articleid=617275; Elizabeth G. Nabel and Eugene Braunwald, M.D., "A Tale of Coronary Artery Disease and Myocardial Infarction," *New England Journal of Medicine* 366 (January 5, 2012): 54–63: http://www.nejm.org/doi/full/10.1056/NEJMra1112570; Harlan M. Krumholz, M.D., et al. "Lack of Association Between Cholesterol and Coronary Heart Disease Mortality and Morbidity and All-Cause Mortality in Persons Older Than 70 Years," *JAMA* 272, no. 17 (1994): 1335–40: http://jama.jamanetwork.com/article.aspx?articleid=381733.

10. Peter Gøtzsche, "Psychiatric drugs are doing us more harm than good," *The Guardian* (April 30, 2014): http://www.theguardian.com/commentisfree/2014/apr/30/psychiatric-drugs-harm-than-good-ssri-antidepressants-benzodiazepines.

11. Scott Glover and Lisa Girion, "Counties sue narcotics makers, alleging 'campaign of deception,'" *Los Angeles Times* (May 21, 2014): http://www.latimes.com/local/la-me-rx-big-pharma-suit-20140522-story.html#page=1.

12. Watchdog, "Dying for Relief: A *Times* Investigation," *Los Angeles Times* (May 21, 2014): http://www.latimes.com/science/la-sg-dying-for-relief-times-investigation-storygallery.html.

13. Joseph Hooper, "When to Say No to Your Doctor," *Men's Journal* (October 2014): http://www.mensjournal.com/magazine/when-to-say-no-to-your-doctor-20140919.

14. Maggie Fox, "More Drugs Do Not Always Mean Better Care: Studies," Reuters (November 3, 2010): http://www.reuters.com/article/2010/11/03/us-usa-healthcare-spending-idUSTRE6A27SO20101103.

15. Jane E. Brody, "Too Many Pills for Aging Patients," *New York Times* (April 16, 2012): http://well.blogs.nytimes.com/2012/04/16/too-many-pills-for-aging-patients/?_r=0; American Society of Consultant Pharmacists, "ASCP Fact Sheet," https://www.ascp.com/articles/about-ascp/ascp-fact-sheet.

Chapter 9

1. Phillippe Autier, M.D., and Sara Gandini, Ph.D., "Vitamin D Supplementation and Total Mortality, A Meta-analysis of Randomized Controlled Trials," *Archives of Internal Medicine* 167, no. 16 (2007):1730–37.

2. David Nayor, "Magnesium: Widespread Deficiency with Deadly Consequences," *Life Extension Magazine* (May 2008): http://www.lef.org/Magazine/2008/5/Magnesium-Widespread-Deficiency-With-Deadly-Consequences/Page-01; Carolyn Dean, M.D., N.D., "The Miracle of Magnesium," Mercola.com (August 2004): http://articles.mercola.com/sites/articles/archive/2004/08/07/miracle-magnesium.aspx; Zahra Barnes, "Magnesium, an invisible deficiency that could be harming your health," CNN.com (December 31, 2014): http://www.cnn.com/2014/12/31/health/magnesium-deficiency-health/.

Chapter 10

1. Corey M. Clark, "Relations Between Social Support and Physical Health," Rochester Institute of Technology, SAPA Project Test, last accessed 3/11/15: http://www.personalityresearch.org/papers/clark.html; Berton H. Kaplan, et al, "Social Support and Health," *Medical Care,* 15, no. 5 (May 1977), Supplement: http://scholar.google.com/scholar?q=social+support++and+health&hl=en&as_sdt=0&as_vis=1&oi=scholart&sa=X&ei=P3_ZU-OuGe3JsQT3_oGQDg&ved=0CBsQgQMwAA; Maija Reblin, M.A., and Bert N. Uchino, Ph.D., "Social and Emotional Support and Its Implications for Health," *Current Opinions in Psychiatry* 21, no 2. (March 2008): 201–5.

INDEX

ACKNOWLEDGMENTS

A book needs a special team, and I have had the most incredible one supporting me.

I am deeply indebted to the brilliant Rachel Kranz, so remarkable and skilled with language, who totally captured my voice and helped me write a succinct and practical book. Her understanding of the most complicated concepts helped me articulate them in ways I could never have done myself. This book would not have been possible without her.

I am extremely grateful to the talented and generous Tricia Williams for the countless hours spent creating the recipe section, a key component of the book. Thanks for always bringing us delicious food and using us as guinea pigs while testing the recipes.

I am particularly appreciative of the lovely Kerry Bajaj, my original Health Coach, who put the program together and who has made it feel like there is a Health Coach supporting the reader along the way.

Many thanks to Dr. Keren Day, for the foam roller fascia release routines, and to Jim Clarry, who created a program of simple but effective exercises.

Sincere thanks to Bobby Clennell, for her exceptional illustrated yoga poses.

Infinite gratitude to my agent, Stephanie Tade, for her love, direction, and guidance.

This book would not have happened without Patty Gift and Reid Tracy from Hay House believing in me and encouraging me to write another book. And much appreciation for Sally Mason, Richelle Fredson, Marlene Robinson, Christy Salinas, Riann Bender, Tricia Breidenthal, Karla Baker, Alexis Seabrook, Sheridan McCarthy, and the entire Hay House team.

Writing a book would also not be possible without my extraordinary, loving, and loyal staff at the Eleven Eleven Wellness Center in New York City. In particular, I am blessed to have Vicky Zodo, who has run the practice like clockwork since we started out together in 1992.

A big shout-out to my incredible team of Health Coaches who continue to amaze me with their ability to help our clients bring health into their lives. You guys have taken my practice to a whole other level and are on the vanguard of a new way of delivering health care.

I am profoundly indebted to the Be Well Team who make life so much easier for me to focus on writing and seeing patients.

A huge thank you to Lindsey Clennell for his invaluable insights, guidance, sense of humor, and wisdom.

Respect and admiration for my mentors, friends, and colleagues in my medical world who for decades have been fighting to change an ailing disease care system into a true health care system.

To my family and friends, too numerous to mention, thank you for all your love, encouragement, and support over the many years.

To my patients who constantly teach me and inspire me to find better ways of getting and keeping them healthy.

Thanks to my beautiful and down to earth daughter, Ali, for always saying it like it is and whose presence is an absolute blessing.

And finally, none of this would have been possible without my wife, Janice. You have been my best friend, lover, partner, personal chef, my rock, and my everything for 40 years. I am eternally grateful for all your love, wisdom, and support (and delicious cooking).

ABOUT THE AUTHOR

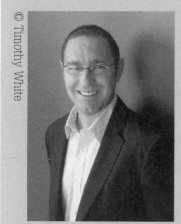

© Timothy White

Dr Frank Lipman is one of the top pioneers in the field of integrative medicine in the USA. A leading international speaker on health and wellness, Dr Lipman is the author of four books, including the *New York Times* bestseller *The New Health Rules*. He has been featured in *Men's Health*, *Vogue*, *Men's Journal*, *Redbook* and *Martha Stewart Living*. He is a regular contributor to *Goop* and *The Huffington Post*, and he writes a weekly blog for his own site.

www.drfranklipman.com

Hay House Titles of Related Interest

YOU CAN HEAL YOUR LIFE, the movie,
starring Louise Hay & Friends
(available as a 1-DVD programme and an expanded 2-DVD set)
Watch the trailer at: www.LouiseHayMovie.com

THE SHIFT, the movie,
starring Dr Wayne W. Dyer
(available as a 1-DVD programme and an expanded 2-DVD set)
Watch the trailer at: www.DyerMovie.com

CULTURED FOOD FOR LIFE: How to Make and Serve Delicious Probiotic Foods for Better Health and Wellness, by Donna Schwenk

GODDESSES NEVER AGE: The Secret Prescription for Radiance, Vitality and Wellbeing, by Dr Christiane Northrup

LOVING YOURSELF TO GREAT HEALTH: Thoughts & Food – The Ultimate Diet, by Louise Hay, Ahlea Khadro and Heather Dane

MIND OVER MEDICINE: Scientific Proof That You Can Heal Yourself, by Dr Lissa Rankin

THE TAPPING SOLUTION: A Revolutionary System for Stress-Free Living, by Nick Ortner

All of the above are available at your local bookstore,
or may be ordered by contacting Hay House (see last page).

NOTES

NOTES

NOTES

NOTES

NOTES

NOTES

NOTES

NOTES

NOTES